the Unofficial Guide to Surviving Breast Cancer

Stacie Zoe Berg
with Richard Theriault,
D.O., M.B.A.

IDG Books Worldwide, Inc.

IDG Books Worldwide, Inc.
An International Data Group Company
919 E. Hillsdale Boulevard
Suite 400
Foster City, CA 94404

For general information on IDG Books Worldwide's books in the U.S., please call our Consumer Customer Service department at 800-762-2974. For reseller information, including discounts and previous sales, please call our Reseller Customer Service department at 800-434-3422.

ISBN: 0-02-863491-8

Manufactured in the United States of America

10 9 8 7 6 5 4 3 2 1

First edition

To my grandmother, Lily Berg, a strong
and loving woman who made
such a difference in my life.

Acknowledgments

I want to thank my co-author, Richard L. Theriault, D.O., Associate Professor, Department of Breast Medical Oncology, The University of Texas M. D. Anderson Cancer Center, for his important contributions to this book, and the Unofficial Panel of Experts—Richard Arenas, Assistant Professor of Surgery and Attending Surgeon at the Breast Center at the University of Chicago; Marsha D. McNeese, M.D., Associate Professor of Radiation Oncology at the University of Texas M. D. Anderson Cancer Center; and Gay McFarland, breast cancer survivor—for their thoughtful reviews of the manuscript.

I'd also like to thank all of the experts interviewed for this book: Eric Winer, M.D., Director, Breast Oncology Center at Dana-Farber Cancer Institute and Associate Professor of Medicine at Harvard Medical School and Paul Richardson, M.D., Attending Physician, Breast Oncology Center, Department of Adult Oncology, Dana Farber Cancer Institute, Boston, Mass., for their generous contributions; Susan Tannenbaum, a Fellow with the College of American Pathologists and a pathologist at United Pathology Associates, in Port Chester, New York; Clifford Hudis, M.D., Chief of Breast Cancer Medicine Service at Memorial Sloan-Kettering in New York; Jeanne Petrek, M.D., Surgical Director at Memorial Sloan-Kettering's Breast Cancer Center in New York; William Berg, M.D., Clinical Assistant Physician, Division of Solid Tumor Oncology, Department of Medicine at Memorial Sloan-Kettering Cancer Center and Instructor in Medicine at Weill Medical College of Cornell University; Robert Schmidt, M.D.,

Associate Professor of Radiology at NYU School of Medicine; John Durant, M.D., Executive Vice President of the American Society of Clinical Oncologists (ASCO); Lyndsay Harris, M.D., Assistant Professor in the Multidisciplinary Breast Program at Duke University; Arthur Hartz, M.D., Professor of Family Medicine at the University of Iowa; Anne Coscorelli, Ph.D, Director of Rhonda Fleming Mann Resource Center for Women with Cancer at the Jonsson Comprehensive Cancer Center at UCLA in Los Angeles, California; Caroline Fife, M.D., Director of the Hermann Lymphedema Center in Houston, Texas; Edward Clifford, M.D., Chief of the General Surgery Section at St. Paul Medical Center in Dallas, Texas, and Clinical Assistant Professor of Surgery at the University of Texas Southwestern Medical School; Yang Liu, Ph.D., Kurtz Chair and Professor of Pathology at Ohio State University's Comprehensive Cancer Center; Mary L. Disis, M.D., Associate Professor of Medicine, Division of Oncology, at the University of Washington in Seattle, Washington; Lu Ann Aday, Ph.D., Professor of Behavioral Sciences at the University of Texas School of Public Health; George Sledge, M.D., Ballvélantero Professor of Oncology at Indiana University in Indianapolis, Indiana; Sandra Haber, Ph.D, in New York City; Mary Jane Massie, M.D., Director of the Barbara White Fishman Center for Psychological Counseling at Memorial Sloan-Kettering Cancer Center's Breast Center in New York City; Stephen A. Feig, M.D., Director of Breast the Imaging Center at Thomas Jefferson University Hospital in Philadelphia, Pennsylvania, and professor of radiology at Jefferson Medical College; Barrie Cassilleth, Ph.D., Chief of Integrative Medicine at Memorial Sloan-Kettering Cancer Center in New York; Samuel D. Benjamin, M.D., Director of the University Center for Complementary and Alternative Medicine at SUNY Stony Brook School of Medicine, Stony Brook, New York; Karen Koffler, M.D, a fellow at the University of Arizona program in integrative medicine; Jeffrey White, M.D., Director of the Office of Cancer Complementary and Alternative Medicine at the National Cancer Institute; Yuri Parisky, Associate Professor of Radiology at University of Southern California School of Medicine in Los Angeles, California; Karen Donahey, Ph.D., Director of the Sex and Marital Therapy program at Northwest University Medical School in Chicago, Illinois; Donald Lannin, M.D., Professor of Surgery and Director of the Leo W. Jenkins Cancer Center at East Carolina University School of Medicine in Greenville, N.C; Judith M. Ford, M.D., Ph.D., Assistant Professor, Department of Radiation Oncology at UCLA and Jonsson Cancer Center; Lee Rosen, M.D., Assistant Professor of Medicine and Director of the Cancer Therapy Development Program at UCLA's Jonsson Cancer Center; John Glaspy, M.D., Medical Director of the Oncology Clinic at UCLA's Jonsson Cancer Center; Lee Berk, DRPH, MPH, a neuroimmunologist and Associate Director of the Center for Neuroimmunology at Loma Linda University's School of Medicine in Loma Linda, California; Blair Justice, Ph.D., Professor of Psychology at the University of Texas Health Science Center; Carol Fred, licensed clinical social worker at the Rhonda Flemming Mann Resource Center for Women with Cancer, part of the Jonsson Comprehensive Cancer Center at UCLA;

Laura Kramer, R.D., at Massachusetts General Hospital in Boston; Connie Dahlin, N.P. at Massachusetts General in Boston; Marsha Oakley, R.N., B.S.N., Breast Center at Mercy Medical Center in Baltimore, Maryland; Sandra Cooley, cancer survivor; Linda Larva, L.S.W., at the Cancer Caring Center in Pittsburgh, Pennsylvania; Jane Hill, a cancer comedian and breast cancer survivor; Audrey Selden, Associate Commissioner for Consumer Protection at the Texas Department of Insurance; Mary Jo Deering, Ph.D., Director, Health Communication and Telehealth at the U.S. Department of Health and Human Services in Washington, D.C.; Mike D. Oppenheim, M.D.; and Julie Durmis, Manager of the Friends Boutique at the Dana-Farber Cancer Institute in Boston for their time and expertise.

A special thanks to the editorial team for all of their hard work. This top-notch team of editors includes Randy Ladenheim-Gil, former Senior Editor; Amy Zavatto, Development Editor; Jennifer Perillo, former Managing Editor; Mary Lou Hurley, Copy Editor; Andrea M. Harris, Layout and Production; Brice Gosnell, Managing Editor; and Jessica Faust, Senior Editor.

I'd like to thank Alicia Kim, Media Coordinator in the public affairs office at Memorial Sloan-Kettering Cancer Center in New York; Kim Irwin, Director for Public Information at UCLA's Jonsson Cancer Center at UCLA, and other media relations officers for serving as my link to the best and the brightest breast cancer clinicians and researchers.

Finally, I'd like to thank my family, especially my wonderful husband for his support throughout and his technical expertise on computers and computer security in Chapter 17; my father Gerald Berg, Ph.D., and cousin William Berg, M.D., for providing answers to my tough questions in immunology and oncology; my brother Michel Berg, M.D., for playing backup, fielding questions when no one else was around; my mother, Lila J. Berg, for her command of the English language and for her incredible resourcefulness; and my uncle, Melvin J. Berg, J.D., for his advice on the tough stuff.

Contents

We Give You More Than the Official Line

Welcome to the *Unofficial Guide* series of Lifestyles titles—books that deliver critical, unbiased information that other books can't or won't reveal—the inside scoop. Our goal is to provide you with the most accessible, useful information and advice possible. The recommendations we offer in these pages are not influenced by the corporate line of any organization or industry; we give you the hard facts, whether those institutions like them or not. If something is ill-advised or will cause a loss of time and/or money, we'll give you ample warning. And if it a worthwhile option, we'll let you know that, too.

Armed and Ready

Our hand-picked authors confidently and critically report on a wide range of topics that matter to smart readers like you. Our authors are passionate about their subjects, but have distanced themselves enough from them to help you be armed and protected, and help make you educated decisions as you go through the process. It is our intent that, from having read this book, you will avoid the pitfalls everyone else falls into and get it right the first time.

Don't be fooled by cheap imitations; this is the genuine article *Unofficial Guide* series from IDG Books. You may be familiar with our proven track record of the travel *Unofficial Guides*, which have more than three million copies in print. Each year thousands of travelers—new and old—are armed with a brand new, fully updated edition of the flagship *Unofficial Guide* to Walt Disney World, by Bob Sehlinger. It is our intention here to provide you with the same level of objective authority that Mr. Sehlinger does in his brainchild.

The Unofficial Panel of Experts

Every work in the Lifestyle *Unofficial Guides* is intensively inspected by a team of three top professionals in their fields. These experts review the manuscript for factual accuracy, comprehensiveness, and an insider's determination as to whether the manuscript fulfills the credo in this Reader's Bill of rights. In other words, our Panel ensures that you are, in fact, getting "the inside scoop."

Our Pledge

The authors, the editorial staff, and the Unofficial Panel of Experts assembled for *Unofficial Guides* are determined to lay out the most valuable alternatives available for our readers. This dictum means that our writers must be explicit, prescriptive, and above all, direct. We strive to be thorough and complete, but our goal is not necessarily to have the "most" or "all" of the information on a topic; this is not, after all, an encyclopedia. Our objective is to help you narrow down your options to the best of what is available, unbiased by affiliation with any industry or organization.

In each *Unofficial Guide* we give you:

- Comprehensive coverage of necessary and vital information
- Authoritative, rigidly fact-checked data
- The most up-to-date insights into trends
- Savvy, sophisticated writing that's also readable.
- Sensible, applicable facts and secrets that only an insider knows

Special Features

Every book in our series offers the following six special sidebars in the margins that were devised to help you get things done cheaply, efficiently, and smartly.

1. **Timesaver**—tips and shortcuts that save you time
2. **Moneysaver**—tips and shortcuts that save you money
3. **Watch Out!**—more serious cautions and warnings
4. **Bright Idea**—general tips and shortcuts to help you find and easier or smarter way to do something
5. **Quote**—statements from real people that are intended to be prescriptive and valuable to you
6. **Unofficial...**—an insider's fact or anecdote

We also recognize your need to have quick information at your fingertips, and have thus provided the following comprehensive sections at the back of the book:

1. **Glossary**—definitions of complicated terminology and jargon
2. **Resource Guide**—lists of relevant agencies,

associations, institutions, web sites, etc.

3. **Recommended Reading List**—suggested titles that can help you get more in-depth information on related topics

4. **Important Documents**—"official" pieces of information you need to refer to, such as government forms

5. **Index**

Letters, Comments, Questions from Readers

We strive to continually improve the *Unofficial* series, and input from our readers is a valuable way for us to do that.

Many of those who have used the *Unofficial Guide* travel books write to the authors to ask questions, make comments, or share their own discoveries and lessons. For Lifestyle *Unofficial Guides*, we would also appreciate all such correspondence—both positive and critical—and we will make best efforts to incorporate appropriate readers' feedback and comments in revised editions of this work.

How to write us:
Unofficial Guides
Lifestyle Guides
IDG Books
1633 Broadway
New York, NY 10019
Attention: Reader's Comments

About the Authors

Stacie Zoe Berg, author of *The Unofficial Guide to Surviving Breast Cancer* and two other *Unofficial Guides*, is a freelance journalist who writes frequently about health and medicine.

Ms. Berg is a member of the American Society of Journalists and Authors and Washington Independent Writers. Over the years she has been associated with other professional organizations, including Women in Communications, for which she is a former board member and newsletter assistant editor, and Women in Museums (sponsored by the Smithsonian Institution). Ms. Berg also is an award-winning Toastmaster.

Richard Theriault, co-author of the *Unofficial Guide to Surviving Breast Cancer*, is a Professor of Medicine in the Department of Breast Medical Oncology at the University of Texas M. D. Anderson Cancer Center in Houston, Texas. For the past twelve years his practice has been limited to care for women with breast cancer. In addition to clinical responsibilities he is a clinical and translational research physician specializing in breast cancer. These activities have included development of new drug treatments, adjunctive treatments for bone disease and treatment evaluation programs for women who are pregnant and have breast cancer.

From 1993 to 1996, Dr. Theriault was Clinic Chief for Breast Medical Oncology and from 1996 to 1999, he was the Medical Director of the Nellie B. Connally Breast Center at M. D. Anderson Cancer Center. At present, he serves as the Medical Director of the M. D. Anderson Physician's Network. In addition to numerous peer-reviewed publications, he has authored or co-authored more than 20 book chapters on breast cancer and breast cancer treatment. Dr. Theriault is also a nationally and internationally recognized speaker and authority on breast cancer in women and has appeared on a number of nationally broadcast television programs.

Dr. Theriault's professional activities include membership in The American Society of Clinical Oncology, American Association for Cancer Research, Fellow of American College of Physicians (F.A.C.P.), and the American College of Physicians–American Society of Internal Medicine. He is also a member of the National Comprehensive Cancer Network Breast Cancer Guidelines panel and Breast Cancer Database Outcomes Committee.

The Unofficial Guide Panel of Experts

The *Unofficial* editorial team recognizes that you've purchased this book with the expectation of getting the most authoritative, carefully inspected information currently available. Toward that end, on each and every title in this series, we have selected a minimum of two "official" experts comprising the Unofficial Panel who painstakingly review the manuscripts to ensure the following: factual accuracy of all data; inclusion of the most up-to-date and relevant information; and that, from an insider's perspective, the authors have armed you with all the necessary facts you need—but that the institutions don't want you to know.

For *The Unofficial Guide to Surviving Breast Cancer,* we are proud to introduce the following panel of experts:

Dr. Richard Arenas is Assistant Professor of Surgery and Attending Surgeon at The Breast Center at the University of Chicago. A medical graduate of the UMDNJ-Robert Wood Johnson Medical School in New Jersey, Dr. Arenas completed his residency training in general surgery at the Hospital of Saint Rafael in New Haven, Connecticut and the UMDNJ-New Jersey Medical School. He later went on to complete a fellowship in surgical oncology at the University of Chicago where he has been on faculty since 1994. His clinical practice specializes in the surgical management of breast and gastrointestinal diseases.

In addition to his clinical activities, Dr. Arenas maintains laboratory interests in the molecular biology of cancers, specifically studying the role of tumor suppressor genes and the feasibility of gene replacement therapy in certain hereditary cancers. He is also the site principle investigator for the recently publicized NSABP Breast Cancer Prevention Trial and for the proposed Study Comparing Tamoxifen and Raloxifene (STAR) Trial. Dr. Arenas is also coordinating efforts to better understand and encourage the recruitment of minority women onto each of these breast cancer prevention trials. Dr. Arenas is active in several organizations including The Society of Surgical Oncology, The American Society of Clinical Oncology, and the Y-ME Breast Cancer Organization.

Dr. Marsha McNeese, a native of Louisiana, attended Louisiana State University undergraduate and medical school prior to moving to Texas in 1974 for her post-graduate training. After she completed her residency training in Radiation Oncology at the University of Texas M. D. Anderson Cancer Center, she joined the faculty, doing clinical research in the areas of electron beam therapy and breast cancer. She is now an Associate Professor of Radiation Oncology and

Chief of the Breast Cancer Radiotherapy Section since 1987. In this role, she sees hundreds of women with breast cancer each year. Her special interest is in extending the options of breast-preserving therapy to more women diagnosed with breast cancer, and in refining treatment techniques and results for the best possible cure rate and cosmetic outcome for these patients. She is an active participant on committees of several national organizations, including the Public Education Campaign for the American Society of Therapeutic Radiology (ASTRO), Radiation Therapy Monitoring Committee for the National Surgical Adjuvant Breast Project (NSABP), the Education Committee for the Southern Association of Oncology, and the Breast Cancer Task Force and Patterns of Care Study Committees for the American College of Radiology.

Gay McFarland-Scarborough, a breast cancer survivor since 1990, is a former newspaper writer and syndicated columnist. Currently, she serves as the Senior News Service Manager for the Office of Public Affairs at The University of Texas-Houston Health Science Center where she facilitates the exchange of medical knowledge from healthcare professionals to both media and the community. She devotes much of her free time to making presentations to cancer survivor groups, answering cancer patients' questions about personal issues, and writing about the challenges and blessings of being a survivor. She is also vitally interested in mental health issues, especially autism and Asperger's Syndrome. McFarland holds an M.A. in creative writing and is the mother of one son.

Introduction

When diagnosed with a potentially life-threatening disease such as breast cancer, you want to talk to the best and brightest in the field. That is exactly what we have done for you. Throughout this book, experts at top cancer centers share their extensive knowledge about breast cancer—causes, treatments, and other important information—to help you better understand the disease and your treatment alternatives.

Observing and treating cancer goes back to at least 3000 BC in ancient Egypt. In 1775, Percivall Pott observed the cancer-causing potential of chemicals by observing the high rate of cancer among chimney sweeps. By the mid-1800s Italian and French researchers observed that women died from cancer more frequently than men. They also noted that the incidence of cancer increased with age, that cancer is found more in the city than in the country, and that single people are more likely to develop the disease.

Between 1900 and the early 1940s there were important advancements in the field of medical science. Researchers began to understand the structures, functions, and chemistry of living organisms. Cancer research began in cell structure, chemical carcinogens, diagnostic techniques, and chemotherapy. It was discovered that x-rays harmed rapidly dividing cells in animals, and a theory arose that cancer was due to abnormal chromosomes. Viral-initiated cancer was documented in chickens in 1911. In addition, both chemical and physical carcinogens were identified, and chromosomal abnormalities were investigated as a possible cause of cancer. In 1915, experiments confirmed that chemicals could induce cancer. In 1930 the NCI was founded in response to public pressure.

Nearly 5,000 years after the first known attempts to treat cancer, the war on cancer had begun.

In recent years, research has progressed so rapidly that a cure for cancer has become an attainable goal. In fact, most early-stage breast cancers are considered curable—and in many cases, breast cancer has become preventable. Doctors are now able to identify women at high risk of developing the disease and are placing them on drugs that have been proven effective at blocking the development of cancer at a molecular level. Furthermore, for women who are not at high risk of developing breast cancer, scientists have discovered many risk factors that can be avoided, such as certain dietary elements, exposure to carcinogens, and much more that help reduce their chances even further.

For all women, early detection is the key to survival. Modern technology has provided us with eyes that can see deep into our tissues, detecting minute cancerous masses that do not become detectable by touch for many years. At such an early stage, these breast cancers are curable.

With the advancement of science and medical techniques and an understanding of the various types of breast cancers and their characteristics, radical mastectomies have become much less common. This disfiguring surgical procedure has been replaced by lumpectomies in most cases.

In recent years, investigators have been able to isolate mutated genes that can cause breast cancer; they have been able to isolate normal genes with a greater than normal presence that overexpress (produce too many) proteins and thereby cause breast cancer; and they have been able to determine that certain hormones can cause breast cancer to grow. Researchers also have been able to isolate immune responses to some breast cancers. All of these discoveries have had, and continue to have, important implications on the causes of and possible cures for breast cancer.

Chemotherapy is an important weapon in the war against cancer. But like radiation therapy, it attacks healthy cells, causing severe side effects that affect the quality of life, and in some cases, death. As a result of all that has been learned about breast cancer up to this point, researchers are adding new weapons to their arsenal that may prove more effective in eradicating cancer and less toxic to the breast cancer patient.

The future looks promising. Scientists are taking varied approaches to controlling and eradicating breast cancer. Researchers are developing molecular markers to detect signs of breast cancer in the blood, urine, and nipple fluid. By being able to identify the characteristics of each specific breast cancer, more appropriate treatments may be used.

More focus is being given to the inheritance of genetic mutations. The National Cancer Institute (NCI) has established the Cancer Genetics Network, a national network of centers specializing in the study of inherited predisposition to cancer. This network will support collaborative investigations into the genetic basis of cancer susceptibility.

NCI is also funding studies on computer-assisted interpretations of digitized mammography images, and on long-distance image transmission technology (teleradiology) for clinical consultations.

If you or someone you love has been diagnosed with breast cancer, remember that there are an estimated 2 million breast cancer survivors in the United States. But until there is a cure, the war on cancer must continue. Breast cancer ranks just behind lung cancer as the leading cause of cancer deaths among women in the United States. In 1994, 183,000 women received their first diagnosis of breast cancer, and an estimated 46,000 women and 300 men died from breast cancer that year, according to NCI. It is the leading cause of cancer deaths among women between the ages of 15 and 54, according to NCI. (However, the incidence of breast cancer among younger women is lower than that for older women.) There is also a disparity among races. African American women are more likely to die from breast cancer. Unfortunately, they seek medical help at more advanced stages of the disease. Education is the key to action, and that is what this book is all about.

Chapter 1 explains the process of how healthy cells become cancerous, reviews the different types of breast cancer, and talks about the symptoms of breast cancer. A key component of this chapter for some women will be the discussion of the myths and facts about breast cancer. For example, many women believe that if breast cancer doesn't run in their families, they won't get it. In fact, about 80% of women who develop breast cancer do not have a family history of it. There are also other worries women contend with, such as being afraid that their boyfriend or husband will leave them if they're scarred, which causes women to bypass screening or to ignore symptoms of breast cancer. Some women have the mistaken belief that mammograms are painful or that the radiation levels are unsafe. The list of myths and concerns goes on and on, and it is these myths and worries, in part, that keep women from getting mammogram screenings. Remember, the key to survival is early detection.

Chapter 2 delves into the immune system. Unlike bacteria and viruses, which are foreign intruders and which trigger an immune response, cancer comes from within. It develops from a healthy cell whose DNA has been mutated. As a result, it grows uncontrollably. Because it is derived from healthy cells, the immune system doesn't always recognize its presence and therefore does not launch an immune response, or at least not a strong enough immune response. In contrast, bacteria and other microbes are distinctly foreign, so antibiotics and other medications have an easy target. The immune system is discussed in more detail in this chapter, and tips are included on how you can boost your immune system. This important chapter also discusses adoptive immunotherapy and cancer vaccines. Both of these new treatments use the body's own defenses to boost the immune response and hold promise for the future.

Treatments result from many years of hard work under extreme scrutiny. That process is detailed in Chapter 3. The ideas begin in the laboratory in a petri dish under a microscope. The ideas that show scientific, not just theoretical, promise move on to animal studies. Promising results from animal studies are tested on a small number of human subjects in phase I clinical trials. Once safety and dosing have been established, testing moves on to phase II clinical trials where another small group of human subjects are tested to see if the treatment has positive benefits. Promising results in animal studies do not always translate into success in human studies, and promising results seen in phase I and II trials don't always pan out in phase III trials, which test treatments on a more general and larger population. But there are some victories along the way, and wars are won by the victories of many small battles.

Chapter 3 has another important purpose. Many women who have been diagnosed with breast cancer want to take an active role in their treatment decisions and turn to research on which to base their decisions. This chapter is designed to teach you how to discriminate among different levels of studies (phase I, phase II, and phase III) and to teach you about the strengths and weaknesses of study designs (for example, a phase II trial doesn't have the strength of a phase III trial because a phase II trial looks at only a small number of subjects who are generally healthy whereas a phase III trial looks at large numbers of subjects whose health is more reflective of the general population) as well as the importance of the replication of results by other investigators.

Everyone is at risk for breast cancer. But how much risk are you actually at? Chapter 4 discusses the known risk factors, including family history. Because of the relatively recent discovery of the BRCA1 and BRCA2 genes and their impact on familial breast cancers, Chapter 5 includes a discussion on the pros and cons of genetic testing. Chapter 5 also focuses on prevention—what you can actively do to protect yourself against developing breast cancer. While changing your lifestyle won't guarantee that you won't develop breast cancer, it will reduce your chances. This chapter presents some little publicized information on prevention, such as why you need to stay hydrated, and why fruits and vegetables may protect you against cancer but vitamin pills may not.

Mammography screenings play an important role in the early detection of breast cancer. However, many women think that if they're screened once or twice, that's enough. They then may wait years before going in for another screening, which they may do at another center. There are several problems inherent in this strategy, and they are discussed in more detail in Chapter 6. First, a radiologist uses the annual "snapshots" to compare against earlier snapshots, in order to see any changes. Therefore, you need routine pictures. Second, you need to get the mammogram taken at the same place each time (or take your earlier x-rays along with you to your new screening center) because they need to be compared. Radiologists look for changes as well as idiosyncrasies. Third, research indicates that not all radiologists are equally skilled at reading mammographies. Therefore, the more frequently you get a mammogram, the more likely it is you'll find a radiologist who detects a malignancy, if one exists. Of course, as this chapter notes, you can increase your chances of getting a radiologist skilled at reading mammograms by going to a center that specializes in mammography.

While mammography plays an important role in early breast cancer detection, self-exams play a vital role. Most breast cancers are discovered by women themselves. Chapter 6 gives detailed instructions on how to perform a breast self-exam.

Breast tissue is filled with natural lumps and bumps. In fact, one out of two women will receive a false-positive result on their annual mammogram during a 10-year period. As a result, nearly 20% of those women will have unnecessary biopsies. Knowing information like this, which is also noted in Chapter 6, might help calm your nerves if a questionable mass is detected on your mammogram. It is clear that more advanced technology with higher rates of accuracy is needed. Future technology is also discussed in this chapter.

Sometimes biopsies (taking a sample of the tissue) are necessary. There are several types of biopsies, some more invasive than others. These are also reviewed in Chapter 6.

There are three primary treatments for breast cancer: surgery, chemotherapy, and radiation therapy.

The treatment for breast cancer depends on the stage of disease—whether the cancer is localized, metastatic, or somewhere in between. Chapter 7 summarizes conventional treatment strategies stage by stage. It also describes the different surgical methods and cancer characteristics associated with the different stages of disease.

Most women are cured after surgery but undergo chemotherapy treatment in case cancerous cells have traveled to another part of the body, where they grow into metastatic cancer if left untreated. Unfortunately, doctors cannot see these microscopic cells, and therefore must treat all women as if they are in this small group.

Getting through treatment is not easy. Chapter 8 tells you how you can get through treatments without extreme anxiety (for example, listening to books on tape or doing relaxation exercises), how you can control physical symptoms through diet (ginger reduces nausea, for example), and how to prevent or control lymphedema, a chronic swelling condition that can occur when lymph nodes are removed under the arm.

While breast tumors rarely cause any pain, many women experience pain as a result of the treatments or because of the spread of the disease. Both radiation and chemotherapy cause fluid accumulation and swelling (called *edema*), irritate or destroy healthy tissue, which causes pain and inflammation, and, possibly, sensitize nerve endings, which also causes pain. If the cancer spreads, the pressure of a growing tumor can cause pain, as can the infiltration of tumor cells into other organs. Chapter 8 tells how pain can be treated effectively.

Chapter 9 discusses a highly controversial treatment: high-dose chemotherapy supported by autologous stem cell transplants or bone marrow transplants. (Stem cell or bone marrow transplants are necessary after this type of treatment because the high doses of chemotherapy kill off these blood-producing cells.) The theory behind high dose chemotherapy treatment is to overcome the drug-resistant cancer cells that often develop after undergoing standard chemotherapy regimens, and to kill off any microscopic cells that might remain behind. But several recent phase III trials have suggested that this therapy might not be any more effective than lower-dose chemotherapy therapy, and should not be recommended as a form of standard therapy. There was, however, one promising study that used a different approach—the study participants received high-dose chemotherapy before receiving a comparable standard regimen. This study must be replicated before it is considered valid.

The phase III trials are reviewed in Chapter 9, and the strengths and weaknesses of these studies are discussed. In this chapter we also note that these study results are preliminary, that not all drugs or drug combinations were tested, and that the strategy may still hold hope for a certain subset of women with breast cancer. We strongly suggest women choosing to undergo this aggressive form of therapy enter a well designed clinical trial.

Chapter 10 is an exciting chapter to read. It reviews new therapies—from hormone treatments to angiogenesis inhibitors to cancer vaccines. Hormone treatments, such as tamoxifen, block estrogen cell receptors. Estrogen causes some cancer cells to grow, and by blocking these receptors, cancer growth is halted. Another approach, called angiogenesis inhibitors, cuts off the blood supply tumors need to grow—again, stopping cancer in its tracks. Cancer vaccines are being used in research trials to boost the body's own defenses in recognizing cancer cells and eradicating them.

Another biological therapy discussed in Chapter 10 is Herceptin, which targets HER-2/neu proteins. HER-2 (human epidermal growth factor receptor 2) is a gene that everyone has but extra copies are found in about 20 percent to 30 percent of women with breast cancer. Those extra copies usually lead to extra copies of the receptor. The HER-2 gene produces a protein on the cell's surface, which signals it to grow. An overabundance of the gene translates to out-of-control growth, which means an aggressive cancer that spreads rapidly. Herceptin is an antibody that was developed to target breast cancer cells overexpressing the HER-2/neu protein.

Many women, like those who choose to undergo high dose chemotherapy, join clinical trials in the hopes of benefiting from a new treatment or contributing information to science. In Chapter 11 we describe experimental treatment methods and we discuss what benefits you can gain from participating in a study, in addition to what drawbacks there are to being in a study. We also provide you with a list of questions to ask the study investigators before joining a study and then tell you how to locate current trials.

Trials for some treatments, those outside of mainstream medicine, have been lacking. But consumer demand is changing that. Cancer patients have turned to alternative medicine practices, which view the body as a whole rather than separate parts, and treat disease and symptoms through mostly nontoxic modalities, such as mind-body therapy, acupuncture, music, nutrition, and more. This chapter reviews alternative and integrative therapies and discusses the politics and scientific challenges that have limited the research of these practices. Note that while some alternative methods offer promise and may eventually be incorporated into conventional medicine, others are toxic and dangerous. Some alternative treatment become dangerous when added to conventional treatments. In Chapter 12, we give you tips about exploring these treatment methods, as well as warnings on watch out for. We also strongly suggest you include your physician in all your treatment decisions.

Cancer also can affect your job and personal relationships. Some women are welcomed back to the office with open arms, and others are shunned as a result of myths in the workplace. In Chapter 14, we'll discuss these reactions and present some options for you to consider if you're in that situation.

In addition, during and for a time after treatment you may be tired and unable to put in a full day at work. We'll tell you about your legal rights and resources that may help you make your job more accommodating during this interim period so you can continue to be a productive worker in the short- and long-term.

Cancer wreaks havoc on the emotions, and has an especially strong impact on relationships. Also in Chapter 14, we discuss how to look and feel better during and after treatment, dating again, sex after surgery, and how to tell your children you have breast cancer. We'll also tell you why it might not be safe to get pregnant after being diagnosed with breast cancer, as well as present studies showing that women who have been previously diagnosed with breast cancer can have healthy babies safely.

After your initial diagnoses, the first thing you must do is find a good doctor, one who specializes in breast cancer. Finding a good doctor might not be so easy. In chapter 15, we tell you why "Best Doctor" surveys may not be a good way to find top-notch doctors. We don't leave you hanging. We give you tips on how to find a good breast oncologist and we tell you how to choose a good hospital. We also tell you ways to cut the insurance paper chase.

Many women turn to the Internet to research breast cancer. Cyberspace is filled with useful sites. But it is also littered with quackery. In Chapter 16, we tell you how to tell the difference between a good and a bad web site. We also give you scores of sites to see.

This book is designed to give you more than a

basic understanding of breast cancer and its treatments in terms you can understand. It's filled with information from the leaders in breast cancer research and clinical practice, those doctors other doctors turn to in order to better understand the disease and treatments. It's filled with practical tips to help you get through treatments. And, it's filled with what you need to know about this disease, which may help to increase your chances of surviving breast cancer. Breast cancer is a frightening disease. But there are good treatments available, good doctors to administer them, good resources for support, and good researchers designing new and better treatments— good reason for hope.

What Is Breast Cancer?

PART I

GET THE SCOOP ON...
How healthy cells become cancerous ▪ The
different types of breast cancer ▪ Breast cancer
facts and statistics ▪ Symptoms of breast
cancer ▪ Myths and facts about breast cancer

The Lowdown on Breast Cancer

Chapter 1

Breast cancer—the very words are frightening, but even more so when softly spoken by a doctor who relays your diagnosis or that of a cherished family member or friend. Often, the words are so shocking you may have difficulty comprehending much more of what's said after that. Leaving the doctor's office dazed, your only thought may be, "Why me?" But soon your thoughts turn to a more important issue: surviving. You begin to think, "What can I do to increase my chances of survival? What treatment options are available? How effective are they? What do the finest oncologists in this country say about the different treatment protocols and current research?" Or, you may not have been diagnosed with cancer, but are among many women who are related to someone who has, or are simply concerned about getting it and want to know about risk factors and what you can do to reduce your risk of getting breast cancer.

We've addressed all of these questions and concerns in this book. To better understand the issues, you must first understand the disease itself. In addition to other issues covered in this chapter, we'll tell you what happens to healthy cells to make them cancerous, give you the lowdown on breast cancer statistics, and set you straight on some of the myths about breast cancer.

What is cancer?

An estimated 8.2 million Americans alive today (in 1999) have been diagnosed with cancer, according to the National Cancer Institute (NCI). Some are considered cured, and others still have evidence of disease, and thus may develop a recurrence. Approximately 1,221,800 new cancer cases were expected to be diagnosed in 1999 and 563,100 Americans were expected to die of cancer in 1999.

Cancer is not just one disease. The term "cancer" refers to a collection of more than 100 different diseases that have one thing in common—the uncontrolled growth of cells resulting from gene mutations. The causes vary, not just among the different types of cancers (lung cancer versus breast cancer, for example), but even within the same type of cancer. For example, most lung cancers result from smoking, but a small percentage of cases (seen in agricultural workers) are believed to be linked to inhaling asbestos in industrial settings and grain dusts in storage and processing areas on farms. Not only do the causes vary, but gene mutations within the same cancer types vary as well. For instance, some breast cancers are the result of a mutation of the p53 gene (which normally inhibits the growth of tumors and can prevent or slow the spread of cancer) while others result from an inherited mutation of the BRCA1 gene (Breast Cancer Gene 1).

To better understand how cancer occurs, however, you need a quick lesson in biology.

Biology 101

The body is made up of 100 trillion cells, which are the smallest elements of life. Although small, the cell is packed with important information and tools. It contains enzymes, lipids, hormones, and other biochemical molecules and systems. Each cell has a nucleus, which holds a genetic formula encoded in long DNA strands divided into 46 chromosomes, 23 from each parent. (Each gene is a segment of DNA made up of many codons. Each codon codes for one of 20 amino acids, the building blocks of proteins.)

This genetic formula gives instructions to the cell so it can perform its job of producing specific proteins to do specific jobs in the body. There are about 50,000 different proteins, each with its own genetic code. Each protein has a specific formulation (the number and ordering of amino acids), configuration (the shape of the molecule—how the amino acids are fitted together), and function. The instructions encoded in the genes determine the protein's job description. Each cell links together amino acids in specific sequences to form specific proteins (in varying quantities) to do specific jobs.

The sequence of amino acids in a protein is determined by the sequence of codons on a gene. The gene also determines when the production of the protein starts and stops. If there is an error in just one codon, the wrong amino acid may be selected, and therefore the wrong protein may be formed. (Abnormal proteins can be detected chemically in the tissues that are affected by a cancer. Then the gene that codes for it can be determined.) If part of a codon is missing or wrong, the whole genetic sequence is thrown off base, and no protein or a wrong protein may be formed.

Each individual cell contains all of the genes needed to perform any function in the human body. Each cell type, however, doesn't need all the genes to perform its specific function, so not all of the genes in each cell are activated. The active and inactive gene specifications vary by cell type and function. For instance, a skin cell doesn't need all of the proteins produced in a liver cell to make skin, so those genes and others are permanently turned off in that cell. Only those genes needed by skin cells are permanently on. However, there are other genes that the cell may only need at certain times, and those genes are capable of being turned on and off.

Cancer occurs when the switches stop working right. This sometimes happens when a gene mutates—altering the protein for which it codes—kind of like a typographical error in the genetic sequence. The new structure affects the amount of the gene's product or activity.

Not all mutations cause cancer. And even if a gene does mutate, remember, you have two copies of every gene. So the second copy, in many cases, takes over to keep the cell alive and functional. The trouble arises when both genes are seriously damaged by a mutation. If the activity of the protein produced by that gene is no longer present, the cell loses one of its functions. Still, that's not enough to cause cancer.

Breaking the body's lines of defense

The body has many protective measures in place. Consider them disaster prevention plans. When the immune system gets wind of a genetic malfunction, it hones in and destroys the mutant. Other times, a failing cell goes through a process called *apoptosis*, a programmed death. Still, other mutations don't have a significant effect on the protein production. In those

Timesaver
If you have questions about breast cancer or any other cancer, call the National Cancer Institute's Cancer Information Service toll-free at 800/4-CANCER or the American Cancer Society at 800/ACS-2345 to speak to a cancer information specialist. Both NCI and the ACS will send you publications about cancer and NCI will send you copies of some scientific studies. These services are free.

cases, the mutant gene is considered a "variant." Variants have played a significant role in evolution. However, when the change reduces the activity or the amount of protein the gene produces, the change is usually referred to as a mutation.

Here's where the problem arises: Genetic mutations play a key role in cancer when they affect genes that regulate cell growth. (Remember, cancer is the unregulated growth of cells.) Normally, cells multiply by dividing in two. As the process begins, the cell grows, makes a copy of its chromosomes (which contain DNA, the genetic material), and divides in two. Each of the two cells, called daughter cells, contain identical chromosomes. Some cells grow and divide routinely while others wait for signals to do so. Either way, under normal circumstances, the cycle is regulated carefully by the body.

There are hundreds of genes that produce proteins that regulate cell division, growth, development, and differentiation. Oncogenes, mutated genes that are capable of causing normal cells to transform into cancer cells, involve these growth "promoter" genes. There are also tumor "suppressor" genes, which act to prevent uncontrolled cell growth, and thus are able to keep cancers from forming. If the promoter gene works without the balance of the suppressor gene, cell growth is uncontrolled. In other words, cell growth goes unchecked when both copies of a tumor-suppressor gene are mutated. A person who has inherited or developed a defective tumor-suppressor gene, such as the BRCA1 gene, lacks one of the body's best defenses against cancer. Scientists have identified at least 20 defective genes that sometimes instruct cells to grow unchecked. Scientists believe that both pairs of several genes must be mutated in order to develop cancer. Generally, a single genetic mutation isn't enough to cause cancer. However, they may make a cell vulnerable to becoming malignant from environmental exposures.

The road to cancer

A cell must go through three steps to become a cancer, a fourth before it becomes a cancer that spreads, and a fifth before it becomes a *metastatic* cancer:

1. *Hyperplasia*—The cell still appears clinically normal, but it is dividing too rapidly.

2. *Dysplasia*—To get to this stage, the gene must mutate again. Under the microscope, the cell's shape or position is no longer normal.

3. *In-situ cancer*—The cell has continued to replicate with further mutations to reach this stage. Now a cancer, the cells are still *localized*, that is, they are confined to the tissue from which they originated.

4. *Invasive cancer*—Another mutation must occur to reach this stage of erratic cell development. "Invasive" means that, under the microscope, the primary tumor has invaded the surrounding tissue and has the potential to travel through the lymphatic system or the blood system and spread to other organs, such as the bones, liver, lungs, and, rarely, the brain in the case of breast cancer. If the cancer spreads to other areas, these new growths are called *metastases*.

5. *Metastatic cancer*—Metastatic means the cancer has spread to another site. Whereas the original tissue growth is referred to as the *primary site*, metastases are called *secondary sites* or *distant sites*. A metastatic tumor in the lung or bone (or

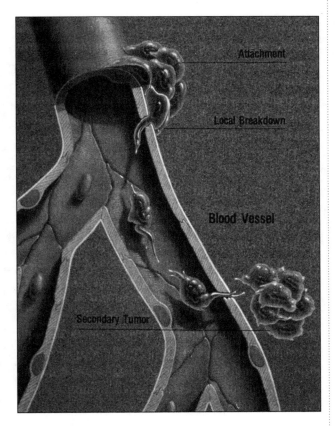

Figure 1.1
How cancer
spreads

other organ) is different from a tumor that originally developed in those organs. So while a person might originally be diagnosed with breast cancer and subsequently diagnosed with lung or bone cancer, under a microscope the pathologist can see that the tumor cells look like the original breast cancer. The cancer cells have traveled through the lymph system or the blood system to the affected organ. A metastatic tumor is not a new cancer.

See Figure 1.1 to see how cancer spreads through the lymphatic system.

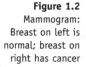

Figure 1.2
Mammogram:
Breast on left is
normal; breast on
right has cancer

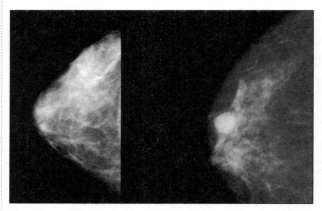

Note: You can have dysplasia without progression just as you can hyperplasia that doesn't progress to in situ cancer, and in situ cancer that doesn't become invasive cancer. Many women have invasive cancer in the breast that never spreads elsewhere. Also of note, most cancer results from a series of mutations that have taken place over many years.

The scoop on breast cancer

Breast cancer, the uncontrolled growth of cells in the breast tissues caused by one of several mutated genes, is the most common cancer among women (except skin cancer) and is the second major cause of cancer deaths among women; lung cancer is the first. (See Figure 1.2 to see a healthy breast versus a breast with cancer.)

How do healthy breast cells become cancerous?

In order for a healthy cell to become cancerous, one or more genes must mutate. As more mutations occur, they overwhelm the body's defenses against unrestrained cell growth. Sometimes the cause is an inherited genetic defect, but most of the time it's not. Defective breast cancer genes BRCA1 and BRCA2, both suppressor genes, are thought to be involved in only about 5 percent of all breast cancers (and a higher percentage of breast cancers affecting women under 45). So it is only a small group that has a strong inherited susceptibility to breast cancer. (Diagnostic testing is available to test for inherited bad copies of BRCA1 and BRCA2 genes. When defective, these genes are also believed to be responsible for hereditary ovarian cancer.)

What about the other 95 percent of breast cancers? They may be triggered, caused, or influenced by environmental factors that either affect levels of the female hormone estrogen or mimic estrogen.

Many experts believe that estrogen plays a role in normal breast cell growth and development by stimulating the release of proteins called growth factors. Growth factors, in turn, deliver a signal to the breast cells that instructs them to divide and specialize, so that normal maturation of the breast can occur.

Estrogen controls breast cell growth by attaching to proteins called estrogen receptors. But estrogens can also cause genetically altered breast cells to divide more rapidly than normal cells, a process that can result in a tumor. This can happen when there are excessive amounts of estrogens present or as a result of being exposed to chemicals that mimic some of the roles of estrogen.

Many environmental estrogens can attach to the estrogen receptors. By doing so, they fool the body or tissues by giving them an "estrogen" signal. Environmental estrogens, according to the National Institute of Environmental Health Sciences (NIEHS), one of the branches of the National Institutes of Health, include a variety of synthetic chemicals and natural plant compounds thought to mimic estrogen or block the natural hormone.

Bright Idea
MAMM magazine provides information on how to live healthier and happier lives for women who have been diagnosed with cancer. You can find more information about this magazine at www.mamm.com.

Watch Out!
Men are not immune from breast cancer. Though rare, it still occurs. During 1999, NCI expected 1,300 new cases of breast cancer in men, and an estimated 400 men were expected to die from it that year.

Environmental estrogens are found in our food, drinks, and even the air, according to NIEHS. The interactions between a woman's genes and several possible environmental factors including diet, tobacco, alcohol use, and chemical pollutants are not completely understood. But there does appear to be an important relationship. In animal studies, according to NIEHS, chemicals known to cause breast cancer don't produce a significant increase in tumors unless the female hormone estrogen is present.

The female hormone estrogen is also likely to be an important factor in male breast cancer, according to a study published in the journal *Occupational and Environmental Medicine* (September 1998). In men, estrogen develops in fatty tissue and from the conversion of the male hormone testosterone. This further supports the belief that lifestyle and occupational (that is, environmental) factors affect the production and metabolism of hormones and that environmental factors may be important in men just as they are in women, the authors suggest.

Recent studies have focused on pesticides and other "environmental estrogens," so called because they "mimic" some of the properties of the female sex hormone. NIEHS and NCI are both funding research on this subject. The Long Island (NY) Breast Cancer Study Project is focusing on the possible links between breast cancer development and environmental exposures, including water and air pollutants, electric and magnetic fields, pesticides and other toxic chemicals, and hazardous and municipal wastes. The Northeast Mid-Atlantic Breast Cancer Program is exploring the relationship between pesticide exposure and breast cancer incidence in women who live in areas where breast cancer rates are higher than the norm.

Is timing everything?

Puberty is a time of awkward moments, social embarrassments, and rapid mood swings. Blame it on hormones. These hormonal changes, in part, contribute to the growth of breast tissue, marked by rapid cell division and differentiation, in young women. During this time, breast tissue may be especially sensitive to the effects of cancer-causing agents, according to NIEHS. For example, when "adolescent" female rats were exposed to aromatic hydrocarbons, typically found in exhaust fumes, almost all of the rats developed breast cancer. And young Japanese females who were exposed to radiation from the atomic bomb during World War II developed breast cancer more often than those who were exposed at an older age.

But there's a flip side to this finding. Exposures to environmental estrogens at some ages can have a protective effect against breast cancer, according to research results from NIEHS grantees. When laboratory animals were fed genestein, a plant product high in estrogen, during neonatal or prepubertal periods, they experienced a temporary increase in cell growth and differentiation. Once these animals reached maturity, these effects were no longer evident. But when these same animals as adults were exposed to known *carcinogens*, cancer-causing agents, they were less likely than animals who were not fed genestein to develop breast cancer later in life. This finding led researchers to believe that this environmental estrogen might have a protective effect. Additional studies are being conducted to confirm this relationship. (Genestein-rich foods include soybeans and other soy proteins.) Interestingly, studies also show that Japanese women's diets are higher in soy compared with American women's diets, and Japanese women have a lower rate of breast cancer.

Types of breast cancer

Breast cancer can be caused by several tumor types. To understand this better, you need a quick primer on breast anatomy.

Inside the breast are *acini*, small sacs clustered in *lobules*, and *ducts*, where milk is produced. Each breast has 15-20 sections called *lobes*, made up of these lobules. Both the lobes and lobules are connected by large ducts, thin tubes that transport milk to the nipple. The lobules and ducts are supported by fibrous tissue and fat called *stroma*. These structures are involved in the production and secretion of milk.

Unofficially...
LCIS is a precancer; DCIS is cancer.

In order to determine treatment when a woman is diagnosed, the *pathologist,* a physician who specializes in studying cells under a microscope, must examine and classify the cancer. The most common tumor types are ductal and lobular. *Ductal cancer,* the most common type of breast cancer, is so named because it is found in the cells of the ducts. Cancer originating in the lobes or lobules is called *lobular cancer.* This type of breast cancer is the second most common of the invasive cancers.

While that is a general overview, you may want to know specifics. Here's the scoop: An *in situ tumor* is a proliferation of malignant epithelial cells that is confined to the ducts and/or lobules. That is, it hasn't spread beyond where it originated. There are two types of in situ carcinomas.

1. ***Lobular carcinoma in situ (LCIS)*—**Considered pre-invasive and pre-malignant, lobular carcinoma in situ is a strong predictor of future new breast cancer in either breast, with a 20 to 25 percent lifetime risk. LCIS increases the risk of

invasive cancer to both breasts, but any histology (microscopic cellular change) can occur. It does not have to be completely excised.

2. ***Ductal carcinoma in situ (DCIS) (also known as intraductal carcinoma or noninvasive ductal carcinoma)***—DCIS is an actual cancer, and it is considered pre-invasive, that is, given time many of these tumors would become invasive. Therefore, it must be completely excised. DCIS is usually diagnosed by mammography. About 15 to 20 percent of all newly diagnosed cancers are DCIS.

(Note: sometimes overlaps exist between lobular-carcinoma in situ and ductal carcinoma in situ.) Sometimes malignant cells migrate outside of the duct or lobules and invade the stroma. This is called *invasive* or *infiltrating* mammary carcinomas. There are three common types of invasive tumors:

1. Infiltrating mammary duct carcinoma (ductal)

2. Infiltrating lobular carcinoma (lobular)

3. Medullary (typical and atypical)

There are a variety of infiltrating ductal carcinoma types, including those where no special histological features are designated. "Good" variants include tubular, mucinous, and papillary. "Bad" variants include carcinosarcomas and sarcomas. Ductal carcinoma in situ is the most common type of noninvasive breast cancer. Infiltrating (invasive) ductal carcinoma accounts for about 80 percent of all breast cancers, according to the American Cancer Society. Invasive ductal carcinoma tumors feel like stones (although they are not always palpable) and commonly metastasize.

Invasive lobular carcinoma accounts for 10-15 percent of invasive breast cancers, according to the

Unofficially...
Breast cancer was expected to cause an estimated 43,300 deaths in women in 1999 and more than 500,000 during the 1990s.

American Cancer Society. (The numbers of infiltrating lobular carcinoma compared with infiltrating ductal carcinoma may be shifting due to earlier detection as a result of mammography screenings.) Rather than feeling like a round pebble, these tumors are more likely to present as thickened areas of the breast because the cancerous cells tend to grow around the ducts and lobules. (However, sometimes lobular cancers do form lumps.) The typical prognosis for infiltrating lobular carcinomas is similar to infiltrating ductal carcinomas.

Medullary carcinomas, which account for 3 to 5 percent of all breast cancers, have only low-grade infiltrative properties. Some studies show that medullary carcinomas have a more favorable prognosis than those with no special histological features while others show a worse prognosis.

(Note: There are rare forms of breast cancer, including squamous, adenocystic, papillary, secretory, and carcinosarcoma (metaplastic duct carcinoma). Many of the more common ductal carcinomas contain small areas of these rarer tumor types.)

Malignant cells that migrate from the duct or lobules may spread beyond the breast to adjacent lymph nodes. They can then travel through the blood or lymph to distant sites and become secondary cancers, that is, breast cancer growing in the bone or lung, for example. As mentioned earlier, this is referred to as *metastatic cancer*.

There are two more rare types of breast cancer—inflammatory breast cancer and Paget's disease—discussed later in this chapter.

Breast cancer facts and figures

In 1999, an estimated 176,300 new cases of breast cancer were expected to be diagnosed in the United

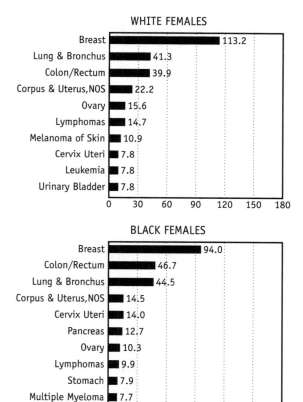

WHITE FEMALES

Breast	113.2
Lung & Bronchus	41.3
Colon/Rectum	39.9
Corpus & Uterus, NOS	22.2
Ovary	15.6
Lymphomas	14.7
Melanoma of Skin	10.9
Cervix Uteri	7.8
Leukemia	7.8
Urinary Bladder	7.8

BLACK FEMALES

Breast	94.0
Colon/Rectum	46.7
Lung & Bronchus	44.5
Corpus & Uterus, NOS	14.5
Cervix Uteri	14.0
Pancreas	12.7
Ovary	10.3
Lymphomas	9.9
Stomach	7.9
Multiple Myeloma	7.7

Figure 1.3

Source: SEER Program, National Cancer Institute, based on an approximate 10 percent sample of the U.S. population

States, 1,300 of them among men. Women living in the United States have a one in eight chance of developing breast cancer in their lifetime by age 95, and one out of every 28 women is at risk of dying from it. In fact, breast cancer is the most common cancer among both Caucasian and African-American women in the United States, although the rate among African-American women (94.0 per 100,000) is lower than that for Caucasian women (113.2 per 100,000), according to the NCI. (See Figure 1.3) When comparing women younger than age 45, more

African-American women develop breast cancer than Caucasian women. Economics, combined with culture, also plays a role in stage at diagnosis. Three times as many low-income, African-American women are diagnosed with advanced disease than high-income women in general. Furthermore, African-American women, compared with Caucasian women, are more reluctant to seek medical attention when they discover a lump. As a result, the current survival rate for Caucasian women is more than 10 percentage points higher than for African-American women, according to NCI statistics.

Breast cancer incidence among women is on the rise. Rates increased from 88.6 per 100,000 in the early 1970s to 109.8 in the early 1990s, according to data from the NCI's Surveillance, Epidemiology, and End Results (SEER) Program. Despite the higher incidence of breast cancer, more Caucasian women die from lung cancer. For African-American women, however, breast cancer mortality is slightly higher than that of lung cancer. But the incidence of lung cancer is also on the rise, so lung cancer deaths may eventually surpass breast cancer mortality for African-American women, too.

Not only are there variations in cancer incidence and mortality rates among women by race, there are also wide geographic variations. According to the World Health organization the incidence rates for breast cancer in women were highest (104.2 per 100,000) among Caucasian women in the San Francisco Bay, California area and lowest (3.4 per 100,000) among women in The Gambia. In a listing compiled by the World Health Organization (see Table 1.1), the breast cancer rates are low and deaths from it are rare in Asian countries. Breast cancer death rates are highest

TABLE 1.1 INTERNATIONAL BREAST CANCER MORTALITY RANKINGS

1.	England & Wales	26.	Sweden
2.	Denmark	27.	Finland
3.	Scotland	28.	Germany, Dem
4.	Ireland	29.	Portugal
5.	Northern Ireland	30.	Spain
6.	Belgium	31.	Cuba
7.	New Zealand	32.	Greece
8.	Netherlands	33.	Poland
9.	Malta	34.	Yugoslavia
10.	Luxembourg	35.	Bulgaria
11.	Uruguay	36.	Singapore
12.	Switzerland	37.	Puerto Rico
13.	Canada	38.	Costa Rica
14.	Germany, Fed	39.	USSR
15.	Israel	40.	Chile
16.	United States	41.	Kuwait
17.	Austria	42.	Venezuela
18.	Hungary	43.	Hong Kong
19.	Australia	44.	Panama
20.	Italy	45.	Mexico
21.	Argentina	46.	Japan
22.	Iceland	47.	Ecuador
23.	Czechoslovakia	48.	China
24.	France	49.	Korea Republic
25.	Norway	50.	Thailand

Source: World Health Organization data as adapted by the American Cancer Society, 1992.

in England and Wales, followed by Denmark, Scotland, Ireland, and Northern Ireland. The United States ranks 16th. Some of the disparity may have to do with environmental factors, including diet, and some may have to do with genes. Screening, detection, and treatment may also play a role.

You may be in a high-risk group for breast cancer because of your nationality, culture, or age. The rate of breast cancer is rising faster in Hispanic women than in other women. American Indian and Alaskan Native women have higher breast cancer incidence rates and lower survival rates than some other groups and several studies suggest that cancer rates increase among Asian and Pacific Islander women as they become Westernized. Two specific gene mutations are higher among Ashkanazi Jewish women than other women. African-American women are more likely than other women to die from breast cancer. And, as you age, your chances of getting breast cancer increase.

But with the increased use of mammography, inthe United States, breast cancers are being detected earlier, when they are in less advanced stages. In fact, mammograms may detect cancerous growths up to two years before a lump is palpable.

Partly because of the increased use of mammograms, and partly due to advances in treatment, more women are being diagnosed early and surviving breast cancer. After increasing about 4 percent per year in the 1980s, breast cancer incidence rates in women have leveled off in recent years to about 110 cases per 100,000. And the five-year relative survival rate is rising.

The five-year relative survival rate for localized breast cancer was 97 percent in 1999, up 25 percent from 72 percent in the early 1940s. For breast cancer that has spread regionally (to neighboring organs or lymph nodes), the survival rate is 77 percent. For women with distant metastases, that rate drops to 22 percent, and survival after diagnoses of breast cancer continues to decline after five years. But 69 percent of women diagnosed with breast cancer survive 10 years, and 57 percent survive 15 years.

(The 5-year relative survival rate is defined as the observed survival rate for a group of individuals with

TABLE 1.2   INCREASE IN SURVIVAL RATES FOR BREAST CANCER.

1974-76	1977-79	1980-82	1983-90
74.3	74.5	76.2	80.4

Source: National Cancer Institute

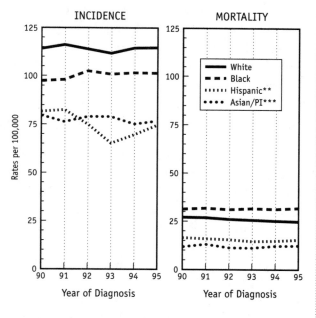

Figure 1.4
Breast Cancer
Rates from
1990-1995

*Source: National
Cancer Institute*

***Asian and Pacific Islanders and population estimates based on unadjusted Census Bureau estimates

**Hispanic is not mutually exclusive from whites, blacks, and Asian and Pacific Islanders

Death rates exclude deaths that occurred in Connecticut, Louisiana, New Hampshire, and Oklahoma

Rates are per 100,000 and age-adjusted to 1970 U.S. Standard Million. Source: NCI, based on SEER, NCHS, and Census data cancer compared with other people in the general population who are similar to the cancer group in age, gender, race, and calendar year of diagnosis. This number is adjusted for other causes of death and will be higher than the observed survival rate because, for example, if you have breast cancer and die in a car accident, the observed survival rate does not truly reflect how long you would have lived.)

The most recent data from NCI indicate that overall 82 percent of women who are diagnosed with breast cancer will survive their disease for more than five years. Incidence and mortality rates from 1974 to 1990 can be seen in Table 1.2 and those from 1990 to 1995 can be seen in Figure 1.4.

And there's hope for even better prognoses among all breast cancers. Scientists worldwide are working around the clock to get a better understanding of this disease and consequently to devise better diagnostic tools and treatments.

Statistics need to be put in context, however. Though it is estimated that one in eight women will be diagnosed with breast cancer in their lifetime, it does not mean that if you and seven other women are sitting in a gynecologist's waiting room, that one of you will leave with bad news. The one in eight figure (approximately 12.6 percent) includes all age groups in five-year intervals (based on the proportion of the population living to that age) up to an open-ended interval of 95 years and over, according to the NCI. (In other words, this assumes all women will live to age 95 without dying of other causes, such as heart disease.) But, the NCI points out, assessing cancer risk at a specific point in time, that is, age-specific probabilities, rather than over a lifetime, is more appropriate. For example, at age 50, an African-

❝
Coronary artery disease is the leading cause of death in women, with six times as many women dying of heart disease than of breast cancer.
—The American Heart Association
❞

American woman actually has only about a 2 percent chance of developing breast cancer by age 60, and a Caucasian woman has about a 2.5 percent chance.

Another problem with using the one-in-eight statistic is that it is hard to predict what the breast cancer incidence rates will be in the future, so that probability is a hypothetical number. Therefore, as noted, your actual risk is probably better reflected in conditional probabilities over one or two decades. Furthermore, these probabilities are based on population averages. Your actual risk may be higher or lower, depending on a variety of factors, including your family history, reproductive history, environmental exposures, and other factors yet to be identified.

Chances for recovery from breast cancer

Once a woman is diagnosed with breast cancer, her first thoughts most likely center around the prognosis—what are her chances for recovery? Recovery is often measured in five-year survival rates.

The chance of recovery (as well as the treatment methods) depends on many factors including:

- The stage of the cancer. That is, at what point in its evolution the cancer is found. Cancer that hasn't spread (localized) is much easier to treat than cancer that has spread (metastasized).

- The type of breast cancer.

- Characteristics of the cancer cells.

- Whether cancer also is found in the other breast.

- The woman's age.

- The woman's menstrual/menopausal status.

- The woman's general health.

More specifically, prognostic indicators most

Unofficially...
Histologic grade looks at the cell as a whole while nuclear grade looks at the nucleus.

commonly used are:

1. *Lymph node involvement (node positive)*—
   Breast cancer commonly spreads to lymph nodes
   in the underarm (*axillary lymph nodes*). Women
   with positive nodes have a greater risk of having
   a recurrence of breast cancer than women with
   negative nodes because once it has spread to the
   lymph nodes it's more difficult to eradicate
   every single microscopic cell.

2. *Tumor size*—Generally, small tumors have a better prognosis than do large tumors.

3. *Histologic grade (how closely the tumor cells
   resemble normal cells when viewed under the
   microscope)*—The grading scale ranges from 1 to
   3 with grade 1 tumors composed of cells that
   closely resemble normal ones and grade 3 tumors
   composed of abnormal-looking and rapidly growing cancer cells.

4. *Nuclear grade (how closely the cell's nucleus
   resembles that of a normal cell)*—The grading
   scale ranges from 1 to 3. Grade 1 means that the
   nuclei of the cells in a tumor are not too abnormal with regard to density, shape, size, irregularity, etc. Grade 3 means the features of the nucleus are markedly abnormal with regard to those
   same criteria.

5. *Mitotic index*—A third criterion used in grading
   a tumor. It is an estimate of the number of cells
   undergoing division in the tumor. With a low
   score of 1+1+1=3 and a high score of 3+3+3=9,
   tumors are graded on a scale of 3 to 9—3 is low-
   grade (least aggressive) and 9 is high grade (most
   aggressive), explains Susan Tannenbaum, M.D.,
   a fellow with the College of American Pathologists and a pathologist at United Pathology

Associates, in Port Chester, New York.

6. *Hormone receptors*—Breast cells contain receptors for the hormones estrogen and progesterone. As noted earlier, these receptors regulate breast tissue growth and change in response to changing hormone levels. About two-thirds of all breast cancers contain high levels of estrogen receptors. (They are called ER+ tumors.) And two-thirds of ER+ tumors have receptors to progesterone and are therefore PR+. (PR+ tumors require an intact estrogen receptor.) Tumors with high levels of estrogen receptors tend to grow less aggressively and respond well to hormone therapy, resulting in a better prognosis.

7. *Proliferative capacity of a tumor*—The rate at which cancer cells proliferate (divide to form more cells) determines, in part, how aggressive the tumor is. The proliferative capacity of a tumor correlates with nuclear grade.

8. *Oncogene expression and amplification*—As noted earlier, oncogenes can either promote or suppress cell growth. Tumor cells that contain certain oncogenes are associated with a higher risk of recurrence after the cancer is apparently eradicated. (HER-2/neu is a good example of this. The HER-2/neu gene produces a protein on the cell's surface. This protein receives biological signals to grow. An overabundance of the gene or protein translates to out-of-control growth, which means an aggressive cancer that spreads rapidly.)

Signs and symptoms of breast cancer

The early stages of breast cancer usually aren't associated with pain. In fact, there may be no symptoms

Unofficially...
Inflammatory breast cancer is a clinical diagnosis, a determination based on the clinical features of a disease, other than histology, a diagnosies made after studying cells and tissue under a microscope.

at all. There may not even be a palpable lump, which is why getting a routine screening mammogram is so important. But as the cancer grows, you may experience one or all of the following symptoms (though these symptoms are not always a sign of breast cancer):

- A painless, palpable, or visible lump
- Unexplained pain in the breast (without presence of a lump)
- A thickening of breast or surrounding tissue
- A thickening of the tissue in the underarm area
- A change in the shape or size of the breast
- A discharge from the nipple (bloody or clear and sticky), although this is rare

There are two exceptions: symptoms vary for both inflammatory breast cancer and Paget's disease.

Inflammatory breast cancer

Inflammatory breast cancer, which may or may not be present with an obvious lump, is a rare form of breast cancer—it only accounts for between 1 to 4 percent of all diagnoses. It grows and spreads quickly, blocking the lymph vessels in the breast and skin and resulting in possible symptoms that include:

- Red, warm, swollen breast
- Skin ridges

Of course, these same symptoms can occur with benign breast problems. A palpable mass (one you can feel with your hands) is not detected in about half of those women eventually diagnosed with inflammatory breast cancer. Survival rates are rising because of improving treatments. However, the prognosis is considered poor, even if the disease appears to be localized.

Paget's disease

Paget's disease is a rare, slow-growing cancer of the nipple that accounts for about 1 percent of all breast cancers. It's usually associated with an underlying DCIS. The disease originates in the milk ducts of the nipple. In fact, the nipple skin often contains tumor cells, which cause the symptoms. This type of breast cancer is characterized by a change in the nipple. Symptoms also include itching, burning, oozing, crusting, and bleeding or a combination of these symptoms. Paget's disease may also present as a sore that won't heal, and remains an open wound. Because the symptoms mimic that of an infection or skin inflammation (it typically affects only one nipple), detection is often delayed.

More than one-half of Paget's disease patients can feel the tumor. To diagnose it, the doctor takes a sample of the tissue and sends it to the lab for a biopsy. The doctor will also take a mammogram of both breasts to see if other tumors are present. If the cancer is localized to the nipple, treatment may consist of removing the affected nipple and surrounding tissue or radiation therapy. But if a more extensive tumor is found in the breast, treatment may consist of surgery, chemotherapy, and radiation. The prognosis for Paget's disease depends on the type of tumor involved and whether or not it is associated with an underlying invasive breast cancer.

Don't blame the messenger

Breast cancer often takes center stage in the media. Prevention methods are recited over and over again. Early detection through self-examinations and mammography are stressed, so much so that many women believe that if they reduce their risk factors as much as possible and have routine exams, they won't get breast cancer.

Distorted information, which may result from the slant of stories relayed by the media, also plays a role. Consider this excerpt from a recently released news story: "Women—especially those who don't smoke, exercise, stay lean, and eat their vegetables—can still develop the disease, even if they have no family history." In fact, as noted earlier, most women who get breast cancer don't have a family history of it. Furthermore, most women who develop breast cancer have no known risk factors, except gender and age.

So it should come as no surprise that there are many women, along with their family and friends, who are extremely angry when they've followed "the rules."

There's a danger in promising women that doing everything right will prevent them from getting breast cancer. It doesn't, says Donald Lannin, M.D., professor of surgery and director of the Leo W. Jenkins Cancer Center at East Carolina University School of Medicine in Greenville, N.C. A large percentage of women develop breast cancer even though they receive routine screenings and maintain a healthy lifestyle, he says. So, they think if they did everything right, someone else must have done something wrong, he says. That someone is the radiologist or primary care physician.

Prevention and screening will not completely eliminate deaths from breast cancer. Studies conclude that screening reduces the breast cancer death rate by one-third. Therefore, two-thirds of those who would have died without screening would have died despite being screened, according to Lannin.

The problem lies in technology and costs,

according to Lannin. About 75 percent of breast cancers show up in mammograms, he says. That means 25 percent of breast cancers don't. It's not always the failure of the machine, technician, or radiologist reading the X-ray. Rather, in some women with false-negative mammogram readings (those whose tumor wasn't picked up on the X-ray), the density of the breast tissue may have been the same density as that of the tumor.

Mammograms and physical examinations are not as good a diagnostic tool for many younger women, according to Lannin, because their breasts are denser and cystic. A lot of women who did everything right—got routine mammograms—and were misdiagnosed as healthy are younger: under age 50. However, although these screenings are not perfect, they are important, and all women should perform breast self exams, get clinical breast exams, and, if they're 40 or older, get screening mammograms.

It's just not a perfect system, Lannin says. "We need better techniques for diagnoses and certainly better techniques for treatment," he adds. However, better technology is costly. Appendix D lists pending legislation affecting cancer research funding and an Internet address in which to find your senators' and representatives' e-mail addresses as well as the phone number to the Capitol.

However, sometimes the radiologist is at fault. Another team of researchers has demonstrated that, in fact, many radiologists are not skilled at reading mammograms. This makes it even more important for women to get screened routinely. (If a cancer is missed one year, another radiologist may find it the following year.) Initial findings from their study are discussed in Chapter 6.

Myths and facts about cancer

There are many myths about breast cancer. They can be dangerous because they may make women less diligent about performing breast self exams, scheduling clinical exams, and getting mammograms. They also may prevent women from either seeking medical care early or accepting medical care after the diagnosis is made.

For example, some women think that finding a lump in the breast isn't important if it's small and doesn't hurt, Lannin says. This can be a dangerous belief because it delays seeking medical attention. "That's the time you want to catch it if it's a cancer," he explains.

Many women seem to have the mistaken belief that if breast cancer doesn't run in their families, they don't have to worry much about getting it. In fact, most breast cancers are not linked to a family history. According to the NCI, 80 percent of women who develop breast cancer have no family history of it.

Some women also believe that if they had one normal mammogram or their doctor didn't recommend they get one that they're exempt from needing this cancer screening test. Not so! Once is not enough for those who have had a mammogram. The first test is used as a *baseline*—it shows the technician and radiologist what your breast looks like under normal (not cancerous) conditions and is used for comparison if later tests find questionable features. If your doctor hasn't made a recommendation and you're over age 40, talk to him or her about getting one. Doctors have busy schedules, and while this is not a good excuse, it is a reason why they might neglect to instruct you to get screened.

Furthermore, some women believe that radiation

levels associated with mammography are unsafe. No one wants to expose herself unnecessarily to radiation, but the levels of radiation emitted during mammography are extremely low. So in this case, the benefits of low doses of radiation far outweigh the risks of missing the opportunity for an early diagnosis.

Some women may know all of this but still avoid screening because they've heard that mammography is painful. While it may not be a day at the park, it's not painful. The pressure may cause some discomfort (and embarrassment, like any physical exam where you have to undress), but discomfort is not the same as pain. Again, the benefits far outweigh the potential discomfort. And keep in mind, the discomfort and possible embarrassment only last a few minutes.

Another misconception: some women who have been diagnosed with breast cancer think they did something to cause it. Typically that "something" is bumping or bruising the breast. There is no scientific evidence to support this supposition. Nor is there any scientific evidence that stress can cause breast cancer.

According to the NCI, some women think they can "catch" breast cancer from other women who have the disease. Breast cancer is not contagious.

Another concern for some women is that wearing a bra increases their risk of getting breast cancer. There's no scientific evidence to support this idea.

Lannin, along with five other researchers, investigated the influence of cultural factors and racial differences among women. Their findings were published in the *Journal of the American Medical Association* (June 1998). They found that a large number of cultural beliefs were significant predictors of late stage at diagnosis. One such finding was the belief that women who have breast surgery are no longer attractive to men.

One myth that researchers found interesting is the belief that air that comes into contact with the tumor during surgery causes cancer to grow or spread. This belief prohibits some women from getting a biopsy.

It is true that rare abdominal tumors can rupture during surgery, causing the cancer to spread. But neither the tumor characteristics of breast cancers nor the surrounding environment share the same characteristics that could make that type of spread possible. (Breast tumors are solid. They are surrounded by tissue. In contrast, the abdomen is a cavity, so it's harder to contain the spread of a punctured cystic tumor.) It does not appear that this folk belief resulted from this finding, but it may be perpetuated by it, Lannin says.

Fundamentalist religious beliefs also play a role in the myths that abound, according to Lannin. As a result of their religion, some women have a fatalistic view of life (their belief system dictates that their developing breast cancer was meant to be) that prevents them from seeking medical help, according to Lannin.

The study found that many of these same people believed that herbal remedies, over-the-counter medications, and chiropractic regimens are effective treatments for breast cancer. These beliefs had a positive correlation with late-stage disease.

Cultural differences are not limited to patients. In a study reported in the British medical journal *Lancet* (March 1999), medical policy analysts at Johns Hopkins in Baltimore, Maryland, and in France reveal how strong a role culture may play on physicians' views in determining the medical care patients receive. The differences arise in the gray areas, such as preventive mastectomies for women with the BRCA1 or BRCA2 genes.

In both countries, the operation is an option for women in that high-risk group. But in France, physicians strongly oppose it for women younger than 30, referring to it in a public consensus statement as "a mutilation." In fact, French surgeons are prevented by law from performing the surgery unless it's clearly therapeutic. In contrast, surgeons in the United States only need the woman's informed consent.

Just the facts

- There are more than 100 different types of cancer.
- Cancer is caused by genetic mutations.
- Breast cancer can be caused by environmental factors (most of which are not well characterized) or inherited.
- There are different types of breast cancer, depending on which cells have the genetic mutation.
- Breast cancer is the leading cause of cancer (except for skin cancer) among women as a group; some cultures and races have higher and lower rates than the norm.
- Bruises and other traumas to the breast don't cause breast cancer.

GET THE SCOOP ON...
How your immune system functions ▪ How cancer
often escapes detection by the immune system ▪ How
scientists are developing therapies that use the
immune system ▪ Ways you can boost your immunity

The Immune System

T he body is amazing. You don't have to know anything about infectious disease to fight off germs. Your body constantly battles off these microscopic intruders and repairs or kills off malfunctioning cells all day and all night. Your body is never in perfect health, but always trying to reach the optimum level to allow it to function well. That is your immune system at work. It's a system so complex that even the brightest scientists have not yet figured out how it works.

But with cancer, something goes awry with the immune system. Just like mammals and reptiles have developed in ways to adapt to and survive in their environment, cancer has evolved to escape detection and eradication by the body's best internal defenses. But that's not the whole picture. Some cancers do elicit a small immune response from the body, and some scientists theorize that many people have cancerous cells, but the body kills them so that tumors never develop and the cancerous cells are never detected by physicians.

In this chapter, you'll learn about the immune

system and how it works. We introduce many technical terms and concepts that are difficult to understand. They will be useful to you as you read this book and even more so if you decide to do your own research. Next, we address the question of why, in some cases, the immune system isn't killing the cancer. Finally, we tell you how scientists are using the immune system to eradicate cancer.

Fighting back

The immune system defends the body against attacks from foreign invaders—bacteria, viruses, fungi, and parasites. It is an elaborate network of specialized cells and organs located throughout the body. Access into the body can happen anywhere, though the mouth, nose, and eyes are key points of entry.

"War and peace"—Identification tags

The immune system must be able to distinguish healthy cells in the body from foreign invaders. That is, they must be able to differentiate between self and non-self. Each cell in your body carries a self-marker, a molecular identification tag. (Molecules identifying a cell as self are encoded by a group of genes contained in a section of a specific chromosome— *major histocompatibility complex* (MHC).) This allows immune cells and all other body cells to recognize each other and co-exist peacefully. This state of peaceful coexistence is called *self-tolerance.*

So, while the right ID tag allows peaceful coexistence, the wrong ID tag ignites war. Foreign invaders (antigens) carry IDs as well. Their identification is in the form of epitopes, characteristic shapes that protrude from their surface, much like a puzzle piece. This molecular region on the surface of the antigen elicits a quick and forceful response from the

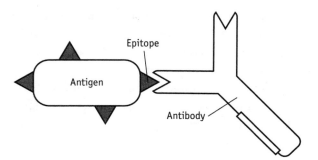

Epitope

Antigen

Antibody

Figure 2.1
Antigens (foreign invaders) have characteristic shapes, called epitopes, that protrude from their surfaces. The immune system produces a tailor-made antibody to combine with the antigen in a perfect puzzle-piece fit.

Illustration: Articulate Graphics

immune system, which produces a tailor-made antibody to combine with this antigen in a perfect puzzle piece fit. (See Figure 2.1.)

Amazingly, the immune system can recognize countless non-self molecules and make matching antibody-antigen fits to rid the body of these foreign invaders. And once infected with a virus, the immune system, incredibly, develops a memory for that virus. Subsequent infections with that same virus—even many years later—result in an antibody response so rapid that illness is prevented. More amazing immune system characteristics are listed in the bulleted list on page 38.

Long-term immunity also can be stimulated by vaccines made of inactivated viruses or from minute amounts of the microbe (germ). Vaccines are also being designed for cancer, which is discussed later in this chapter.

The immune system is made up of lymphoid organs throughout the body. The organs grow, develop, and deploy white blood cells called *lymphocytes,* which are the primary fighting agents. The lymphoid organs are connected together with other organs in the body through a vast array of lymphatic vessels through which lymph, a clear fluid, travels. Along this lymphatic network are lymph nodes, which have special compartments where immune cells gather. The lymph nodes also strain out foreign matter from the lymph returning from the tissues. Hence, the lymph nodes are where some of the battles against infection takes place.

The amazing immune system—what it can do:

- It can distinguish "self" from "non-self," the body from foreign invaders or cells from another body, except an identical twin.

- It has a perfect memory, making its defense so swift against previous invaders that often the body never gets sick from them again. The body, having already been exposed to an antigen, responds slowly to produce antibodies. But subsequently, if that antigen is ever encountered again, the antibody production response is quick, making other bodily responses unnecessary or minimal.

- It displays enormous diversity and incredible specificity in its ability to attack such a vast array of enemies.

- It has a highly sophisticated array of weapons, including fever, antibodies, cells that engulf foreign substances (phagocytic cells), and more.

Weaponry

The skin serves as the body's first line of defense. But if invading molecules rush the gates and gain entry, the immune system has a vast array of weapons specialized to match up to each foe and rid it from the body.

The system is made up of a sophisticated and dynamic communications network that regulates millions of cells that are organized into sets and subsets. These cells pass information back and forth.

Like all blood cells, immune cells arise from stem

cells in the bone marrow. Consider this the trunk of the immune system family tree. (See Figure 2.2.) There are two offspring: myeloid cells and lymphoid precursors.

Myeloid cells are large white blood cells known as *phagocytes*, which can engulf and digest foreign invaders. Phagocytes include the following:

- **Monocytes**—These large phagocytes circulate in the blood, enter the tissue, and develop into a macrophage.

- **Macrophages**—These versatile phagocytes are found in tissues throughout the body. As scavengers, they cleanse the body of old cells and other debris. They digest and process antigens and present them to T cells, initiating the immune response. They also secrete powerful

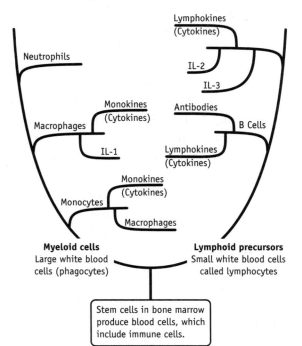

Figure 2.2
The Immune System Family Tree.

Illustration: Articulate Graphics

Figure 2.3
Macrophage
is a cell that is
attracted to the
receptors on the
antibody and will
digest and kill
any cell to which
the antibody is
attached.

*Art source:
Mary L. Disis, M.D.,
associate professor of
medicine, division of
oncology, at the
University of
Washington in
Seattle, Washington.
Illustration:
Articulate Graphics*

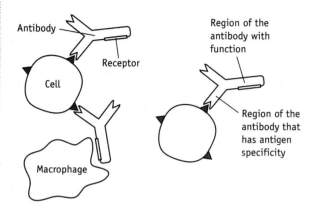

chemicals (monokines) that regulate immune and inflammation responses. See Figure 2.3.

- **Neutrophils**—These phagocytes also circulate in the blood. They move into tissues when they are needed. Neutrophils are not only phagocytes but also granulocytes. That is, they contain granules filled with potent chemicals. Neutrophils kill microbes by ingesting them. These chemicals are used to break down the microbes once ingested. Neutrophils also play a key role in acute inflammations.

Lymphoid precursors occupy the other branch of the family tree. They develop into small white blood cells called lymphocytes. There are two major classes of lymphocytes: B cells and T cells.

B cells (B lymphocytes) secrete immunoglobulins. Each B cell makes one specific antibody; these antibodies are tailor-made to fit each antigen encountered. When a B cell meets its enemy, it, and certain other cells, stimulate the production of plasma cells.

Each plasma cell serves as a factory, producing

that one tailor-made antibody, because in peacetime (when no antigens are present) only a few of these antibodies are stored. During an immune response, millions of antibodies are made and poured into the bloodstream.

Specific antibodies form from *immunoglobulins*, a family of large molecules (proteins) that have two matching heavy chains and two matching light chains that form a Y shape. The section making the open mouth of the Y varies from antibody to antibody. This uniqueness allows for the antibody to identify its matching antigen and lock together like two puzzle pieces, marking it as a target for destruction. The base or stem of the Y is identical in all antibodies in the same class (IgG, IgD, and IgE—short for immunoglobulin G, D, and E) and is used by the antibody to link to other components of the immune defenses.

There are nine chemically distinct classes of human immunoglobulins—four kinds of IgG, two IgAs and IgE, IgD, and IgM. Each class has a distinct role in the battle strategy against foreign invaders.

- **IgG**—This is the predominant immunoglobulin found in the blood and can enter tissue spaces. It coats microorganisms to expedite their uptake by other immune system cells.

- **IgA**—This immunoglobulin has two Ys linked at the base tip of the Ys. It's found mostly in saliva, tears, and respiratory and gastrointestinal tract secretions. Its structure and locations make it able to guard the entrances to the body.

- **IgE**—Normally present in only trace amounts, this immunoglobulin causes allergy symptoms. IgE is often bound to mast cells, which cause allergy symptoms.

- **IgD**—This immunoglobulin is found on the surface of B cells and is thought to play a role in recognizing antigens.

- **IgM**—Typically found in star-shaped clusters, this immunoglobulin often circulates in the blood, killing bacteria.

Whereas B lymphocytes originate in the blood, T cells (T lymphocytes) form in the thymus. Some T cells have the job of commander and help to regulate the immune system operations. Some are *cytotoxic,* killing infected and malignant cells on contact.

Regulatory T cells do two things:

1. They help activate B cells, other T cells, natural killer (NK) cells, and macrophages through helper/inducer T cells.

2. They give the "all's clear" sign to turn off or suppress immune cells.

Cytotoxic T cells (also known as killer cells) also do two things:

1. They help rid the body of virally-infected as well as cancerous cells.

2. They reject non-self cells from tissue and organ grafts.

T cells and B cells secrete lymphokines, a form of cytokine. Cytokines are varied chemical messengers, and include both lymphokines and monokines. While both T and B lymphocytes secrete lymphokines, monocytes and macrophages secrete monokines.

Cytokines bind to receptors on target cells and recruit many other cells and substances to the battlefield.

Cytokines do the following:

- Stimulate cell growth

- Help to activate cells, including those responsible

for an inflammatory response, which results from increased blood flow and a flood of immune cells and secretions to the wounded area

- Direct the flow and direction of cellular traffic

- Destroy target cells, some of which are cancerous

- Activate macrophages

Cytokines that are also interleukins include the following:

- **IL-1 (interleukin-1)**—This cytokine is produced by macrophages and other cells. It plays a role in activating both B and T cells.

- **IL-2 (interleukin-2) (also known as T cell growth factor or TCGF)**—This cytokine is produced by T cells that have been activated by antigens. It fosters the growth or maturation (differentiation) of both B and T cells. It helps to stimulate the immune system by increasing the number of lymphocytes and activating them to make them more effective.

- **IL-3 (interleukin-3)**—This cytokine is derived from T cells and is one family member of the protein mediators called colony-stimulating factors (CSFs). CSFs, in addition to other roles, are responsible for helping immature precursor cells develop into mature blood cells. Treatment with CSFs is sometimes used to help the blood-forming tissue recover from the effects of chemotherapy and radiation therapy.

- **IL-4 (interleukin-4)**—This cytokine helps B cells grow and differentiate. It also has an impact on T cells, macrophages, mast cells (which cause allergy symptoms), and granulocytes (which digest microorganisms or produce inflammatory

Unofficially...
The cytokine lymphotoxin, produced by lymphocytes, and tumor necrosis factor, produced by macrophages, kill malignant (cancerous) tumor cells.

responses).

▪ **IL-5 (interleukin-5)**—This cytokine helps B cells grow and differentiate.

▪ **IL-6 (interleukin-6)**—This cytokine helps B cells grow and differentiate.

Like cytotoxic T cells, NK (natural killer) cells are lymphocytes that kill on contact by binding to their target and delivering a burst of chemicals that make holes in the target cell's membrane, causing the cell to burst. But unlike T cells, NK cells don't need to recognize an antigen to destroy it. NK cells target tumor cells as well as infectious microbes.

Why isn't the immune system responding?

Unofficially...
Several cytokines are being used alone and in combination, linked to toxins, in clinical cancer trials.

Typically, when something goes awry in the body, the body's defense mechanisms respond quickly. And under normal circumstances, the body is quick to respond to mutations in cells by either repairing them or through *apoptosis*, natural cell death. (See Figure 2.4.) But what happens with cancer? What's going on in the mapping room? For reasons not clearly understood, cancerous cells, at least those that eventually grow into a tumor, evade the body's immune response and are therefore permitted to grow uncontrolled.

Although cancerous cells may try to duck and hide from the immune system, they aren't always successful.

When normal cells become cancerous, the transformation changes some of the antigens on the cell's surface. Cytotoxic T cells, NK cells, and macrophages take notice of these "foreign" cells. (See Figure 2.5.) Some scientists believe that these "foreign" cells are continuously being eradicated and that tumors only

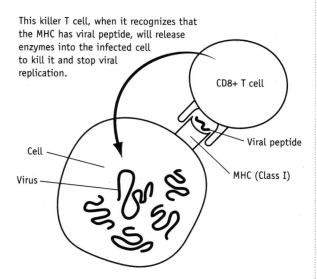

This killer T cell, when it recognizes that the MHC has viral peptide, will release enzymes into the infected cell to kill it and stop viral replication.

CD8+ T cell

Viral peptide

Cell

Virus

MHC (Class I)

Figure 2.4
Apoptosis—natural cell death.

This cell in your body has been infected by a virus. The virus has taken over the cell's "machinery" and is producing more virus. Some of the virus gets chopped up by the cell machinery into peptides and is displayed in the MHC receptor. CD8 and killer T cells can recognize these viral peptides and directly kill the virally infected cell.

Art source: Mary L. Disis, M.D., associate professor of medicine, division of oncology, at the University of Washington in Seattle, Washington. Illustration: Articulate Graphics

develop when the immune surveillance system breaks down or becomes overwhelmed.

But some tumors hide and others elude the immune system by disguising their tumor antigens. Still other tumors may elicit the production of suppressor T cells, which block the cytotoxic T cells that would otherwise attack the growing tumors.

"There are a number of ways cancer can escape recognition by the immune system," explains Mary L. Disis, M.D., associate professor of medicine, division of oncology, at the University of Washington in Seattle, Washington. "First, as cancers grow and spread in the body they can reduce the number of immune recognition molecules they express. Second, there are receptors present on the surface of many cells that activate the immune system and make it function better," Disis says. "Tumors generally don't express those activation molecules," she notes. "In addition, tumors can secrete natural sub-

Figure 2.5
The immune
system response
to a cancer cell.
Some scientists
believe that the
immune system
continuously kills
cancer cells in
healthy individu-
als. In addition,
some cancers are
known to produce
an immune
response.

*Art source:
Mary L. Disis, M.D.,
associate professor of
medicine, division of
oncology, at the
University of
Washington in
Seattle, Washington.
Illustration:
Articulate Graphics*

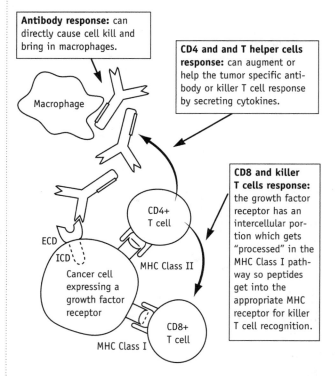

Antibody response: can directly cause cell kill and bring in macrophages.

CD4 and and T helper cells response: can augment or help the tumor specific anti-body or killer T cell response by secreting cytokines.

Macrophage

CD8 and killer T cells response: the growth factor receptor has an intercellular por-tion which gets "processed" in the MHC Class I path-way so peptides get into the appropriate MHC receptor for killer T cell recognition.

CD4+
T cell

ECD

ICD

MHC Class II

Cancer cell
expressing a
growth factor
receptor

CD8+
T cell

MHC Class I

stances that can dampen the immune response. Another potential problem arises when the intercel-lular machinery that chops up proteins displayed in immune recognition molecules is malfunctioning, which often happens in cancer," she explains.

Disis notes that scientists now know what parts of tumors can potentially be recognized by the immune system. Many of these tumor proteins are also pro-teins that are present in normal cells. Because they share many characteristics with normal cells, the immune system may not respond to them fully, but rather generate a weak response.

"The methods cancer uses to dodge the immune system are an area of intense research," Disis says.

Scientists don't know for sure why the immune

system can't "see" breast cancer, says Yang Liu, Ph.D., Kurtz Chair and professor of pathology at Ohio State University's Comprehensive Cancer Center.

But there are theories. Liu presents two:

1. The cancers cells do not turn on T cells.

2. Even if T cells are turned on, cancer cells might be able to hide from them.

There are many reasons why cancer cells do not turn on T cells. For instance, cancer cells may not look different from normal cells in the "eyes" of T cells. As noted earlier in this chapter, self cells are clearly identified so as not to be destroyed by the immune system. Molecules identifying a cell as self are placed on the cell's surface for recognition. These molecules are encoded by a group of genes called the major histocompatibility complex (MHC; human MHC is also called HLA). MHC molecules are produced in the cell and transported to the cell's surface. On the way to the surface, MHC picks up a fragment from another molecule found elsewhere in the cell. That fragment is carried out to the surface and displayed. The displayed fragments are routinely inspected by killer T cells (scientists think killer T cells and NK cells may be the same with different functions or different cells) or cytotoxic lymphocytes. If the fragments, which are composed of a bit of every protein made in the cell, are those proteins normally found in the body, then cytotoxic lymphocytes take no further action. However, if the fragment comes from a foreign protein, that is, one from a virus, the cell is destroyed. Because cancer cells are produced from normal cells, the fragment that T cells check on may not be that different from the collective self. Moreover, cancerous cells may produce substances that actively prevent T cells from being

> **"**
> The most exciting phrase to hear in science, the one that heralds new discoveries, is not 'Eureka!' (I've found it!), but 'That's funny...'
> —Isaac Asimov
> **"**

activated, even if they "see" something different.

The second theory is illustrated by a recent discovery made by Liu and his colleagues and published in the journal *Nature* (November 1998). The team found a gene mutation (in tumors implanted into mice) that destroyed the master switch that controls the MHC system. "The target the T cell [usually] sees is no longer there," Liu says. "They [the cancer cells] know what they're doing." It's their survival mechanism. Specifically, in breast cancers, there is a larger proportion of cancer cells that turn off the target for T cells by turning off HLA, or human leukocyte antigen, the human MHC molecules that are an essential part of the target. (HLA is made of proteins and is located on the surface of white blood cells. HLA plays a critical role in activating the body's immune system to respond to foreign substances. HLA varies from person to person and is therefore considered a genetic fingerprint.) It will be interesting to see if the same mechanism Liu described in mouse models operates in humans, and if so, whether scientists can correct the defects therapeutically. But mouse models don't always translate to humans, he notes.

Science is turning toward the immune system for answers and treatments. In theory, the immune system may make a difference in survival rates among cancer patients diagnosed with the same disease and sharing similar characteristics, both in disease and history. As of yet, there is no scientific support. But there are clues: In some breast cancers there is more inflammation, meaning there is some immune response. Interestingly, in some types of tumors inflammation is associated with a better prognosis, Liu says. This may have to do with the immune system being activated, he suspects. (Note: This does not refer to inflammatory breast cancer. Both the tumor types and inflammation types are different.)

The immune system has weapons to deal with abnormal cells, such as viruses, bacteria, and foreign invaders (the category that cancer fits in). In animal models, if you stimulate the immune system, you can make it eliminate cancers, Liu says. You can push it in many ways. One way is by attaching cytokines (T cell activators, in this case) onto the tumors to get the T cells to fight the cancer cells. Scientists are trying different approaches such as these on humans. Those approaches are collectively referred to as *immunotherapy*.

Boosting the fighting spirit— immunotherapy

People can and do develop antibodies and T cell responses to some tumors. Some of these tumors have an over expression (an overproduction) of normal proteins. In some cases of breast cancer that protein is HER-2/neu, which serves as a tumor antigen. In other cases, the cancerous cells make an abnormal protein, which can also serve as an antigen. So the immune response does exist in some patients.

Scientists are currently developing ways of stripping off cancer cells' camouflage to make tumors more recognizable to the immune system. They are accomplishing this by targeting specific tumor antigens and designing immune-based treatments.

There are four primary categories of immunotherapies being studied:

1. Biological response modifier therapy

2. Monoclonal antibody therapy

3. Adoptive immunotherapy/cellular immune therapy

4. Cancer vaccines

Biological response modifiers

Biological response modifiers, such as interferon and interleukins, are being used experimentally to stimulate or boost the immune system. This cytokine therapy is accomplished in two ways: biological response modifiers are injected into the cancer patient or lymphocytes are transformed in the lab into lymphokine-activated killer (LAK) cells and tumor-infiltrating lymphocytes (TILs) and then injected back into the patient.

Cytokines, as noted earlier in this chapter, are produced in the body and play a role in the immune response.

Monoclonal antibody therapy

Researchers are able to generate specific antibodies to target tumor antigens in mice. These monoclonal antibodies are infused into some people with cancer to target their tumor antigens. A monoclonal antibody is created from a hybridoma, the laboratory fusion of two cells. To make a hybridoma, a mouse is injected with a specific antigen. Antibody-producing plasma cells are produced by the mouse and collected from the mouse's spleen. They are then fused to cancerous plasma cells to produce an antibody to the tumor. This hybrid cell can be cloned again and again and the daughter cells will secrete the immune cell product.

When linked to radioactive substances, monoclonal antibodies can find hidden metastatic cancer cells. Monoclonal antibodies are being used experimentally in their original form to treat cancer or are linked to anticancer drugs, radioactive substances, and natural toxins to enhance their killing power.

Unofficially...
The first genetically-engineered antibody therapy for advanced breast cancer, (trastuzumab) Herceptin®, has been approved by the Food and Drug Administration (FDA).

For example, in breast cancer therapeutic anti-HER-2/neu monoclonal antibodies (Herceptin) are being used on some breast cancer with amplification of the HER-2/neu (c-erbB-2) gene. (See Chapter 10 for more for information on HER-2/neu and Herceptin.)

Adoptive immunotherapy (cellular immune therapy)

Adoptive immunotherapy uses the fighting abilities of T lymphocytes to battle weak tumor responses. T cells, or T lymphocytes, as noted earlier in this chapter, kill cells carrying antigens. In adoptive immunotherapy, T lymphocytes that recognize tumor antigens, that is, those taken from the tumor itself, are multiplied in the laboratory, often to the billions, and stimulated to activate a powerful killer response. In the future, researchers expect to be able to infuse these cells back into the patient to seek out and destroy cancer cells. By doing so, scientists hope to overcome the obstacles of immune response suppression caused by the tumor itself because the infused cells will already be multiplied and stimulated. This approach is still being studied in animal models.

Cancer vaccines

Cancer vaccines have actually been around for more than 100 years, but scientists put their energies into more promising treatments at the time, such as surgery, chemotherapy, and radiation therapy. But now scientists understand enough about the complexities of the immune system to once again concentrate on taking advantage of its anticancer properties. Today, scientists are using the immune system to make customized anticancer "vaccines" from individual tumor cell structures.

Interest in cancer vaccines was regenerated in the 1950s when researchers discovered that mice could be immunized against cancers of the connective tissue caused by exposure to chemicals. Then, in the 1980s, scientists found that T cells could be used to cause tumors to shrink in animals. Currently, there are many clinical studies of cancer vaccines.

Scientists are developing several types of cancer vaccines, and these vaccines are made in different ways. In general, scientists are using proteins found in tumors to prepare the immune system to recognize the cancer cells and produce immune T cells and/or antibodies to attack and destroy the cancerous growth.

The goal for cancer vaccines is to get the cancer patient's immune system to recognize and react to the tumor's presence. Furthermore, vaccines should protect against a recurrence because the immune system has memory.

There are several challenges to developing cancer vaccines:

■ Tumors can secrete cytokines that suppress the immune system. Larger tumors produce more of this substance, making the immune system in patients with larger tumors—which translates to more advanced disease in many patients—less responsive to vaccines.

■ Tumors evade recognition (for the most part) by the immune system.

Today, according to Disis, cancer vaccines are made in two ways:

1. They are made from whole tumor cells or broken up tumor cells (tumor cell lysates) that have been re-engineered in the laboratory to express high levels of HLA molecules or T cell signaling

molecules to make them produce an immune response. (Tumor cell lysates have been used extensively in melanoma vaccines.) Disis calls this the whole tumor cell category.

2. They target a unique protein antigen expressed by the tumor either on or in the cancer cells. (Many tumor antigens are self proteins. So there may be an immune response in some patients, just not a full-fledged functional immune response, Disis says.) She refers to this type of vaccine as the antigen-specific category. "The vaccines can be protein, peptide, or DNA based," Disis explains.

Disis is running a Phase I antigen-specific cancer vaccine trial at the University of Washington for women with Stage III or Stage IV breast and ovarian cancer whose tumors over express the HER-2/neu oncoprotein, the vaccine's target. (For breast cancer staging, see Chapter 6.) These cancer vaccines are generally well-tolerated and have very few side effects, Disis says. (For more information, call 206/616-9538.)

Effective cancer vaccines, if able to be developed, would probably be the most useful in patients who have had their cancer removed or have been treated to the maximum extent with standard therapies. It would not be a first-line treatment. "If you develop a severe pneumonia infection, your doctor wouldn't treat you with a pneumonia vaccine," Disis points out. He or she would give you an antibiotic. "Just as infectious disease vaccines are used to protect against the development of an infection, cancer vaccines' greatest use will [probably] be to protect *against* cancer relapse, not to treat existing cancer," Disis says.

Disis says that it is important to remember that

the recent advances in science have just started to allow us to understand how the immune system recognizes cancer and how cancer evades immune recognition. "Many people believe that the immune system may play a role in fighting cancer, but there is not enough known to choose an immune-based treatment rather than a standard tested therapy, such as chemotherapy or surgery, which has been shown to improve outcome. I hope that we can soon add vaccines to the list of agents we use to treat cancer," Disis says.

Boosting the immune system

Stress plays a key role in the level of immune system response: the more stress, the less immune system response. For years, researchers have suspected that stress increases susceptibility to cancer and infectious diseases. Scientists in the field of psychoneuroimmunology—a field that is generating more and more interest—are exploring the brain-body connection and its influence on health. While there is not conclusive scientific evidence directly linking stress with causing cancer or with impeding the healing process, there is evidence linking stress to a weakened immune response.

It is noted, for example, that there are biological links between the immune system and the central nervous system. Hormones and other chemicals convey messages along nerve cells and communicate with the vast network of immune system cells. And some nerve fiber networks have been noted to connect lymphoid organs, that is, the organs of the immune system.

It appears that there is, in fact, a two-way flow of information from the immune system to the brain and back. Some scientists theorize that immune cells detect foreign invaders and relay that information to the brain through chemical signals. The brain may in turn respond with chemical signals that direct cellular traffic through the lymphoid organs.

Research shows that stress depletes immune resources. Scientists have measured levels of T and B cells, including immunoglobulin A and immune substances like NK cells. They found a drop in both T and B lymphocytes, fewer IgA antibodies, and a weakened NK response after stressful events, including breast cancer.

According to the National Cancer Institute's publication *Understanding the Immune System*, there are three levels of biological links between the immune system and the central nervous system:

1. **The adrenal glands**—When the body is stressed, the adrenal glands respond to stress messages from the brain by releasing corticosteroid hormones (epinephrine/adrenalin) into the blood. This activates the body's fight or flight response. It gives alertness and a quick burst of energy to help a person act quickly in an emergency. It does so by mobilizing the body's energy reserves, which decreases the number and strength of both antibodies and lymphocytes circulating in the blood.

2. **Hormones and neuropeptides**—Hormones and neuropeptides, chemicals released by nerve cells, relay messages to other central nervous system cells and organs throughout the body. In addition, it has been recently noted, they also communicate to immune system cells. Scientists have found that both T cells and macrophages have receptors for certain neuropeptides. NK cells are also in the communication loop. In fact, some activated lymphocytes and macrophages manu-

facture neuropeptides, and some lymphokines, including interferon and interleukins, which are secreted by lymphocytes, are able to transmit information to the nervous system. Furthermore, it is not only T cells produced by the thymus that act on cells in the brain, but other hormones produced by the thymus, as well.

3. **Brain**—The brain sends messages, which may have a direct impact on the immune system, down nerve cells. Nerve fiber networks have been found connected to the thymus gland, spleen, lymph nodes, and bone marrow. Immune function can be altered by destruction of specific areas of the brain.

There are many ways you can decrease stress and boost your immune system, including the following:

- Moderate exercise
- Nutritional diet
- Mirthful laughter

Diet and exercise are covered in Chapter 5 and mirthful laughter in Chapter 14.

Just the facts

- The immune system can detect some cancers, but most of the time has a weak response.
- Cancer has learned many ways to hide from the immune system.
- Scientists are unlocking the secrets of how cancer hides from the immune system and are developing ways to help the body detect and attack it.
- Stressful events, such as being diagnosed with breast cancer, appears to weaken the immune system.

GET THE SCOOP ON...
How treatments are researched ▪ How studies are
designed ▪ What biases exist in study designs that
could alter their findings ▪ What questions you should
ask yourself when reviewing published studies

Research

Many women diagnosed with breast cancer want to understand their disease. They also want to see if any new treatments can offer them more hope or fewer risks than what is currently available. They want to find out if there are new treatments with fewer side effects. In an effort to do so, many women turn to medical journals, the stuff doctors read, to get a better handle on their disease. But these articles are written in highly technical terms and are difficult for lay people to understand. Plus, some studies are poorly designed and others may not deal with the type of breast cancer or the exact stage of the disease they are researching

In this chapter, we'll show you how to navigate through the sea of journal articles that are out there. We'll tell you how scientific studies—which form the basis of these articles—are set up, the strengths and weaknesses of different study designs and study stages (from Phase I animal studies to Phase III clinical trials of large groups of people), the weaknesses of scientific investigations, and where you can access journal articles.

57

Getting a grip on research protocol

Many studies have valid results that tell us a lot about the causes of and treatments for breast cancer. But not all studies are created equal and, therefore, not all results are useful. So what you need is a leg up on how to discriminate among studies that have good data that is of value to you, those that have valid and reliable results but may not apply to you, and those that might be flawed.

There are four levels of studies:

1. **In vitro research**—These are studies using biological substances in the lab on a microscopic level.

2. **Animal studies**—Typically, mice and other rodents are studied to determine how these animals react to different environmental effects to pinpoint causes of cancer or how the tumors in animals react to specific drugs or drug combinations to determine if a treatment may work in humans. These studies may also be used to see how a tumor grows and evolves.

3. **Clinical studies**—These studies look at the effect of treatments on human subjects.

4. **Meta-analyses**—These research studies extract and compare data and other information from many prior studies published in peer-reviewed journal articles in an effort to come to a conclusion and/or a generalization. (The researchers are trying to see "the big picture.") For example, if 10 studies had results showing that Japanese women living in Japan have lower rates of breast cancer than women of Japanese descent living in the United States, the authors of the meta-analysis may conclude that diet plays a strong role in breast cancer development and they may suggest that this finding may apply to all women.

The process of progress

The testing of treatments that hold promise begins in the laboratory under a microscope. The ideas that pass such extraordinary scrutiny move on to the next step—animal testing— to determine how the treatment may actually affect cancer in people and to assess possible harmful effects. If the treatment appears effective and the side effects manageable, the treatment is tested on humans.

These studies on people, called clinical trials, are typically done through cooperative groups, such as the Eastern Cooperative Oncology Group (ECOG), National Surgical Adjuvant Breast and Bowel Project (NSABP), Southwest Oncology Group (SWOG), and European Organization for Research on Treatment of Cancer (EORTC).

Rats!

Animals play a key role in the development and testing of new cancer therapies and in understanding risk factors and prevention. Scientists look to animal models to gain a better understanding of the causes and biology of cancer. Rodents are used in pre-clinical research because their physiology and genetics are well understood and, like humans, they are mammals. In addition, tumors in rodents grow much faster than they do in humans (months versus years), which helps speed up the learning process.

With the development of transgenic mice—those that have a gene from another animal, such as a human, transplanted into them during fetal development—scientists can study specific genes and their influences on tumor development.

But the match of animals to humans is not perfect, so you must review the results of animal studies with caution. Even scientists are careful not to leap

> 66
> It is the mark of an educated mind to be able to entertain a thought without accepting it.
> —Aristotle
> 99

Watch Out!
Treatments that hold promise in laboratory studies or in animals don't always translate to humans. Although animals used in the lab have many biological similarities to humans, there are many important differences, as well, and sometimes those differences appear when treatments that are successful in animals fail in human trials.

to premature conclusions.

There are several important differences between animals and humans. Consider the following:

- Animals and humans differ metabolically, physiologically, and hormonally. The last difference is especially important, because hormones play a key role in the development and treatment of breast cancer.

- Sometimes there are large variations between the way animals and humans deal with carcinogenesis (the process of a healthy cell becoming a cancer cell), so some carcinogens (cancer-causing agents) cause cancer in animals but not in humans, which makes it difficult to determine if certain environmental exposures can lead to cancer in humans. Likewise, certain factors may cause cancer in humans but not in animals.

- Sometimes animal models exaggerate the risk of developing cancer because they are exposed to much higher concentrations of carcinogens in the lab than humans would normally encounter. While this high exposure speeds the process of carcinogenesis and causes cancer to develop in enough animals to make the study feasible, the higher concentrations may not translate to the development of cancer in the real world. Furthermore, because animals and humans are different in how they metabolize carcinogens and in how their cells repair DNA, results from animal studies may not translate to humans.

- Many rodent strains are genetically similar in the laboratory due to inbreeding. In contrast, humans are genetically diverse. As a result, rodents will all have similar responses to a treatment that, in the real world, may work for one person but not for another.

■ In transgenic animal models, all the cells in the animal carry the transplanted mutated gene, so a tumor cell is surrounded by other cells that could also become cancerous. In contrast, a tumor cell in a person is surrounded by healthy cells. As the tumor grows, it overrides normal immune controls. So the process of how cancer spreads differs between some lab animals and humans.

Types of clinical studies

There are primarily three types of human studies: prospective, retrospective, and epidemiological. Each type of study has inherent strengths and weaknesses. All three types of studies are discussed in more detail here.

Prospective studies

Taking what they've learned from laboratory experiments or previous trials, investigators formulate questions that they try to answer in clinical trials. In prospective studies, epidemiological studies in which people are enrolled and followed over time, researchers try to determine the effectiveness of a new treatment, perhaps a new drug, or new treatment method, for example, combining two conventional drugs or changing the timing of administration of the drug or changing the timing of the surgery based on the menstrual cycle. Typically, three phases are used, but when a drug or other treatment has exceptionally promising results and an urgent need, it may gain FDA approval and be used in the general population before completing all three phases. Sometimes a treatment goes through a fourth phase after completing all three phases. Phase IV trials are used for continued evaluation of the drug treatment

Bright Idea
If you don't have online access at home, go to the public library. Many libraries are connected to the Internet. If you go at a time when there aren't many visitors, you may be able to use the computer for a long period of time.

after FDA approval. It is often referred to as post-marketing surveillance.

The use of phases, or steps, gives researchers the opportunity to ask questions to gain a better understanding of the drug, how it works, its safety, and its effectiveness.

As noted earlier, there are three basic standard designs (phases) of prospective studies used to investigate the efficacy and toxicity of new drugs in humans. These study designs are phase I, phase II, and phase III trials.

Phase I trials

When a new drug is developed, a phase I trial is conducted to determine whether or not the drug is safe, and if so, at what dose. That is, the investigators must determine the maximum tolerated dose. The maximum tolerated dose is not necessarily one without side effects, but one in which the side effects are tolerable, according to George Sledge, M.D., Ballvé-Lantero professor of oncology at Indiana University in Indianapolis, Indiana.

The patient population on which drugs in a phase I trial are tested is diverse. For instance, instead of testing the drug only on breast cancer patients, the drug is tested on patients with many different types of cancer, Sledge notes.

To qualify for a phase I trial, your standard therapy must no longer be helpful or useful. In addition, your general health needs to be at least adequate to withstand the treatment. Typically you must have normal cardiac, pulmonary, renal, and liver function, healthy bone marrow, and no major co-morbid conditions such as diabetes, neuropsychological illnesses (because they may interfere with informed consent, which requires a complete understanding of the study from the patient's perspective and is necessary to participate in a trial), etc.

Because patients are given low doses that don't produce a therapeutic response, phase I trials do not show drug efficacy, the effectiveness of the drug. In this study design, patients are given low doses of the drug initially and then are subsequently given higher doses until they reach what is referred to as the dose-limiting toxicity, Sledge says. The dose-limiting toxicity occurs when the side effects are too uncomfortable or too dangerous for the patient to withstand. The side effects are graded using NCI toxicity criteria. The maximum tolerated dose is usually defined as the dose level that is one level lower than that which causes grade III or IV toxicity in two of six patients.

Phase II trials

After a phase I trial is successfully completed, the drug moves on to phase II where investigators see if specific diseases (for example, breast cancer only rather than all cancers) at specific stages of disease respond to a safe dose of the drug or drug combinations being tested. (Phase II trials can test single drugs or a combination of drugs.)

Phase II trials are designed to give response rates—the number of people who respond—to the drug or drug combination. These trials look at relatively healthy patients, so they exclude people who have many diseases found in the general population. For example, if a drug is determined to be safe but excreted through the kidneys, patients whose kidneys are not functioning normally will have a higher grade of toxicity, that is, more of a toxicity, from this drug. In this patient population, if the drug was not excreted, toxic effects on other body systems could

Bright Idea
You can learn more about informed consent at NCI's Cancer Trials site: http://cancertrials.nci.nih.gov.

be severe. Therefore, that population, those with kidney damage from diabetes or high blood pressure, for example, will be excluded from participating in the trial. This patient population selection process has two implications:

1. Phase II trials have a selection bias because the patients selected to participate in these trials are relatively healthy. Patients who are relatively healthy respond better to drugs than those with the same disease or condition, same age group, same sex, etc., but who are less healthy. Therefore, patients taking the drug once it is widely available may not be as healthy as the study participants and may not respond as well to the drug.

2. In the "real world," if a patient has additional health problems that would interfere in some way with the drug, as in the earlier example of kidneys and drug excretion, a patient's physician would reduce the drug dosage to allow that patient to take the drug and, consequently, the patient may receive less benefit than those in the study.

Sledge gives this example of selection bias: In Italy, investigators looked at the effect of the anti-cancer drugs doxorubicin (Adriamycin) and paclitaxel (Taxol) in combination on women with advanced stages of breast cancer. They found a 94 percent response rate. These patients had not been treated previously with chemotherapy. Two trials in the United States found a response rate of about 55 percent. But the patients in the United States had previously undergone chemotherapy. This dramatic different in response rates illustrates the impact of selection bias.

Phase II trials have another weakness besides patient population bias. There is an implied statistical bias because only about 20 to 40 patients participate in these trials. Such a small number of patients is unlikely to reflect the health profile of the majority of patients who may eventually be taking the drug.

There is a way around selection bias, Sledge says—a phase III trial.

Phase III trials

Phase III trials compare the best known conventional therapies to new ones, typically drugs. These trials generally enroll hundreds or thousands of patients in the study. These large numbers of patients balance out the selection bias inherent in phase I and phase II trials, not just by sheer numbers, but by randomization of group assignment. So, for instance, there will be the same number of patients with hormone-sensitive and hormone-insensitive tumors, heart problems, and kidney problems in each arm of the trial, Sledge says. These large numbers and the randomization make this patient population reflective of the general population sharing the disease.

Phase III trials randomly assign patients to a control or experimental group. The control group receives a conventional treatment or placebo, an inert substance (although there are very few placebo-controlled anticancer trials), while the experimental group receives the treatment under investigation. These are referred to as study arms. If the researcher knows which patients are getting which treatment but the patients don't know what they're getting, it is called a single-blinded study. If neither the researchers nor the patients are aware of who is getting which treatment, it is called a double-blinded study. (An administrator knows which patients are receiving which therapy, and the blinds are lifted after the trial ends.) These methods are used to reduce or

Unofficially...
The Food and Drug Administration requires new drugs to go through the trial process to demonstrate their safety and effectiveness.

eliminate any bias.

Phase III trials have another advantage over phase I and phase II trials. Whereas phase I and phase II trials have a single lead investigator who may personally benefit from a successful trial (perhaps because the investigator may have stock in the company that would produce a new drug he or she is developing, for example), thus being subject to another bias, phase III trials have checks and balances built in.

But there are checks built into the system. Trial results, when reported, require a statement from the investigator(s) about the potential conflicts of interest, including financial stakes. Furthermore, peer review is intended to identify bias and bad science. (Note: Most scientists do their best to remain objective.)

Phase III trials often take place at multiple institutions and doctor's offices, so many physicians are involved. These physicians will not personally benefit from the trial's outcome. Their collective focus is on patient outcomes, that is, how well their patients fare. In addition, phase III trials have external reviews in place. While each physician evaluates the response of his or her patients and notes any side effects, patient data is always reviewed by members of the study's central operation office and is also typically reviewed by the investigators running the study. In addition, the data is frequently analyzed in a blinded fashion, so the reviewer does not know which type of therapy the patient underwent.

If you have breast cancer, and you're looking at phase II trial results in a peer-reviewed journal article, you must take the results with a grain of salt, Sledge says. On the other hand, phase III trials are more carefully controlled and better reflect the average breast cancer patient. In phase III trials, response to the drug and toxicity caused by the drug may differ from the results found in a phase II trial because of the differences in the population studied. Large trials also show rare side effects, which can be dangerous, he notes. It is these findings that are an important component of a patient's decision-making process. A good phase III trial provides more data with more reliability than phase I or phase II trials.

Phase IV trials

Phase IV trials examine the long-term safety, effectiveness, and tolerability of a drug after it receives FDA approval. They are also designed to study side effects that become apparent after the completion of the Phase III trial. Patients are followed for years after taking or continuing to take a newly approved drug. Phase IV trials are also referred to as post-marketing surveillance.

For a concise overview of all four phases, see Table 3.1.

TABLE 3.1 PROSPECTIVE STUDY PHASES AT A GLANCE

Phase I trial: Studies safety and dosage levels and sometimes drug pharmacokinetics—absorption, distribution, localization in tissues, biotransformation, and excretion; usually 30 patients

Phase II trial: Focus on tumor response and side effects that may not have appeared in the phase I trial—specific tumor type studied; usually 20-24 patients

Phase III trial: Compares the experimental to the standard treatment - typically large, multiple sites (a multi-center trial); Usually 2,000-3,000 patients

Phase IV trial: Studies side effects that may not have been apparent during the phase III trial

Retrospective studies

While prospective studies try to determine what may happen if a drug is approved for use in a general patient population, retrospective analyses, in contrast, go back and look at a group of patients treated for a specific disease at specific institutions over time. Using this method of analysis, investigators determine if use of the drug over long periods of time provides any insight into its effectiveness. For example, one well-known early study on adjuvant therapy for breast cancer, the CALGB 8541, tested the efficacy of a drug called doxorubicin (Adriamycin). This study was used in a retrospective analysis to determine if higher doses of this drug worked better than lower doses. But what researchers found was that the only patients who benefited from this drug were those women with HER-2/neu positive tumors, according to Sledge.

If a study is designed carefully, investigators can use old data to answer new questions such as "Are there any long-term side effects?" or "Does the drug work better in one group of patients than another?". Or it could also look at tumor characteristics, for example, HER-2/neu and estrogen receptor status. Because the trials weren't originally designed to answer these questions, the results aren't completely clear, so retrospective analyses are considered hypothesis-generating trials, Sledge says. These hypotheses must then be tested in prospective trials to assess their validity.

> 66
> Because of progress made through clinical trials, many people treated for cancer are now living.
> —NCI CancerTrials: Taking Part in Clinical Trials- What Cancer Patients Need to Know
> 99

Epidemiological studies

While phase I, phase II, and phase III trials, as well as retrospective studies, are intervention trials, that is, they provide and analyze treatments, epidemiological studies try to answer the question, "Why did the patient develop breast cancer?" A classic example of an epidemiological trial is the one that linked cigarette smoking to lung cancer in the 1930s and 1940s, according to Sledge. In this study, investigators interviewed people with lung cancer and healthy people about their smoking habits to determine if smoking causes lung cancer. This setup, called a case-control trial, is a retrospective study. It partners case subjects—individuals who have the disease—with control subjects—individuals who do not have the disease—to make comparisons.

Epidemiological studies are sometimes affected by reporting bias, because patients may not answer questions completely or truthfully or they simply may not remember accurately, as is often the case when subjects are questioned about their diets.

In addition to reporting bias, case-control study investigators may hold biases themselves, and consequently may take a more detailed history of those patients they think may provide answers that support their belief about a causal relationship, Sledge says. Furthermore, small case-control studies, like other studies with small numbers of subjects, have statistical biases because they do not necessarily look at a population that reflects the population as a whole.

Another type of epidemiological study is a cohort study. This is a prospective study that compares two groups of people, those with the disease and those without. Researchers look at the development of the disease over time in an attempt to identify such things as risk factors.

Prospective epidemiological trials

Prospective epidemiological trials take large groups of healthy people and ask them questions about their lifestyle and medical history. Study researchers follow patients over time to see who comes down with what disease and then try to determine the cause of disease by looking at the data collected. This is a very effective way of identifying a causal link between lifestyle, environment, diet, and disease. The classic

Bright Idea
A quick way to find out the strengths and weaknesses of a published study is to read the editorial, comments, and correspondence sections of that and subsequent editions of the journal in which the study was published.

Watch Out!
The way a study
is designed can
affect outcome!
For example, the
reduction in risk
of developing
breast cancer that
is associated with
exercise is
observed more
often in case-con-
trol studies than
in cohort studies.

prospective epidemiological trial for breast cancer is the Nurses' Health Study. Researchers at Harvard School of Public Health, Boston, Massachusetts, reviewed the data from this study and found that an increased risk of developing breast cancer associated with alcohol consumption may be reduced by getting adequate folate in the diet. The study results were published in the *Journal of the American Medical Association* (May 1999).

Tools for evaluating scientific studies

One method used to evaluate the worthiness of a study is to look at the external and internal validity.

External validity answers the question, "How generalizable are the findings?," says Lu Ann Aday, Ph.D., professor of behavioral sciences at the University of Texas School of Public Health. This can be determined, at least in part, by looking at who the study subjects were. For example, were they mostly white middle-class women? Can the findings be generalized to African-American women who are at higher risk? (As mentioned in Chapter 1, breast tumors in African-Americans are typically identified at a later stage. These women also seem to have a poorer prognosis stage compared with Caucasians.)

Your next question should be, "Where was the research done," Aday asks. Was it done in a controlled clinical trial or an experimental setting? The answer may relate to the efficacy, she says. Ask yourself if the treatment was used in a real world setting where such issues as physician knowledge and patient compliance could affect the outcome. Keep in mind, with regard to clinical or experimental trials, that there is an underrepresentation of certain populations. All these factors play a role in the outcome. Therefore, Aday says, you should ask yourself,

"How does it apply to me?" Consider your lifestyle factors, culture, diet, race, age, menopausal status, and the like.

Next there is internal validity: Was the study properly designed to determine what might cause the cancer and how it might be treated? Internal validity looks at cause and effect. Research designs differ in their strength and capacity to answer the questions their hypotheses pose, such as, "Does exercise reduce the risk of developing cancer?"

Timesaver
You can find links to more than 100 peer-reviewed medical journals focusing on cancer at www. sciencekomm. at/journals/ medicine/onco. html.

Stages of certainty

There are three main stages of development: descriptive studies, analytical studies, and evaluative studies.

1. **Descriptive studies**—observational and cross-sectional studies—represent the beginning of the investigational process and answer the question, "What is?" These studies may estimate or discover trends of a disease, survey a group of patients, or show vital statistical data. For example, in some of these studies, scientists are trying to find characteristics associated with higher risks of cancer or differences in survival rates, Aday says. In others, scientists may try to describe how characteristics differ among groups. For instance, some women who have relatives with breast cancer have a mutated BRCA1 or BRCA2 gene; others don't. Some women eat a high-fat diet; others don't. Some women go for regular mammography screenings, and others don't.

2. **Analytical studies** answer the question, "Why?," mostly through case-control and prospective studies. This type of study is a hypothesis-testing phase based on descriptive work, according to Aday. It addresses such topics as the role of genetics, the influence of occupational exposure, and

the impact of diet. When setting up analytical studies, scientists should consider whether or not there are enough cases to look at and determine which study design is best. Should the hypothesis be tested through a case-control study or as a prospective study? These studies look at what factors should be examined and controlled. If the results of this type of study show promise, then the study can move on to the evaluative stage, which will look at interventions that might help prevent or treat the disease.

3. **Evaluative studies** are typically done using randomized clinical trials. This type of study addresses the question, "What makes a difference in prevention, treatment, and survival rates?" When a treatment is safe and effective, the studies move the analysis from the cellular level to pharmaceutical therapy in animals to trials on humans, she says. In terms of intervention, it compares groups. For example, with regard to breast cancer, this type of study can be used to determine if education will help with early intervention. One group of women will learn the importance of early intervention while the other will receive no additional education, and behaviors of both groups will be observed and compared. This type of study is difficult to do accurately. For example, if two communities are being compared, they may not be well matched in terms of other characteristics (referred to as selection effect differences), she says. There may be other sources of differences, for example, perhaps the mayor's wife in one community was diagnosed with breast cancer and she has taken a leadership role in educating residents about the dis-

ease, Aday points outs. That community will have a higher awareness of breast cancer. Factors like that can affect study results.

As we move up the chain of the studies from descriptive to analytical to evaluative, the hypotheses get stronger, Aday explains. But with each link in the chain, there are concerns about whether or not there are enough cases to determine if actual differences exist. This is referred to as statistical power. So you must ask yourself, "How much power does the study have to detect a difference, if one is present?" In other words, do the investigators have the capacity to find differences? There are many errors that can be made: In reality, there may be no differences and the investigators find one or there may be a difference and the investigators do not find it, leading them to conclude that there is no difference, Aday explains.

If you read the "Methods" section of a published study, you'll see a P value, the probability that an observed difference was due to chance. Therefore, when designing the study, the investigators must come up with a confidence level. For example, if the investigators don't want to find a difference (that in fact does not exist) more than 5 percent of the time the P value would be would be 5 percent (P = .05) and the confidence level would be 95 percent—the investigators are 95 percent certain that their findings are accurate but they acknowledge that there is a 5 percent chance that they are incorrect.

How rigorously the investigators try to minimize their errors is important when looking at the clinical significance of their findings, Aday explains. If there is a drug with a serious side effect, you want the study to be designed to minimize those types of errors so that the side effect will not come as a surprise when the drug is used in the general marketplace. In this case, the investigators must set up a more conservative study, she says. Look at how often they're willing to be wrong.

You can evaluate the investigator's views of the study's strengths and weaknesses by reading the study limitations that are typically discussed at the end of the article. "The authors should review what the strengths and weakness of their study are, and what the subsequent implications might be in interpreting and applying study results," Aday says. "If there is no such discussion, then 'caveat emptor' should be the message to the reader," she says.

Measurements of reliability and validity data are additional concerns. Reliability is related to variation and validity is related to accuracy. Reliability addresses the question of whether or not a study can be replicated in different settings by different investigators. If it can, it is more likely that the results are true. Reliability depends upon many factors, including how data is gathered. For example, if information is gathered from patients, do the patients fully understand the questions? Are the interviewers leading patients to give certain responses? That's why it is so important to show that the data can be replicated in different studies at different institutions. With regard to reliability, ask yourself, "What is the variability that might exist?" For example, if the study subjects were asked about their diet over the past six months, is it possible that the subjects could have recalled their diets inaccurately? You should also ask yourself, "Is it likely that there is a large variability?" For example, is it likely that the subjects have responded that they drank a full glass of milk each morning when they really drank only a half glass every other day? Finally, you should ask yourself, "Is it likely that the variability is random?" If it's random, it may not have a significant impact on the findings.

The validity of the study pertains to its accuracy—its sensitivity in finding an existing problem, for example, a causal link between exercise and the risk of breast cancer. If the study is examining a diagnostic or screening procedure, for example, the question then becomes will it detect existing abnormalities or will it find abnormalities that don't really exist, that is, a false positive result? A good example of validity pertains to the variability of mammography screening outcomes, discussed in chapter 6. In many cases, the radiologist misses cancerous masses while reading the mammography X-ray, leading to false negative results. In other cases, radiologists detect masses that are not cancerous, possibly leading to false positive results. When you look at a study, ask yourself if the weaknesses in the study design are addressed.

All things considered...

Sometimes journal articles have no meaning because the science they are based on is poor, the results of a study are slanted to fit an industry or political need, or the results are falsified (although falsified results are rare). That's why it's important for both patients and researchers to see if investigators in many institutions can replicate the results of one investigator's initial findings. To get an idea if a study is valid, search for other journal articles on the same subject. Make sure the articles are published in reputable peer-reviewed medical journals such as the *Journal of the National Cancer Institute*, *Cancer*, the *New England Journal of Medicine*, the *Journal of the American Medical*

Association, and the *Lancet*. Sometimes notations are placed on abstracts when data has been known to be falsified. (Not all falsified data impacts results, so some studies may have this note but still have valid results.) This matter is discussed in more detail later in this chapter under the heading "Scientific Misconduct." Another way to determine if a study is valid (and to see its weaknesses) is to read the editorials and correspondence printed in the issue in which the article under question appears and in subsequent issues.

Here's an example of when the results of a study may have been slanted to fit an industry need:

According to the Cancer Prevention Coalition, a January 1999 study found no risk of breast cancer from oral contraceptive use. The study was based on 23,000 healthy women who had "ever used" the pill. They were followed over a 25-year period. The average age at termination of the study was 49, an age when breast cancer is still relatively uncommon. There are at least four problems with this study design:

Unofficially...
Intentionally or unwittingly, personal biases may come into play if a study is not double-blinded.

1. "Ever used" may mean that a woman used the pill for a short period of time. Duration may be the key, if there is a causal relationship.

2. The study was based on healthy women. There are many women who use oral contraceptives who are not healthy.

3. The average age at termination was too young to produce meaningful data. Most breast cancers occur after age 55.

4. Although 23,000 women seems like a large study, the sample size may be too small to draw general conclusions

The study was funded by major international pharmaceutical companies, thus the chance of bias is present, according to the Cancer Prevention Coalition.

In contrast, the Collaborative Group on Hormonal Factors in Breast Cancer completed an comprehensive analysis of 54 epidemiological studies on breast cancer and hormonal contraceptives based on individual data on 53,297 women with breast cancer and 100,239 women without breast cancer. They found that women among taking combined oral contraceptives, and in the 10 years after stopping, there is a small increased risk of having breast cancer. The study was published in the *Lancet* (June 1996).

This illustrates why it's so important to see if investigators in many institutions can replicate the results of another group's initial findings.

Irreconcilable differences?

Different studies sometimes come to different conclusions. In March 1999, the *Journal of the American Medical Association* published research showing no evidence that lower fat intake was associated with a decreased risk of breast cancer, that is, a higher fat intake did not appear to be a risk factor. But there are scores of other studies showing just the opposite, and consequently a high-fat diet has been considered a risk factor for breast cancer. Women and their doctors are now left to draw their own conclusions until more definitive research is available.

It is not at all uncommon for investigators around the world and over time to produce different findings when investigating the cause of a disease or the effectiveness of a specific treatment. Some of the differences in findings can be attributed to the differences in the population studied, biases, study design, and the number of people studied. Nonetheless, it leaves patients and physicians in a position of having

Unofficially...
Only one to two of 1,000 women at age 45 will be diagnosed with breast cancer each year.

to make their decisions or form their views based on inconclusive evidence.

Scientific misconduct

On February 5, 1999, the NCI press office sent out a press release headlined "ORI Reports Fabricated and/or Falsified Data for Three Patients on NCI-Sponsored Studies." It stated that the Federal Government's Office of Research Integrity (ORI) found scientific misconduct by a data manager who worked at hospitals that were participating in breast cancer treatment studies sponsored by the NCI. According to the press release, the data manager fabricated and/or falsified data on three patients, one in each of three different clinical trials.

Because the trials included large numbers of patients and were conducted at many institutions, the falsification of records was not expected to affect the results. Nonetheless, it has happened before and will probably happen again, which is why you can't necessarily believe the findings of every study. It's best to consider studies where the results have been replicated.

Stuff happens

Sometimes mistakes happen unintentionally. MD Anderson's Web site posted a warning to scientists about the authenticity of cell lines. Titled "Do you know whether the cell line you are using in your research is authentic?," this article stated, "Cell line contamination is not an uncommon incident in a laboratory handling more than one cell line." A cell line contamination occurs when one cell line contaminates and then overgrows another as a result of careless handling in the laboratory. Thus, the contaminated cell line is typically another cell line (one that grows faster). Cell lines differ because they have different genetic makeups. But scientists working with purchased or donated cell lines presume the cells are pure and usually do not examine their genetic makeup. As a result, some investigators may be innocently publishing erroneous data with misleading conclusions.

In addition, with regard to breast cancer studies, factors such as the timing of blood specimen collection relative to the menstrual cycle for premenopausal and perimenopausal women may have an impact on study results if the researchers are investigating the impact of estrogen and progesterone on breast cancer and specific treatments because hormone levels fluctuate during the menstrual cycle, for example. The timing of breast cancer surgery may be another good example of how hormone levels during the menstrual cycle impact outcomes. (Outcomes vary based on what phase of the menstrual cycle the surgery was done.)

The gold standards

When you look at a journal article, you'll see that the format is basically the same from journal to journal. The authors begin with an "Introduction," (sometimes presented as "Background" or "Purpose"), which explains why they did the research. Next comes the "Methods" section, which tells how the study was set up and what methods the investigators used to analyze the results. The "Results" section details the study findings, and a "Discussion" section explains how the findings can be applied to the problem described in the introduction. (Sometimes the discussion takes place in the "Results" section.) Finally, the "Conclusion" section summarizes the findings in nontechnical language.

If you want to assure yourself with some certainty

Timesaver
If you don't have
time to read
scores of journal
articles, skim the
text and jump
down to the
conclusions, or
just read the
conclusions in the
abstracts.

about the reliability or validity of outcomes, determine if the studies you are considering use the "gold standards" of study setup and design:

- Double-blinded, randomized, controlled trials are the gold standard used to determine the effectiveness of treatments.

- Cohort or case-control studies are the gold standard used to address the issue of causation; that is, they show a strong causal link.

- Longitudinal cohort studies, those running over a course of time, are the gold standard for looking at prognosis.

- Case reports can be used to see any adverse drug reactions and other incidental findings.

Researching research

One of the easiest ways to research studies on breast cancer is through Medline, an electronic database of information housed at the National Library of Medicine in Bethesda, Maryland. Medline (accessible through Internet Grateful Med at http://igm.nlm.nih.gov) contains more than 11 million journal article abstracts and records dating back to 1966, which can be searched electronically through the Internet. (Full-text articles can be ordered through Loansome Doc or found in many public and medical libraries, which are located in both medical schools and local hospitals. Typically these libraries have hours when the public can access their stacks.)

You can search Medline using keywords, such as "breast cancer," "HER-2/neu," or other topics. Or you can select from about 18,000 Medical Subject Headings (MeSH). However, many articles are not on Medline and many aren't posted until months after they've been published. In addition, some articles on

Medline are misclassified. Some sections of journals are completely left off Medline, so if you want to see the "Comments" section of the *Journal of the National Cancer Institute*, for example, you'll have to get a copy of the publication. Some journals, such as the *Journal of the American Medical Association* (www.ama-assn.org) and the *British Medical Journal* (http://www.bmj.com/index.html), publish the full text of their articles on their Web sites.

Other electronic databases on the Internet include Internet Grateful Med. This database gives you access to such sites as Toxline, which contains information on toxicological effects of drugs.

Another good Web site is Medscape at www.medscape.com. It has coverage of medical conferences as well as articles on timely topics. In addition, Doctor's Guide to the Internet at http://www.docguide.com carries medical news updates. Both Medscape and Doctor's Guide to the Internet offer free e-mail medical news updates.

The paper chase

There are several different formats for journal articles. Each type of article will provide you with different information. The following is a general overview:

- **Cell culture studies**—The first step to developing any treatment starts in the laboratory in a test tube or petri dish and change is noticed under the microscope. This type of paper is used by investigators to report in vitro (laboratory) findings, such as the impact a drug has on a cancer cell. This type of study may give you hope, but there's a long scientific row to hoe before you'll know for sure.

- **Animal trials**—New treatments are tried on animals before they are tried on humans. Some

Watch Out!
When comparing early to more recent studies, keep in mind that radioimmunoassays, the current standard for determining the level of hormones in blood, were not often used in earlier controlled dietary studies, so results may differ based on study design.

prove applicable to humans, but others don't make the transition. (These are phase I trials described earlier in this chapter.)

■ **Basic science reports**—Investigators use this format to report on the mechanisms underlying breast cancer etiology or breast cancer treatment. If you want to learn about the disease or have unanswered questions of why you developed it, these reports may shed some light, but they are highly technical and directed at sophisticated readers.

■ **Clinical trials**—These papers summarize the findings of clinical trials and can be useful as "prognostic indicators" for how well you might fare using that type of treatment.

■ **Epidemiology reports**—Epidemiological studies examine what causes carcinogenesis. This type of report is used to summarize study findings. These reports are useful if you don't have breast cancer and want to take action to prevent it.

■ **Review articles**—Review articles summarize current research to keep physicians up to date. There are two categories of review articles: those that cover a specific disease and those that cover a specific technology. They are a quick and easy way to see what's going on in the field of breast cancer research and technology.

■ **Reports on prognostic studies**—Prognostic studies are usually first retrospective—a hypothesis is generated—and then assessed in prospective fashion. (Findings lead to a hypothesis that is then evaluated in a prospective fashion.) Reports of prognostic studies summarize factors that appear to be associated with prognosis.

(HER-2/neu expression in breast cancer is a good example of this type of study.) Keep in mind that scientists cannot predict the future. There are many unknown factors that play a role in prognosis. Many long-term cancer survivors had been given a poor prognosis. It is also important to note that treatments and treatment strategies have changed in recent years and continue to advance. Therefore, when comparing your stage of disease with the study subjects, you should keep in mind that newer treatments are often associated with longer survival rates.

■ **Case reports**—Using this format, researchers report on a specific case or several cases pertaining to the same situation or disease that is unusual in some way, such as a previously unreported side effect or benefit. Unless you're a perfect match to the cases reported, these papers will not be very useful in your search for information.

Be a critic

As you read through journal articles for answers, try to take a critical view of the study design and results to determine if they are strong enough for you to consider them in your decision-making. Ask yourself the following questions:

■ Were the results published in a peer-reviewed journal, like the *Journal of the National Cancer Institute* or the *Journal of the American Medical Association*?

■ What type of study was conducted—an in vitro (laboratory) or animal study, a clinical trial, or a meta-analysis? If it was a clinical trial, was it a phase I, phase II, or phase III trial?

■ What biases are inherent in that type of study?

- What were the characteristics of the patient population studied? Were they similar to you in terms of health status, dietary intake, environmental exposures, lifestyle, age, menopausal status, weight, or exercise habits?

- How many patients were in the study? Were there enough study subjects (hundreds or thousands) to reflect the general population in terms of health, sex, age, and other important demographics? Were there enough study subjects (hundreds or thousands) to see an effect that may exist in the general population but not in a small group of patients? How many patients completed the study? If patients dropped out of the study, why?

- If the study was a phase III trial, were there similar numbers in the control and experimental arms? Was the study double-blinded?

- Were patients eliminated when the data was analyzed? If so, why?

- Were patients allowed to crossover from the control to experimental treatment arm? If so, were crossover patients included in the data analysis? (Including crossover patients in the data analysis may affect study results.)

- Were patients followed after the study concluded? If so, what were the long-term findings?

- Who funded the study? Is it a reputable organization or educational institution? If the study was funded by private industry, do the investigators who led the study stand to gain financially from the results? (Study funding can often be found in a disclosure at the end of an article.)

Just the facts

- It is difficult to know if a specific promising treatment under study will benefit you.

- Some studies look into the future and some studies look at the past and draw conclusions.

- Studies contain biases that may significantly alter their outcomes.

- When drawing you own conclusions from studies, you must be careful to consider all the study's weaknesses.

What Do We Know About Breast Cancer?

PART II

GET THE SCOOP ON...
What risk factors you may have ▪ How
hormones, pregnancy, dietary fat, and more
affect your risk ▪ Who's at risk for familial
breast cancer ▪ Which relatives count

Risk Factors

Breast cancer is not a given. There are certain things that put a woman at a higher risk for developing this disease. In this chapter, we will tell you about known risk factors. By knowing them, you can take some control over your chances of developing breast cancer. However, knowing these risk factors will not give you complete control, since factors other than age contribute to only about a third of all cases of breast cancer. Scientists have yet to uncover the predominant cause or multitude of causes of breast cancer. However, that does not discount the importance of arming yourself with the facts that are available.

Risky business

Besides inherited gene alterations, there are many factors, known and unknown, that affect your risk of developing breast cancer. Some of the factors include medical history and hormone levels. Breast cancer risk also increases with age. (Note: Scientists don't know what role these risks play in influencing the likelihood of disease in women with BRCA1 or BRCA2 mutations discussed later in this chapter.)

Unofficially...
DNA is continually damaged by both exposure to environmental chemicals and radiation and by events that occur naturally in the cells. As a result, "mismatches" occur between DNA strands as the cells replicate. Normally these mismatches are repaired or removed so the cells continue to function properly. But when the repair or removal mechanism is malfunctioning, such as in the case of a mutated tumor suppressor gene, the mismatch remains and can lead to cancer.

Age

Your risk for breast cancer increases as you age. Most women—80 percent—are older than 50 when diagnosed. Women under age 30 have a lower risk of developing breast cancer than those over 30. Although, as mentioned earlier, women with inherited forms of breast cancer, specifically those with an altered BRCA1 or BRCA2 gene (Breast Cancer Gene 1 and Breast Cancer Gene 2), are among those who have a higher frequency of developing breast cancer before age 50.

Gender

Women have a significantly higher chance of developing breast cancer than do men—99 percent of diagnosed breast cancer cases occur in women.

Race

Caucasian women have a greater risk of developing breast cancer than African-American women. American women have a greater chance of developing breast cancer than women in many other countries, and rank 16th in incidence of breast cancer cases worldwide, as discussed in Chapter 1.

Medical history lesson

Women who have already been diagnosed with a primary breast cancer (one that developed in the breast from breast tissue and not one that resulted from another cancer that traveled to the breast) are at higher risk of developing it again, not just as a recurrence, but as a new primary cancer. In fact, women who have had breast cancer in one breast are five times as likely to develop breast cancer in the other breast as are women who have not had breast cancer. The risk might be even greater for those whose first breast cancer developed before age 50. An estimated

10 to 15 percent of women treated for ductal carcinoma in situ are later diagnosed with a second primary breast cancer, and about 25 percent of women diagnosed with lobular carcinoma in situ develop invasive breast cancer.

Atypical hyperplasia

Women who have an excessive formation of cells (diagnosed during biopsy) have an increased risk of developing breast cancer. The amount of increased risk appears to vary according to the type of atypical hyperplasia and other risk factors.

Researchers at Channing Laboratory, Brigham and Women's Hospital, Boston, Massachusetts, reviewed the medical journal articles and found that women with a history of benign breast biopsies had a fourfold increase in cancer risk if the biopsy showed atypical hyperplasia compared with those women who didn't. Atypia alone, they found, doubles a woman's risk. (These findings and others were published in the journal *Cancer* (February 1993)). Unlike other risk factors, atypia may be a precursor lesion for breast cancer in some women.

The classic paper on this subject was published in the *New England Journal of Medicine* (January 1985). To determine the importance of various breast cancer risk factors in women with benign proliferative breast lesions, the investigators reevaluated 10,366 consecutive breast biopsies performed in women at three Nashville hospitals; for 3,303 women, 1,925 of whom had proliferative disease, were followed for a median of 17 years. They found that 70 percent of the women who underwent breast biopsy for benign disease were not at increased risk of breast cancer. However, women at higher risk can be identified if they have had atypical hyperplasia

Watch Out!
Don't let the absence of risk factors make you less compliant about getting mammograms and breast examinations: most women diagnosed with breast cancer have no risk factors, other than gender and age. Women with more than one risk factor should be especially vigilant.

Watch Out!
Higher than normal estrogen levels and prolonged exposure to estrogen influence breast cancer development.

and a family history of breast cancer. In fact, women with atypia and a family history of breast cancer have a risk 11 times that in women who had non-proliferative lesions and who did not have a family history of breast cancer.

Breast tissue scarring

Women with benign breast disease who have radial scars, a tissue abnormality surrounded by a cluster of ducts radiating outward, are almost twice as likely to develop breast cancer compared with women who don't have that abnormality. Radial scars, however, can be seen only on mammography. Biopsy is necessary to confirm or refute malignancy.

Researchers at Beth Deaconess Medical Center in Boston, Massachusetts, reviewed benign biopsy specimens from 1,396 women. Of those, 99 women had at least one radial scar, and these women had nearly two times the risk of developing breast cancer compared with those without scarring. The study results were published in the *New England Journal of Medicine* (February 1999).

Breast density

Research shows that women age 45 and older who have at least 75 percent dense tissue on a mammogram have a higher risk of developing breast cancer than their counterparts with less dense tissue. The association between breast tissue density and breast cancer risk is not completely understood.

You cannot tell if you have dense breasts by how firm they feel or look. Breast density is not related to breast texture, shape, size, or lumpiness. It is related to the amount of glandular and fibrous tissue that make up the breast and can only be measured by mammography.

Gail Greendale, M.D., research director for the

Unofficially...
The Epstein-Barr virus, which causes mononucleosis, may play a role in the development of some breast cancers, according to research published in the *Journal of the National Cancer Institute* (August 1999). Although interesting, the significance of these findings for clinical care and the implications for future research are not yet clear.

Iris Cantor/UCLA Women's Center, led the PEPI (Postmenopausal Estrogen/Progestin Interventions) trial. Results of this study, published in the *Annals of Internal Medicine* (February 1999), noted that mammographic density may be a risk factor for breast cancer.

Researchers are currently investigating whether there's a genetic component to mammographic density and looking at changes in density as they relate to age, menopausal status, hormone use, and exposure to environmental carcinogens.

The PEPI trial and other studies show that about 25 percent of women who use hormone replacement therapy (HRT) with progestin have increased mammographic breast density. In contrast, according to the PEPI trial, only about 8 percent of women taking estrogen-only HRT had increased breast density. Whether or not this synthetically-induced breast density produces the same risk as naturally dense breast is not known. Of course, there may only appear to be a causal relationship between breast density and breast cancer. Tumors are difficult to detect in dense breasts because the tumor may have the same density as the breast and therefore "disappear" in the background on the mammogram regardless of whether the density is natural or a result of HRT. So what may be happening is that they are discovered later, making it appear that there is an increased risk among women who have dense breasts.

Abortion and breast cancer

The possible causal relationship between abortion and breast cancer has stirred up a lot of controversy. Some scientific studies have found an association between abortion and breast cancer. The theory of at least one of these studies that is as follows: In

Watch Out!
If you have one or more risk factors reviewed in this chapter, be extra vigilant about getting mammograms and breast examinations, but don't let it make you nervous. Many women who have risk factors don't develop breast cancer.

normal pregnancies, breast cells differentiate, that is, they specialize. Without this specialization, lactation couldn't occur and the new mother would not be able to nurse her newborn. But when a woman aborts the fetus, the cells are left in a state of limbo, not fully differentiated, and they are exposed to estrogen.

The ways some of these studies were structured left them vulnerable to reporting bias—that is, some women, particularly those not diagnosed with breast cancer, may have given inaccurate information. "Results from a study that examined the accuracy of reporting abortions indicate that women with breast cancer are more likely to accurately report having had an abortion than women without breast cancer," according to NCI. Furthermore, other lifestyle factors may have played a role, so if there is an association between induced abortion and breast cancer, it may not be a causal association.

But even those studies that showed an association only showed a slight increase in risk. No associations have been found between miscarriage and an increase in breast cancer risk. Investigators theorize that the body takes care of the breast cells that have begun to specialize.

Bottom line? There is no conclusive evidence that induced abortion can increase the risk of breast cancer.

Body shape, body hair, and skin type

Women with excessively oily skin, an apple-shaped body, and excessive body hair may have a greater risk of developing breast cancer than other women, according to researchers at the University at Buffalo. They analyzed women who took part in a study in Northern Italy called HORDET—HORmone and

Timesaver
You can download a computer program from www.oncolink. upenn.edu/ disease/breast/ cause/breastca_ risk that allows you to project your estimated risk for invasive breast cancer over a 5-year period and over your lifetime, up to age 90.

Diet ETiology of Breast Cancer. Their findings were presented in June 1998 at a meeting of the Society for Epidemiologic Research.

Women who have these masculine characteristics have greater levels of male sex hormones—androgens—the most active of which is testosterone. These hormones are produced by the ovaries and the adrenal glands, but in smaller amounts than what is produced in males by the testes. Androgen, like estrogen, is associated with an increased risk of developing breast cancer.

Paula Muti, M.D., an assistant professor of social and preventive medicine at the University of Buffalo, led this investigation. It found no association between excessive body hair and risk of developing breast cancer in premenopausal women, but high amounts of sebum production and an apple-shaped body (i.e., one in which the waist is larger than the hips) appears to be associated with an increased risk for this group of women. In fact, those women who had the highest levels of sebum production had a 2.5 times increased risk compared with those women who had the lowest levels of sebum production. The researchers found the same increased risk for women with apple-shaped bodies compared with women with pear-shaped bodies, those with hips larger than the waist.

Although excessive body hair was not a risk factor for premenopausal women, it does appear to play a role after menopause. In the study, postmenopausal women had a 33 percent increased risk of developing breast cancer compared with women with no excessive body hair. Neither excessive sebum production nor body shape affected risk in this group of women.

Circumstantial evidence—environmental and lifestyle risks

As noted in Chapter 1, contaminants in the environment—air, food, water, soil—sometimes contain environmental estrogens, which may have an effect on estrogen levels or may mimic estrogen. Insecticides are one such chemical being researched. Timing may be a factor in the amount of risk environmental estrogens pose: During adolescence, breast tissue may be especially sensitive to the effects of cancer-causing agents due to the increase in hormone levels and cellular activity (proliferation and differentiation) as the breasts develop.

Lifestyle

Drinking alcohol increases your risk of developing breast cancer. Study results on alcohol consumption and its risk on breast cancer conflict, however. Some researchers believe that alcohol may indirectly affect estrogen levels. If true, there may be a small increase in risk among those women who drink alcoholic beverages. The degree of risk appears to be correlated with the amount of alcohol consumed. But before you decide to be completely dry, consider this: More women die of heart disease than breast cancer, and drinking moderate amounts of alcohol has protective effects against heart disease.

Other lifestyle risk factors include smoking, getting little or no exercise on a regular basis, and gaining a lot of weight after age 18.

Electromagnetic fields

The news that electromagnetic fields may play a role in breast (and other) cancers scared quite a few people several years ago. But data on low-frequency electromagnetic fields found in the environment—specifically, proximity to high voltage electrical lines—are inconclusive.

In fact, according to a report in *The Cancer Letter* (June 30, 1999), the HHS Office of Research Integrity announced that a researcher, Robert Liburdy, falsified and fabricated data and claims about the purported cellular effects of electric and magnetic fields published in the *Annals of the New York Academy of Sciences* (649:74-95, 1992) and *FEBS Letters* (301:53-59, 1992).

If you use electricity to keep warm at night, rest assured you are not increasing your risk of developing breast cancer. A study by researchers at the Columbia School of Public Health, published in the *American Journal of Epidemiology* (September 1998), found that electric blanket use for women under the age of 55, is *not* associated with an increased risk of breast cancer. The investigators found no association for mattress pads or heated water beds, either, regardless of how long they were used or the woman's menopausal status.

Timesaver
Exercise at home while you watch TV. You'll save drive time to and from the gym, you won't miss your favorite shows, and you'll be doing something to improve your health.

Hormonal influences—like watering a plant, they make cancer grow

High levels of natural hormones (those produced by your body) that persist over a longer than average period of time can increase your risk of developing breast cancer. You may be at increased risk if:

- Your menstrual cycle began before age 12. (Most girls begin later.)

- You have your first child after age 30.

- You never have children.

- If you begin menopause after age 55. (Most women begin earlier.)

Estrogen, a female hormone, stimulates the normal growth of breast tissue during adolescence and again during pregnancy when breast cells specialize to produce milk. In between these two events, the breast cells are exposed to estrogen, which is fine unless the exposure is prolonged due to a late first pregnancy. When a women doesn't get pregnant until after she turns 30, or not at all, her breast cells have not yet specialized (differentiated) and become vulnerable over time to becoming cancerous as a result of estrogen exposure in that prolonged state of limbo. (On the flip side of that risk equation, a woman's risk of developing breast cancer appears to be reduced with each pregnancy.)

Pregnancy after age 30 can also be a risk factor because of the explosion of hormones that occurs during this time. But it is not a causal risk; it is a developmental risk. (Scientists theorize that the increase in estrogen exposure does not cause the cancer to develop in these cases. The cancerous cells are already present. The increase in estrogen exposure causes breast cancer to grow more rapidly.) Because of the changes in the breast during pregnancy, breast cancer is often diagnosed at a later stage in pregnant women, but stage for stage, the prognosis and survival rate is the same as for women who are not pregnant.

Higher risk related to hormones is seen in women who had their first menstrual period before age 12, which is considered early, and those who began menopause after age 55, which is considered late.

Scientists think that excessive exposure to estrogen may contribute to breast cancer risk because estrogen stimulates breast cell growth. In this case, the growth is cancerous.

Though synthetic, HRT, which some women use to get relief from symptoms caused by menopause, may be associated with an increased risk of breast cancer, especially when used for more than 10 years, according to numerous studies. However, 50 studies conducted over the past 25 years show conflicting results in general. Bottom line? Currently, scientists do not know whether breast cancer risk is affected by taking fertility drugs, which contain hormones.

There is also controversy over whether women who have had breast cancer should use HRT because increased exposure to a hormone that causes breast cell growth could cause a mutated cell to grow into a tumor. The NCI reports that breast cancer survivors are widely discouraged from using HRT. But some researchers question the validity of this concern because there are no good prospective, randomized trials on the subject.

To determine whether HRT has a causal association with breast cancer, the Women's Health Initiative, a well-known, large study, and other studies are investigating the effects of long-term HRT in postmenopausal women. This 15-year nationwide study is being sponsored by NCI.

Birth control pills

Like hormone replacement therapy, birth control pills are hormone based. Therefore, they may slightly increase a woman's risk of developing breast cancer, especially if she has taken them longer than eight years and began taking them before age 20, or before her first pregnancy. (Again, there is an increased exposure for a prolonged period of time on breast cells that have not yet differentiated.) On the other hand, birth control pills are associated with a decreased risk of ovarian cancer.

DES

DES (diethylstilbestrol) is a synthetic form of estrogen that was prescribed to several million pregnant women between the early 1940s and 1971. While it was used to help with complications during pregnancy, it ended up affecting the development of the baby's reproductive system when taken during the first five months of pregnancy.

Mothers who took DES have a 30 percent increased risk of developing breast cancer compared with women who did not take the drug. So far, research does not indicate an increased risk of breast cancer for DES-exposed daughters, but clear cell cancer of the vagina is a risk.

Some women don't know whether they took DES when they were pregnant. While difficult, there are ways to find and search records:

- Contact the obstetrician or the obstetrician who took over the practice if the attending physician retired.

- Contact the hospital where the delivery took place and ask for your medical records from the archives.

- Contact the county medical society or health department.

- Contact the pharmacy if you know where your family's prescriptions were filled.

- If you, your husband, or your parents were in the military, contact the proper branch. Military medical records are stored for 25 years.

If you were or think you may have been exposed to DES, be sure to tell your doctor and be extra vigilant about breast exams and mammographies.

For more information, referrals, and support, contact:

Watch Out!
Although studies have not shown oral contraceptives or hormone replacement therapy to be unsafe for DES-exposed daughters, if you were or think you were exposed to DES, explore all your options, and weigh the benefits and risks thoroughly before taking them.

- DES Cancer Network, Suite 400,
  514 10th Street N.W., Washington, DC
  20004-1403; 800/DES-NET4, 202/628-6330.
  e-mail: DESNETWRK@ aol.com;
  Web site: www.descancer.org.

- DES Action USA, Suite 510, 1615 Broadway,
  Oakland, CA 94612; 800/DES-9288,
  510/465-4011; e-mail: desact@well.com;
  Web site: http://www.desaction.org.

- The Registry for Research on Hormonal
  Transplacental Carcinogenesis (Clear Cell
  Cancer Registry), University of Chicago,
  MC 2050, 5841 South Maryland Avenue,
  Chicago, IL 60637; 773/702-6671;
  e-mail: registry@babies.bsd.uchicago.edu;
  Web site: http://bio-3.bsd.uchicago.edu/
  ~obgyn/registry.html.

Unofficially...
Overweight, older women appear to have a greater risk of breast cancer than the general population. Obesity is associated with a higher level of estrogen.

Dietary fat

For some time, a high-fat diet has been thought to be associated with an increased risk of developing breast cancer. It's generally been believed that a high-fat diet increases estrogen levels by increasing overall energy intake, resulting in an increase in adipose tissue storage—fat. Fat increases estrogen levels in the body.

But a recent study suggests that the causal link is not there; researchers found no link between a low-fat diet and reduced risk, according to an article published in the *Journal of the American Medical Association* (March 1999). But, a low-fat diet not reducing your risk does not mean a high-fat diet has no risk.

An article published in the *Journal of the National Cancer Institute* (March 1999) sides with the original contention that a low-fat diet reduces the risk of breast cancer. The investigators completed a computerized search of English language literature on estrogen/estradiol and dietary fat intervention studies published from January 1966 through June 1998 using Medline. They found an overall reduction of –13.4 percent (–7.4 percent among premenopausal women and –23.0 percent among postmenopausal women) of estrogen levels in women who ate a reduced fat diet. They concluded that dietary fat reduction may offer an approach to breast cancer prevention.

But the controversy doesn't end there. It may not be fat intake alone that increases or decreases estrogen levels. In an editorial in that same edition of the *Journal of the National Cancer Institute*, other researchers suggested that there may be other factors that cause or contribute to the reduction of hormone levels found in the blood. They note that when people reduce their fat consumption, they may also alter their intake of total calories (which, as noted in chapter 5, affects cellular aging), fiber, carbohydrates, fruits and vegetables, carotenoids and other micronutrients. They also note that in addition to affecting estrogen levels in the blood, these factors may also alter sex steroid metabolism.

The authors of the *Journal* editorial went on to say that variability of an individual's response (people respond differently to caloric intake—for example, some people can eat a lot and not gain weight while others eat much less and do gain weight) to any specific dietary alteration may, in part, explain "the apparent lack of response to dietary fat reduction found in some studies."

The studies on dietary fat intake generally compared people getting 35 to 40 percent energy from fat (the average U.S. diet) with those reducing their dietary fat intake to 18 to 25 percent of total energy.

Charred and fried food

Do you grill a lot? Do you live on fried foods? Women who eat charred or fried, well-done red meat, particularly bacon, hamburger, and steak had a 4.6 times increased risk of developing breast cancer compared with those who ate their meat medium or rare, according to research by Mayo Clinic investigators in Rochester, Minnesota. They studied women between the ages of 55 and 69 and published the results in the *Journal of the National Cancer Institute* (November 1998).

Thomas A. Sellers, Ph.D., an epidemiologist at the Mayo Clinic, led the study. The investigators theorized that protein cooked at extremely high temperatures leads to the formation of chemicals that, when eaten, can mutate DNA.

But don't think this is a message to eat meat that can still moo. In order to protect yourself from *e. coli* and other bacterial contaminants found in meat, cook it thoroughly by baking, broiling, or boiling, the researchers say. You can also avoid charring food by cooking it slowly rather than searing it on a high flame.

Taking control—reducing your risk

The body is not separated by its parts. Staying healthy overall helps to reduce your chance of getting many diseases. You can further reduce your risk of developing many cancers by eating a low-fat diet and five fruits and vegetables a day, according to the NCI. Eating vegetables, fruits, and fiber may help to lower testosterone levels. You also can limit your alcohol intake to less than two drinks a day, and limit your exposure to radiation as much as possible.

While your risk of developing breast cancer is not lowered by getting annual mammograms starting at age 40, regular screening mammograms, a yearly

Watch Out!
Because most research has looked at large families with a strong family history of breast cancer—that is, many family members who have been diagnosed with the disease—the estimates generally cited for the risk of developing breast cancers in women carrying altered BRCA1 or BRCA2 genes may be artificially inflated. Recent studies of groups more representative of the general population have found a somewhat lower risk.

clinical breast examination, and monthly breast self examinations each month increase your chances of survival because the earlier that breast cancer is detected, the easier it is to treat.

Family history—the genetic link in the cancer chain

Contrary to popular belief, most breast cancer is not hereditary. In fact, only 5 to 10 percent of all breast cancer cases are inherited, although that percentage is much higher for early-onset (before age 40) breast cancer.

While it may increase your risk, a family history of breast cancer doesn't mean you will definitely develop breast cancer. It's just one risk factor. An altered gene alone doesn't cause cancer.

Scientists simply don't know all the reasons why people get cancer. In fact, you can have a mutated gene and not get cancer, just as you can have genes for blue eyes and have brown eyes.

Of those 5 to 10 percent of hereditary breast cancer cases, it is believed that somewhere between 30 to 70 percent involve mutations in the BRCA1 and BRCA2 genes. Of the small percentage of breast cancers that are familial, about 40 percent are associated with BRCA1 gene mutations and between 40 to 45 percent are linked to the BRCA2 gene. Scientists believe that the remaining 10 to 15 percent of cases are attributable to a yet to be discovered gene or group of genes, referred to as BRCA3.

Both men and women have BRCA1 and BRCA2 genes. The risk of developing breast cancer as a result of an inherited mutation is highest for those women with one or more family members with ovarian cancer and among those of Ashkenazi (Eastern European) Jewish descent of whom 2.5 percent (20 out of 800) will have an altered BRCA1 or BRCA2 gene. In the general population, that number drops to about 1 in 800, according to the NCI. Scientist do not know if Ashkenazi Jewish women have a higher incidence rate of breast cancer compared with the general population.

At most, 1 in 10 breast cancer cases involves an inherited altered gene, and not all inherited breast cancer involves the BRCA1 or BRCA2 gene. It is likely that more breast cancer genes will be discovered in the future, according to the NCI.

Which relatives count?

Though not all relatives count when figuring out your risk for inherited forms of breast cancer, surprisingly, fathers, brothers, uncles, and grandfathers count just as much as mothers, sisters, aunts, and grandmothers.

In order to be considered at risk for inherited breast cancer, you must have a *significant* family history, which is defined as the following:

1. You have two or more close family members who have had breast and/or ovarian cancer. A close family member can be your mother, sister, aunt (both your mother's sister and father's sister), grandparent on either your mother's or father's side, brother, or uncle. Family members may also include your daughter or son.

2. Those breast cancers were diagnosed before those relatives turned 50.

Your risk is increased if your relative's cancer affected both breasts and/or developed before menopause. Also, the more significant family members you have who have been diagnosed with breast cancer, the greater your risk. You also have an increased risk of breast cancer if you or a member of your family has

Unofficially...
Men with an altered BRCA2 gene have higher rates of breast cancer than men without an altered gene. The BRCA2 gene appears to account for many of the familial breast cancers in men. However, breast cancer in men is rare. In fact, it accounts for just 1 percent of all breast cancer cases.

had ovarian, colon, or uterine cancer.

P-TEN and Cowden's Syndrome

Another breast cancer susceptibility gene is the
P-TEN, named after a mutation on chromosome 10,
which has been known to play a role in various spo-
radic cancers, according to a study published in the
American Journal of Human Genetics (November 1997).
Also called MMAC1, a P-TEN mutation can increase
a woman's risk of developing breast cancer. Like the
BRCA1 and BRCA2 genes and p53 gene, the P-TEN
appears to be a tumor suppressor gene. The gene is
believed to be the genetic basis of Cowden's
Syndrome, an uncommon dermatological disorder
that causes skin rashes, tiny wart-like bumps, thyroid
disease, and severe benign fibrocystic disease during
adolescence. Between 50 and 75 percent of women
with Cowden's Syndrome develop breast cancer in
their forties.

Cowden's Syndrome often goes unrecognized by
the medical community, says lead investigator Monica
Peacocke, M.D., associate professor of medicine and
dermatology at the Columbia-Presbyterian Medical
Center in New York.

Cowden's Syndrome may also increase the risk of
developing endometrial cancer (as well as benign
and malignant tumors in the thyroid, brain, and
skin). Therefore, women who develop breast cancer
and who have a P-TEN mutation may not be good
candidates for treatment with tamoxifen, a drug
used to control and prevent breast cancer, because
tamoxifen also can increase the risk of endometrial
cancer. However, there have not been any prospective or retrospective studies of women with Cowden's
Syndrome that examined this issue.

Watch Out!
Risk estimates
can be useful for
considering risk in
large groups of
people; they
cannot provide a
precise cancer risk
for an individual.

Just the facts

- Prolonged exposure to estrogen increases your chances of getting breast cancer.

- Most women with breast cancer have no known risk factors other than gender and age.

- It appears that weak electromagnetic fields do not cause breast cancer.

- Family history increases the risk of breast cancer among a small group of women and men.

Prevention Techniques

Chapter 5

You can take control and reduce your risk of developing breast cancer. Diet, exercise, and environmental exposures to carcinogens (cancer-causing agents), as well as genes, all have an impact on the health of your breast epithelial cells. While you can't change your genetic makeup, you can take action to reduce your chances that those genes won't mutate and grow uncontrollably.

In this chapter, we'll tell you what scientific investigators have learned about the role diet, exercise, the environment, and inherited factors play in breast cancer development and how you can use that information to protect yourself. We also discuss genetic testing and possible preventive strategies for those women who test positive.

Risk reduction strategies

Most women diagnosed with breast cancer don't have any of the risk factors noted in Chapter 4, except age. (The vast majority of women who develop breast cancer are older than 50.) While you may think there's not much you can do about getting older, there is scientific evidence showing a healthy, low-caloric diet may play a role in slowing the aging process. A healthy diet will also do a lot more for you than just give you an edge on age—you can impact other breast cancer risk factors as well. Here's how: Diet—not just how much, but what you eat—plays a large role in cancer etiology, and, therefore, prevention. It appears exercise may play a direct role, too. Both diet and exercise affect the immune system, and a boosted immune system may help to repair cells before they mutate. In some instances, the immune system may actually attack and eradicate mutated cells.

There are other, more extreme measures, some women can take to reduce their chances of developing breast cancer. A small percentage of women have an increased risk of developing breast cancer as a result of inheriting a mutated BRCA1 or BRCA2 gene (Breast Cancer Gene 1 and Breast Cancer Gene 2). These women can get a genetic test to see if they have these genes and can make choices if they test positive. Choices include chemoprevention (medicine used to prevent the development of breast cancer in women who are at high risk of developing breast cancer, but there are no data published yet showing the effectiveness on this strategy) and prophylactic double mastectomies (surgical removal of both breasts to help prevent breast cancer, although this does not modify ovarian cancer risk, which is also associated with BRCA1 and BRCA2).

What's food got to do with it?

Scientists believe that diet contributes to more than one-third of all cancer deaths in the Western world, according to a report published in the *Journal of the*

National Cancer Institute (June 1981). Another study, this one published in the journal *Mutation Research* (May 1998), backs up that statistic specifically for the United States. Some food and drink contain mutagens (something that causes cells to mutate) and carcinogens (cancer-causing agents) as well as antimutagens/anticarcinogens. The investigators state that there is overwhelming evidence that a diet high in fruits and vegetables and low in certain fats, together with moderate caloric intake and exercise, is associated with reduced cancer risk. But the authors go one step further, noting that these observations are supported by studies using "complex" food, such as fruits and vegetables, as well as fats. Those studies focusing on only single compounds (vitamins or antioxidants) generally have not produced the same findings. The bottom line: Supplementing your diet with vitamin pills will not have the same result as getting your nutrition from fruits, vegetables, and grains.

As noted in Chapter 1, some countries have much lower breast cancer rates than the United States, and cultures within the United States have different incidence levels. For example, Mexico has a very low incidence rate of breast cancer, and in the United States, Hispanic women have the lowest incidence rate. The traditional Hispanic diet is high in fiber compared with other groups, which may explain the lower incidence of breast cancer among some Hispanic populations, according to results of a study published in *Annals of the New York Academy of Sciences* (December 1997). The diet is also rich in fruits, vegetables, grains, and beans, which reduce estrogen levels.

Japanese women living in Japan also have a low rate of breast cancer. Soy appears to have a protective effect against breast cancer. Researchers note an

Unofficially...
A diet high in fruits and vegetables (at least five a day), combined with routine physical activity, can reduce cancer incidence by 30-40 percent, which translates to 3-4 million few cases per year around the world, according to the Produce for Better Health Foundation.

Watch Out!
While a restricted number of calories appears to have a protective effect against cancer, it's important to fill your diet with food and nutrients known to have beneficial effects on cancer and good health in general. Check with a nutritionist to find out how many calories you should get on a daily basis in order to maintain or achieve a healthy weight.

association between soy intake and levels of estradiol (a potent estrogen) and sex hormone-binding globulin in Japanese women. They believe that the results, if causal, suggest that eating soy lowers breast cancer risk by modifying estrogen metabolism. The report was published in *Nutrition and Cancer* (Volume 20, Issue 3, 1997).

One key factor explaining these differences in breast cancer incidence rates among different cultures appears to be diet.

Drinking from the Fountain of Youth

Scientists know there is an increased risk of developing breast cancer due to aging, and you might think that's a risk factor you simply can't control. Think again. Both diet and exercise appear to slow the aging process.

Studies over the past 30 years have shown calorie-restricted diets may prevent cancer or slow its growth. Animals on calorie-restricted diets have less cancer and fewer signs of aging.

Restricting calories by 40 percent reduces oxidative stress and increases life span in animals, according to research published in *Annals of the New York Academy of Sciences* (November 1998). It also appears to reduce the incidence of many cancers, which investigators say could be due to a reduction of mitogenesis, that is, a reduction in cell reproduction. However, there are currently no specific human correlates.

Investigators at the National Institute of Environmental Health Sciences (NIEHS), one branch of the National Institutes of Health, have discovered the mechanism involved in this phenomenon. The NIEHS researchers (J. Carl Barrett, Ph.D., Sandra Dunn, Ph.D., Frank Kari, Ph.D., and Jeff French, Ph.D., along with other colleagues) reported in the

Unofficially...
The generation of cancer is multifactorial.

journal *Cancer Research* (November 1997) that calorie restriction delays tumor progression by reducing the amount of insulin-like growth factor 1 (IGF-1), a hormone in the blood and body.

Such a decrease had been shown to reduce the development of spontaneous cancers in an earlier study reported in *Cancer Research* (June 1993). In this study, scientists demonstrated that the growth of established bladder cancers in mice was greatly reduced and then increased by reducing and adding IGF-1. The mice were genetically modified to be like cancer-prone humans, deficient in the p53 gene, which is associated with several cancers, including bladder and some breast cancers. The scientists believe their findings apply to cancer in general.

Further research shows that if you block the IGF receptor in laboratory mice, you can block the spread of breast cancer while it's still localized, Dunn says. (Human breast cancer cells were used in the mouse models.) Results from that study were published in *Cancer Research* (August 1998).

In contrast, excessive weight, because it affects estrogen levels, can adversely affect your risk of developing breast cancer.

Eat, drink, and be merry

While a poor diet filled with fried and charred foods may increase your chances of developing cancer, a diet filled with certain nutrients can help prevent cancer.

The NCI urges people to eat five fruits and vegetables a day. Eating fruits, vegetables, and fiber may help lower testosterone levels, and testosterone and other hormones play a key role in the development of breast cancer.

It appears that nutrients may work alongside

Bright Idea
Learn about the biology of breast cancer from experts in the field through the National Breast Cancer Coalition Project LEAD (Leadership Education Advocacy and Development). For more information visit their Web site at http://www. natlbcc.org/ trainingindx.asp. (Click on Project LEAD.)

Bright Idea
Don't forget to eat your brussels sprouts, broccoli, and cabbage because they contain substances that may protect against cancer. Among substances present in these three vegetables are phytochemicals, chemicals produced by plants that are thought to reduce the incidence of cancer.

TABLE 5.1   EAT HEALTHY! FRESH FRUITS AND VEGETABLES CONTAIN A WEALTH OF VITAMINS AND MINERALS, AND SOME ARE A GOOD SOURCE OF FIBER

Apples	High in fiber. Also contain vitamin A, vitamin C, and iron.
Apricots	High in vitamin A, vitamin C, potassium. (Dried apricots lose their vitamin C.)
Artichokes	High in vitamin C, folate, and magnesium and a good source of fiber.
Asparagus	High in vitamin C, a good source of folate. Also contains vitamin A, calcium, and iron.
Bananas	High in fiber. High in vitamin C and potassium.
Bell peppers	High in vitamin C. Also contain vitamin A, calcium, and iron.
Blueberries	High in vitamin C. Good source of fiber. Also contain calcium and iron.
Broccoli	Vitamin C, folate, vitamin A, iron, and calcium.
Brussels sprouts	High in fiber. High in vitamin C. Good source of folate.
Cabbage	High in vitamin C.
Cantaloupe	High in vitamin A and vitamin C. A good source of folate. Also contains calcium and iron.
Carrots	High in vitamin A. High in fiber. Also contains vitamin C and calcium.
Cauliflower	High in vitamin C and folate. Also contain calcium and iron.
Celery	Good source of vitamin C. Also contains vitamin A, calcium, and iron.
Cherries	Good source of vitamin C and fiber.
Corn	Good source of vitamin C.
Grapefruit	High in vitamin C and fiber. Good source of vitamin A. Also contains calcium.
Grapes	Good source of vitamin C. Also contain vitamin A, iron, and calcium.
Honeydew melon	High in vitamin C. Also contains vitamin A and iron.
Kiwifruit	High in vitamin C and fiber. A good source of potassium and vitamin E.
Romaine lettuce	High in vitamin A. Good source of folate.

Mangos	High in vitamin A and vitamin C.
Oranges	High in fiber. High in vitamin C. Also contain vitamin A, calcium, and iron.
Summer squash	High in vitamin C. Also contains vitamin A, calcium, and iron.
Sweet potatoes	High in fiber. High in vitamin A and vitamin C. Also contains calcium and iron.
Tangerines	High in vitamin C. High in fiber. Also contains calcium.
Tomatoes	High in vitamin A and vitamin C. Also contain calcium and iron.
Watermelons	High in vitamin A and vitamin C. Also contain calcium and iron.

each other or together in a complex interaction. So rather than taking a single vitamin, which contains no fiber, scientific evidences shows it's wiser to eat fruits and vegetables, which contain fiber and a mix of vitamins and minerals. (See Table 5.1 to find out the basics on which vitamins and minerals are found in selected fresh fruits as well as which fruits and vegetables are high in fiber.) Some fruits and vegetables contain antioxidants (vitamins C and E and beta carotene) that may help prevent damage to cells caused by free radicals, unstable forms of certain chemicals that react with other chemicals and produce mutations. Folic acid may also help prevent cells from mutating and appears to play a role in strengthening the immune system. Fruits, vegetables, and grains also contain phytochemicals, plant chemicals that appear to have a protective effect against some cancers and inhibit the spread of already malignant cells.

Understanding the value of vitamins, minerals, antioxidants, and phytochemicals is one thing. Getting them into your diet is another. Here are some quick and easy ways to include five fruits and vegetables a day into your diet:

Unofficially...
Eating vegetables from the cabbage family, including broccoli, cauliflower, brussels sprouts, kale, bok choy, collards, turnips, mustard greens, kohlrabi, and watercress, may lower the risk of hormone-related cancers. Some breast cancers have hormone receptors. Eating foods from the cabbage family may also help protect DNA, and boost the body's ability to fight off cancer, according to the Produce for Better Health Foundation.

Unofficially...
One-quarter cup of dried fruit equals one five a day serving. So does one-half cup of cooked or canned vegetables. Generally, a fruit or vegetable serving is about the size of your fist. However, a serving of leafy greens is larger than your fist, and a serving of dried fruit is smaller than your fist.

Timesaver
If you don't have time to make a pie, bake an apple. Simply core and fill with raisins, sprinkle with cinnamon, and microwave or bake until soft. Or bake bananas until black, and slice open. Sprinkle with brown sugar or cocoa. It makes a delicious custard-like treat.

- Drink a glass of orange juice or grapefruit juice with your meals and for a quick thirst quencher.

- Slice bananas, strawberries, or peaches into your cereal or toss in a few raisins or blueberries.

- Buy prewashed, precut carrots for quick snacks and premade salad mixes for an easy meal, snack, or appetizer.

- Keep dried fruit handy for a quick, sweet snack.

- Toss grapes, raisins, apple slices, orange slices, or pineapple chunks into chicken or tuna salad.

- Freeze seedless grapes, cantaloupe balls, or watermelon balls for a refreshing, cool snack.

- Make fruit into dessert. Make pies or crisps with an oatmeal crust.

- Add bell pepper, broccoli, cauliflower, zucchini, yellow squash, or peas to pasta dinners for a tasty meal and colorful presentation.

- In addition to lettuce, tomato, and onion, add bell pepper rings, and cucumber slices to your sandwiches.

- Add grated carrots or other vegetables like zucchini to potato, tuna, or chicken salad. Add grapes, raisins, apples, and oranges to salads for a sweet twist.

- Add sliced bananas or other fruit to plain yogurt or cottage cheese.

- Mix tomato, cucumber, and onion slices with vinegar, salt, pepper, and parsley for a relish salad that will improve in flavor each day. This salad will stay fresh for about a week in your refrigerator.

While most discussions about diet focus only on food, it should come as no surprise that many people forget about the importance of hydration. According to research published in the *Journal of the American Dietetic Association* (February 1999), water is an essential but overlooked nutrient. The authors note that new research indicates hydration, water consumption in particular, can lower the risk of developing breast cancer as well as other cancers and other medical conditions.

To be well-hydrated, the average sedentary adult woman needs at least nine cups of noncaffeinated, nonalcoholic, fluid per day. (According to the Mayo Clinic Women's HealthSource, you should divide your weight in half to determine the appropriate number of ounces of water you need daily. If you exercise or are otherwise physically active enough to sweat, you'll need more water. Caffeinated and alcoholic beverages are dehydrating and don't count toward your daily water intake.) The authors of the study note that dehydration, measured as a 2 percent loss of body weight, can impair physiological and performance responses.

Getting a jump on it

You can try to keep one step ahead of cancer by getting regular exercise. The majority of epidemiological studies suggest that physical activity offers a protective effect against breast cancer.

The optimum protective response of cancer defense mechanisms is gained from moderate levels of energy expenditure, according to investigators whose work was published in *Critical Reviews in Oncogenesis* (Vol. 8, Nos.2&3 1997). There appears to be a dose-response relationship: The less you exercise, the less you're protected from cancer, and the more you exercise, the more protected you are.

How exactly does exercise help to prevent breast cancer? Researchers have developed many theories

Unofficially...
Orange-colored vegetables such as carrots, sweet potatoes, and winter squash as well as orange-colored fruit including cantaloupe, papaya, and mango are good sources of the antioxidant beta carotene.

66
Walking is man's best medicine.
—Hippocrates
99

Watch Out! Studies show that stressful levels of exercise, such as marathon running, have an adverse impact on immune responses.

including:

- Physical activity may reduce the number of ovulatory menstrual cycles, thereby decreasing the cumulative exposure to both progesterone and estrogen (*Sports Medicine*, September 1998).

- In addition to lowering estrogen levels, exercise may lower insulin levels, which, when elevated, are also associated with an increased risk of developing cancer in general (*European Journal of Cancer Prevention*, June 1998).

- Exercise may delay age at menarche (the date of your first menstrual period) (*Cancer*, August 1998).

- Exercise results in a higher energy expenditure, possibly reducing your weight (*Cancer*, August 1998).

- Exercise enhances your immune system (*Cancer*, August 1998).

In contrast, obesity seems to be a major component in the exercise-cancer relationship, according to a report published in *Sports Medicine* (November 1998). In addition to facilitating the synthesis of estrogen, obesity appears to alter the pathways of estradiol metabolism and decreases estradiol binding. Estrogen, as noted in other sections of this chapter and throughout this book, plays an important role in the process of breast cell carcinogenesis, the generation of cancer from normal cells.

Watch Out! Risk estimates can be useful for assessing risk in large groups, but they cannot provide a precise cancer risk for an individual.

Further research is needed to determine which, if any of these theories, are of practical importance.

Taking a dip in the genetic pool

About 5 to 10 percent of all women in the United States carry the BRCA1 or BRCA2 gene, placing them in a high-risk group of developing breast (and ovarian) cancer. These genetic mutations account for less than half of all inherited breast cancer cases. Knowing that you fit into this group may be unsettling. But keep in mind that being in a high-risk group is a far stretch from an actual diagnosis of breast cancer. Many women have these genes and don't develop breast cancer.

When they're healthy, BRCA genes actually protect against cancer. Both the BRCA1 and BRCA2 genes appear to be tumor suppressor genes, which produce a protein that protects against uncontrolled cell division.

But it takes more than just the mutation of these genes to cause cancer. Other factors, including your reproductive history (your age at first live birth), your age, and if your cells have and continue to repair or rid your body of any broken strands of DNA, all effect your risk.

Are you really a good candidate for genetic screening?

It's easy to get carried away with the fear cancer elicits. Even though it's more likely that you won't ever develop breast cancer than you will develop it, it's hard to feel that way, and as a result, many women want reassurance.

Keep in mind when making your decision about getting tested that most women who are diagnosed with an inherited form of breast cancer, caused by a mutated BRCA1 or BRCA2 gene, have a significant family history of the disease. Remember, significant family history is defined by the NCI as:

1. You have two or more close family members who have had breast and/or ovarian cancer. A close family member can be your mother, sister, aunt (both you mother's sister and father's sister),

Unofficially...
Before undergoing genetic testing, there are many factors to consider. For example, how will it affect your daughters, sisters, aunts, and mother if you test positive for one of the genes? The results may indicate that they, too, are a carrier, and they may not want to know if they have a genetic predisposition to developing breast cancer. Furthermore, give some thoughtful consideration as to how you might *really* feel if you test positive for a gene that may cause breast cancer.

Unofficially...
At present, altered genes cannot be repaired. But some day it may be possible to fix or manipulate the genes or sets of genes that cause or increase your risk of developing cancer and other illnesses.

grandparent on either your mother's or father's side, brother, or uncle.

2. Those breast cancers were diagnosed before your relatives turned 50.

"Knowledge is power," says Mary Jane Massie, M.D., director of the Barbara White Fishman Center for Psychological Counseling at Memorial Sloan-Kettering Cancer Center's Breast Center in New York City. If you're worried, ask your doctor if you fall into the high-risk group. Because the vast majority of women don't, you'll probably leave the visit with a sense of relief, she says.

Drawbacks—think twice about getting tested

There are some significant drawbacks to getting tested. There is the risk of getting a false positive test result, which could cause you unnecessary distress. It may also cause you to make radical decisions, such as getting a double mastectomy or taking tamoxifen, based on wrong information. A false negative reading is also possible. That could lead you to become less vigilant in your surveillance.

Genetic testing can affect relationships with family members. If you end up testing positive, you will probably need a lot of emotional support from your family, Massie says. While some families are interested in knowing their risks and will rally around the relative who gets tested or even get tested as a group, other people would rather not know if they have the gene and may react with anger rather than support. Therefore, you may want to consider asking your family what they think of your desire to get tested before you make your decision, she says. At least that way you'll know whether or not to expect support from them.

Getting tested

If you have a significant family history, genetic testing is an option you can consider. Your test results may rule out any worries you might have or determine that you have one of the genes. Even so, it is not a certainty that it will mutate and cause cancer. Knowing that you have the gene may spur you on to get mammograms routinely, do breast self-exams monthly, and see your doctor as scheduled. If a cancer did develop, you would have a better chance at catching it in its earliest stage. However, it may also fill you and your family with unnecessary anxiety. On the other hand, a negative result may relieve you and your family of unnecessary worry.

Genetic testing has another benefit. For the small group of women who test positive for the genes, there are options. These women can consider taking tamoxifen or raloxifene for chemotherapeutic prevention or undergo risk-reducing surgery.

No studying necessary

While genetic tests are high tech, all that's needed from you is a simple blood test (no studying, no No. 2 pencils required). Remember, as noted in Chapter 1, each cell in the human body contains an individual's entire genetic makeup, so mutations can be detected in your white blood cells. (White blood cells have nuclei, red blood cells in circulation do not. Nuclei are required for DNA analysis.) You'll have to sit tight for a while, though—it can take several weeks or even months to get your test results. The price of testing varies and can be expensive, ranging from several hundred to more than a thousand dollars, depending on the number of mutations the lab must look for.

Before getting tested consider the following:

Bright Idea
If you are thinking about genetic testing, discuss it with your doctor, a genetic counselor, and possibly your family. To get a referral to centers that have health care professionals trained in genetics, call 1/800-4-CANCER.

Unofficially...
Genetic tests may not be covered by health insurance, but you may not want your insurance company to know you were tested because they may consider you a high risk if you test positive.

1. The limitations of the test. The test cannot tell you if you'll develop breast cancer, or that you won't. Furthermore, the testing is for a specific gene only. Remember, most breast cancer is not a result of an inherited form of it. Either way, you still need to take proper precautions such as doing self-exams, getting clinical exams, and mammograms starting at age 40 or before if your doctor believes it's necessary.

2. How you will cope if you find you're at an increased risk of developing breast cancer.

A balancing act: weighing pros and cons of getting tested

There are many advantages and disadvantages to getting tested. Table 5.2 addresses many of the issues.

Protecting your privacy

If you get tested for altered genes, more eyes than just yours and those of your healthcare team may see your results. The results may be placed in your medical records, regardless of whether you or your insurance company pays for the test. The inclusion of the results in your medical records may prevent you from getting insurance: When you apply for medical, life, or disability insurance, you may be asked to sign forms that give an insurance company permission to access your medical records. A positive test result may cause the insurance company to turn down your application because of the costs it may incur down the road should you develop cancer.

If you want to keep the results private, ask your physician to keep them out of your medical records. Some physicians will comply. (Others worry that the insurance company will charge them with fraud for the omission.) If you're tested as a part of a study, ask to see if it's possible to keep the records private. (This

TABLE 5.2   WHAT ARE THE ADVANTAGES AND DISADVANTAGES OF TESTING?

Advantages of Testing

Make medical and lifestyle choices.

Find out that you do not have an altered gene.

Cope with your cancer risk.

Decide whether or not to have prophylactic surgery.

Give other family members useful information (if you choose to share your test results).

Contribute to research.

Disadvantages of Testing

There is no proven way to reduce cancer risk.

There is no guarantee that test results will remain private.

You may face discrimination for health insurance, life insurance, or employment.

You may find it harder to cope with your cancer risk when you know your test results.

Negative test results may provide a false sense of security because you think you have no chance of getting cancer. You would still have the same risk as women in the general population and need to take the proper precautions.

Source: National Cancer Institute

Moneysaver
If you're a member of a high-risk family, you can reduce the costs of genetic testing by testing a member of the family who has already been diagnosed with breast cancer. Then you and other members of the family can be tested only for that specific mutation.

is an important issue not yet resolved by the Office for Protection from Research Risks (OPRR) at the National Institutes of Health.)

In addition, consider paying with cash or a money order and use code names on your blood specimens. You will have to arrange with the clinic in order to use a code name so they will know which specimen belongs to you.

If you don't plan to foot the bill, check with your insurance company before getting tested. Insurance policies vary with regard to whether the cost of genetic testing is covered.

Even if you are able to get your medical records sealed, insurance companies and employers can gain access to your results simply by asking you to provide the information. Failure to tell the whole truth is considered fraud and can cost you your insurance coverage or job. The amount of insurance and employment discrimination protection varies from state to state, so keep in mind that a decision you make today may have repercussions in the future if you move to another state with lesser protections.

Other insurance problems may arise when you seek a new job. In addition to health insurance coverage, it may be difficult to get life and disability insurance. If you do qualify, you may have to pay higher premiums or settle for less coverage.

A positive test result exposes you to potential employment discrimination as well as insurance discrimination. You may, however, have some protection from discrimination from the Americans with Disabilities Act (ADA). Though the Equal Employment Opportunity Commission (EEOC) has expanded the definition of disabled to include people who carry genes that put them at higher risk for genetic disorders, the extent of this protection has not yet been tested in the courts.

But even if your test results are kept private, insurance still may prove troublesome. If you test positive and decide to increase surveillance, get surgery, or take drugs, you must justify these moves to the insurance company. If you have a strong family history of the disease, you'll have a much stronger case. If you don't, you could encounter difficulty. (However, if you don't have a strong family history of breast cancer, you may not want to get tested.)

Testing positive—one test you don't want to "ace"

While no one wants to pass this test, if you do find out you have an altered gene, you can use that information to take measures to help reduce your risk of getting cancer. You can start by being vigilant about detection. Ask your doctor if you should get more frequent mammograms and clinical breast exams, be more vigilant about performing monthly breast self-exams, and get an ultrasound of your ovaries, since BRCA gene alterations also increase your risk of ovarian cancer.

You can also join a research study as an added protective measure. The study may entail changing your diet, reducing the amount of alcohol you drink, or trying new drugs to reduce the risk of cancer. (If the study involves taking medication, you should find out everything you can about the drug, possible side effects, long-term effects, etc.) By taking part in a study, you also will be contributing information to science. You can find out about NCI-funded studies that are currently open by calling the Cancer Information Center at 800/4-CANCER and other studies via the Internet. For more information about joining a study and where to locate one, read Chapter 11.

Tamoxifen

Although it seemed like a new drug with the flurry of news reports in 1998, tamoxifen has actually been used for more than 20 years. Tamoxifen was introduced in the United States in 1978. In 1985, tamoxifen was given, along with conventional chemotherapy, to postmenopausal women whose breast cancer had spread to the axillary (underarm) lymph nodes. By 1989, it was given to premenopausal women with advanced breast cancer. In the early 1990s, tamoxifen was prescribed for node-negative breast cancer in women and advanced breast cancer in men. On October 29, 1998, tamoxifen was approved by the FDA to be used to reduce the incidence of breast cancer in women who are at high risk for developing the disease.

Tamoxifen, which is in pill form, interferes with the activity of estrogen (a female hormone). Tamoxifen continues to be studied for the prevention of breast cancer. It is also being studied in the treatment of several other types of cancer.

This drug works, in part, by interfering with the effects of estrogen, which promotes breast cancer cell growth. Hence, it's often referred to as an *antiestrogen*.

Initial trial results of a study of tamoxifen by the National Surgical Adjuvant Breast and Bowel Project (NSABP), a Pittsburgh-based research network, found a 45 percent reduction of breast cancer cases among healthy women who took tamoxifen over a four-year period. A follow-up report published in the *Journal of the National Cancer Institute* (September 1998) showed a 49 percent reduction in breast cancer incidence among women at increased risk of developing breast cancer who took tamoxifen for five years. (A total of 13,388 women participated in the trial: 6,707 women received a placebo and 6,681 received tamoxifen.)

While tamoxifen holds promise for keeping cancer at bay, it does have some very serious possible side effects, particularly for women over 50. In the study, tamoxifen increased the women's chances of endometrial cancer (cancer of the uterine lining), pulmonary embolism (a blood clot in the lung), and deep vein thrombosis (a blood clot in a major vein). There were 33 cases of endometrial cancer in the tamoxifen group and only 14 in the placebo group, 17 cases of pulmonary embolism in the tamoxifen group compared with six in the placebo group, and 30 cases of deep vein thrombosis in the tamoxifen group versus 19 in the placebo group.

On a more positive note, there wasn't any difference in the number of heart attacks between the tamoxifen and placebo group, and women taking tamoxifen had significantly fewer bone fractures of the hip, wrist, and spine—there were 47 cases in the tamoxifen group versus 71 cases in the placebo group. And those under age 50 didn't appear to have any excess risk of incurring such adverse effects as deep vein thrombosis and endometrial cancer.

Because of the possible side effects, you and your physician will have to consider the following factors: your age, medical history, and family medical history. Women who are pregnant are advised to not take this drug.

The final results may not be so final

In the British journal *The Lancet* (July 10, 1998), two research groups report that tamoxifen did not appear to prevent breast cancer in their studies. The differences in findings may be the result of variations in trial design. There was a significant difference in the number of women who participated in these studies, a difference in their ages (the women in the U.S. study were older), and variations in risk factors.

In the first trial, 5,408 women who had hysterectomies were selected to participate in the trial because they would not be susceptible to endometrial cancer, a side effect of tamoxifen noted earlier. The women were randomly assigned to either the tamoxifen or placebo group. The study was lead by Umberto Veronesi, M.D. and colleagues from Milan and Bologna, Italy (the Italian Tamoxifen Prevention Study). The study results showed that after nearly four years, there was no significant difference in the number of women who developed breast cancer.

Watch Out!
If you are at increased risk of developing blood clots, taking a blood thinner, or are pregnant or plan to become pregnant you shouldn't take tamoxifen, according to the manufacturer. Tamoxifen used during pregnancy may harm the fetus, according to animal studies. If you're taking birth control pills or hormone replacement therapy, you must stop them before taking tamoxifen and use another form of birth control.

There were 19 diagnoses of breast cancer in the tamoxifen group and 22 in the placebo group. However, how many women actually took the drug and for what duration is questioned by other scientists.

The second study involved 2,494 women with a family history of breast cancer. After nearly six years, there was no difference in the overall breast cancer rates between the two groups. This study was led by Trevor Powles, M.D., and colleagues from London, England.

However, some scientists question whether a number of these women also took HRT, didn't fill their prescriptions, and had no risk assessment prior to enrolling.

So far, these negative studies have had little or no impact in the medical community. The Study of Tamoxifen and Raloxifene (STAR) trial, with more than 20,000 participants, will help clarify the results. (Note: Raloxifene is available only in the STAR trial as chemoprevention for breast cancer. To find out STAR trial site locations, call 800/4-CANCER.)

Raloxifene

Another drug, raloxifene, an osteoporosis drug, has also shown potential in reducing the likelihood of developing breast cancer. However, it is not yet approved for this type of use. Initial studies by University of California-San Francisco (UCSF) researchers found that raloxifene reduced the risk of breast cancer by 70 percent in the group of women studied and that it didn't increase the risk of endometrial cancer as does tamoxifen.

According to Abby Sinnott, a news service staff member, there is not enough data to determine if some women will fair better on one drug or the other.

She also notes that the 70 percent outcome from their study and the 49 percent outcome from the tamoxifen study cannot be compared because investigators studied different groups of women. "[The] main difference at this point seems to be that raloxifene does not seem to increase the risk of endometrial cancer the way tamoxifen does," she says.

If you're postmenopausal, 35 or older, or at increased risk of developing breast cancer, you may be eligible to participate in the STAR trial, a study that will compare the two drugs. For more information, contact the National Surgical Adjuvant Breast and Bowel Project, Box 21, Pittsburgh, PA. 15261; Web site: www.nsabp.pitt.edu, call NCI's Cancer Information Service at 800/4-CANCER, or speak with a cancer information specialist at the American Cancer Society by calling 800/ACS-2345.

Oophrectomies

Estrogen, the female sex hormone that plays a key role in the development of breast cancer, is produced by the ovaries. Removal of the ovaries (artificial menopause) has been shown to reduce risk. However, this option should only be considered by women at high-risk of developing breast cancer. Removal of the ovaries can cause other health problems, since estrogen has an important protective effect on the heart and bones. The incidence of heart attacks rises after menopause as does the incidence of osteoporosis. As a women ages, hip fractures become more common and sometimes can have complications that can be fatal: There's a one-year mortality of 20 to 25 percent.

If you're considering this type of surgery, you may want to talk about the benefits and drawbacks of your decision with a therapist who specializes in breast cancer. Give yourself plenty of time to make a

Unofficially...
Both tamoxifen and raloxifene are selective estrogen receptor modulators (SERMs). This class of drug blocks the actions of estrogen in breast and certain other tissues while mimicking estrogen's actions in bones and other tissues. Therefore, SERMs help to prevent osteoporosis or deter its progress in post-menopausal women. Their effect on bone in premenopausal women is unclear.

Unofficially...
A prophylactic mastectomy removes all breast tissue but does not remove muscles or lymph nodes.

thoughtful, well-informed decision.

Prophylactic double mastectomies

The *New England Journal of Medicine* (January 1999) published a retrospective study by researchers at the Mayo Clinic in Rochester, Minnesota. Their findings suggest that prophylactic double mastectomies, surgically removing both breasts as a preventive measure, reduces a woman's risk of developing breast cancer by about 90 percent for those at moderate to high risk.

(Note: Prophylactic double mastectomies will only benefit a small group of women who are at high risk of developing breast cancer.)

In addition to reducing your risk of developing breast cancer, surgery may also reduce your worries. But losing body parts can be traumatic. The change in your physical features may result in a deep sense of loss. And, many women who consider this type of surgery end up experiencing severe anxiety. Furthermore, the surgery cannot remove all of the breast tissue. Some women in the Mayo study later developed breast cancer in the tissue that was left behind.

If you're at a high risk of developing breast cancer and are considering such a radical preventive measure, you may want to explore the benefits and drawbacks of your decision with a therapist who specializes in breast cancer. Be sure to give yourself plenty of time to make a thoughtful, well-informed decision.

Watch Out!
Preventive mastectomy carries with it a greater risk than preventive tamoxifen use because of the risks associated with general anesthesia.

Just the facts

- Diet and exercise may play a role in the prevention of breast cancer.

- Genetic testing may relieve you of worry or may result in cause for concern.

- Tamoxifen and raloxifene both appear to have protective effects against breast cancer development. Only tamoxifen has been tested and approved.

- Oophrectomies and prophylactic double mastectomies are very serious measures to use as prevention. Think seriously before undertaking them and talk about all concerns with your physician.

Unofficially...
Breast tissue is not confined to the breast. Breast tissue is distributed over the chest wall, up to the collarbone, over into the armpit, and down to the abdominal wall.

Diagnosis And Prognosis

GET THE SCOOP ON...
How to perform a breast self-exam ▪ How mammography
works and the different types used ▪ Why you should be
cautious when choosing a radiologist ▪ What types of tests
might be done if a suspicious mass is detected ▪ What
happens in the laboratory when a lump is found

Diagnosis
Techniques

I t's dreadful to have a diagnosis of breast cancer. But a cancerous growth caught in the early stages is the easiest to treat and usually has the best prognosis.

In this chapter, we'll teach you how to examine your own breasts to detect any abnormalities early, and we'll discuss other monitoring and detection techniques. We'll also review the procedures used to determine if a mass is cancerous and explain how treatment options and a prognosis are determined.

Detection—a three-pronged approach

Detection is the first step to getting a diagnosis and prognosis. It is also the first step to recovery. Typically, the earlier a cancerous growth is detected, the better the prognosis. That's why it's a good idea for you to monitor your breast tissue. There are three components to monitoring your breasts:

1. Breast self-exam

2. Clinical breast exam

3. Mammography

135

The American Cancer Society recommends the following schedule: Between the ages of 20-39, you should perform a monthly breast self-exam and get a clinical breast exam every two years. Between the ages of 40 to 49, you should perform a monthly breast self-exam and get a clinical exam and mammogram annually. National Cancer Institute (NCI) guidelines, however, recommend mammograms every one to two years in the over-40 age group for women with no unusual risk factors. (Women at high risk should stick to annual mammograms.) Women ages 50 and older should perform a monthly self-exam and get a clinical exam and mammogram every year. (If you're under 40 and have a significant family history of breast cancer, talk to you doctor about how often you should get a mammogram and clinical breast exam.)

Do-it-yourself breast exams

Some studies show that more than 90 percent of breast cancers are found by women themselves. That's a pretty strong argument for performing breast self-exams, even if they do make you nervous.

If you're premenopausal, you should examine your breasts one week following the end of menstruation. If you have irregular periods or skip from time to time, then you should perform the exam on the same day every month. If you're postmenopausal, pick one day of the month for self-examination. By examining your breasts every month, you will become familiar with the "terrain" and be better able to detect changes.

Here's how to perform a breast self-examination:

Step 1. Stand in front of a mirror, hands on your hips, and visually examine your breasts.

Next, stand with your hands behind your head,

Unofficially...
Mammography, ultrasound, and magnetic resonance imaging (MRI) are now used during diagnosis, sparing some women surgical biopsies.

Source: National Cancer Institute

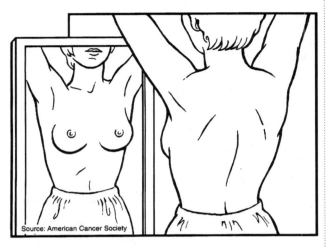
Source: American Cancer Society

Figure 6.1
Breast self exam
mirror check.

*Source: American
Cancer Society.*

fingers interwoven. (See Figure 6.1.)

Look for lumps, changes in size, color, shape or contour, dimples or puckering, or inverted nipples.

Step 2: Press each nipple to see if there is a discharge.

Step 3: Lie down with a pillow under your left shoulder or stand in a shower. Place your left hand under your head if lying down, and above your head if standing. Using your right hand, fingers flattened together to form a pad, press on the top portion of the left breast in a circular (clockwise or counterclockwise) motion to examine the entire outer, then inner circle of the breast, including the areola and nipple. You can use powder or lotion to make the surface smooth. Perform this process using three different pressures. On the first run, use light pressure to gently feel the area under the skin's surface and then add more pressure to feel halfway into the flesh. On the third round, use deep pressure to feel down to the ribs. Examine your breast and chest area under your armpit up to your collarbone, and over

Figure 6.2
Breast self-exam
—standing up in
a shower or lying
on a bed.

*Source: American
Cancer Society.*

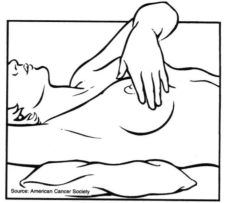

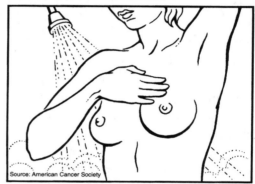

Figure 6.3
Breast self-exam
patterns.

*Source: American
Cancer Society.*

Figure 6.4
Finger pads.

*Source: American
Cancer Society.*

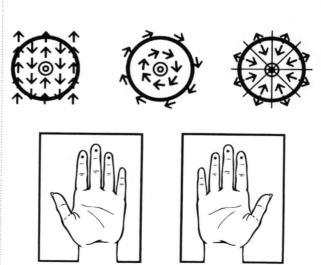

to your shoulder. Repeat on the right side, examining the right breast with the left hand. (See Figures 6.2, 6.3, and 6.4.)

You should be feeling for lumps and thickening areas. Of course, if you find a lump, thickening of the skin, puckering, or discharge, call your doctor.

A cautionary note

While it's important to do self-examinations every month, it's also important not to be overly vigilant. A team of British researchers reported in the journal *Psychosomatic Medicine* (March 1999) that too many breast self-examinations can be counterproductive for women with a family history of breast cancer. Doing breast self-examinations every day or every week doesn't improve detection. In fact, it may reduce the effectiveness of the procedure because these women may be substituting frequent, less thorough exams for less frequent, more thorough ones. The high frequency can also lead to more false-positive findings. Also, very frequent exams may not allow you to notice subtle, gradual changes.

Interestingly, the investigators found anxiety about getting cancer was lowest among women who examined themselves least often and highest among those who examined themselves most often.

A helping hand

Another, perhaps easier, way to perform a breast self-exam is by using an aid, in addition to bear-hand self-examination, called Sensability (Becton-Dickenson). (See Figure 6.5.) It is made of two thin, round latex-free plastic sheets with a liquid lubricant sealed in between them. The pad measures about 10 inches in diameter. It is designed so your hands will glide smoothly across your breasts during a self-examination to help detect a lump. The pad comes with an

Timesaver
Make the first mammography appointment of the day. This way, you can cut down on the time you spend in the waiting room.

Figure 6.5
The Sensability
(Becton-Dickenson)
pad magnifies the
feel of very small
growths. It is
available without
a prescription at
drug stores.

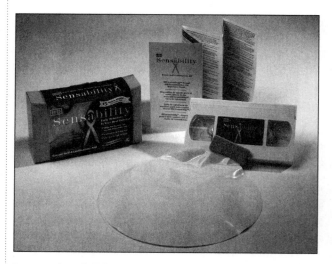

instructional videotape in English and Spanish as well as written instruction in a variety of languages.

The doctor is in...clinical breast exams

Clinical breast exams should take place during your annual gynecological examination. During this exam, you will have one hand tucked under your head (the right hand while your right breast is being examined and your left hand while your left breast is being examined). Your physician will place pressure on your breasts in a circular motion using the pads of his or her fingers. This exam does not hurt but may cause some discomfort if your breasts are tender.

Mammograms—detecting what you can't

Mammography has the ability to detect a cancerous growth up to two years before it can be felt by a manual exam. Mammography is an X-ray image of the breast. There are two types of tissue in the breast: fat tissue and fibroglandular tissue. The two types of tissue look different on the film. Breast cancer may be seen as a mass (a lesion that could not be a tumor, blood vessel malformation, tissue overgrowth, etc.), calcifications, or as a distortion of normal breast architectural markings, according to Stephen A. Feig, M.D., director of the Breast Imaging Center at Thomas Jefferson University Hospital in Philadelphia, Pennsylvania, and professor of radiology at Jefferson Medical College. He says the markings are analogous to looking at branches on a tree in the winter—if you see a branch at an abnormal angle, it might be broken. Masses and calcifications can be either benign or malignant. Most are benign. Most distortions detected by mammography are also benign.

Breast calcifications are made of minute amounts of calcium that cannot be detected by self or clinical breast exams. They can only be detected by mammography and, in some cases recent research shows (*JAMA*, January 1999), by ultrasound. There are two categories of breast calcifications: macrocalcifications and microcalcifications:

1. Macrocalcifications are often associated with injuries, inflammation, and aging of the breast arteries—benign conditions.

2. Microcalcifications are typically located in areas filled with rapidly dividing cells. When microcalcifications are seen in clusters, they may indicate a small cancerous growth. About 50 percent of the cancers detected by mammography are detected by the appearance of a microcalcification cluster. Microcalcification clusters, however, do not always indicate a cancerous growth.

As noted earlier, masses and calcifications can be either benign or malignant. Most are benign. Even so, there tends to be some panic about the American Cancer Society statistic that one out of every eight women will get cancer. One in eight is based on actuarial life projections (mathematical computations of average life spans), not that one in eight women who get screened walk away with a diagnosis of breast cancer, according to Robert Schmidt, M.D., associate professor of radiology at New York University School of Medicine. "For example, at age 45 in a screened population, only one to two women per one thousand will be diagnosed with breast cancer each year," he says.

In addition, the old debate on when to get a baseline fuels more fear. Unless you're in a high-risk group, getting a baseline at age 35 is not a good idea, Schmidt says. At that age, breast tissues have a lot of lumps and tissue tends to be too dense to get an accurate picture. Furthermore, only 1 to 2 percent of all breast cancers are in that age group.

Unless you're in a high-risk group, the NCI recommends women get their first screening at age 40.

Some mammography screening trials have shown a 30 to 45 percent reduction in deaths, according to Feig. A lot has to do with the quality of the images, the quality of the interpretation, and how frequently the screening is performed, he says.

Not all mammography equipment is equal, Feig says. That's a hard obstacle for a patient to overcome. It's difficult for a patient to tell if the equipment is good. It depends on how well-maintained the equipment is, he says, as well as other quality factors, such as how well the technician positions the breast and how skilled the radiologist is at interpretation.

Although mammography centers are certified by the FDA, not every radiologist is equal in his or her ability to read the X-rays. How do you know who the best ones are? A good radiologist should be perform-

Unofficially...
Some hospitals throw out mammographies after five years, as advancements in technology make it difficult to compare films at future screenings. Readings are based, in part, on changes. So, don't skip! Get a mammogram as scheduled if you're over 40.

ing at least 10 mammograms a day and should be interpreting at least that many per day, according to Feig.

Screening and diagnostic mammography

In many instances, a radiologist can make a prediction on the likelihood a lesion is malignant based on a screening mammogram, Feig says. If the radiologist is concerned about a mass or microcalcification, he or she may order extra mammographic views or an ultrasound examination. Based on this second set of pictures, the radiologist can make a more accurate prediction as to the likelihood of cancer. Additional tests are just extra views to reduce false positives, Feig stresses, noting that the extra workups will result in earlier detection if there is a cancer present. Feig also notes that among women who get mammograms routinely, only about 5 percent need to get additional views. Of those, some are normal. Others need biopsies to determine if the suspicious area is benign or malignant. Less than 1 percent of women getting a screening mammogram will need a biopsy.

Diagnostic mammographies, used for women who already have symptoms suggestive of breast cancer (a palpable lump, for example), are the same as screening mammographies, except they include additional views. They are used to determine the nature of the woman's symptoms.

What you can expect

Mammograms may sometimes cause discomfort because the breasts must be compressed until the skin is taut. (See Figure 6.6 to see how a mammogram is done.) A mammogram has to involve compression of the breast for two reasons:

1. By decreasing the thickness of the breast through compression, a lower radiation dose can be used.

Watch Out!
Mammography may not be able to detect a growth in dense breast tissue, the type of tissue often seen in young women's breasts.

Figure 6.6
During a
mammogram
the breasts are
compressed.
Mammography
compression
should not be
painful, though it
may cause some
discomfort.

*Source: American
Cancer Society.*

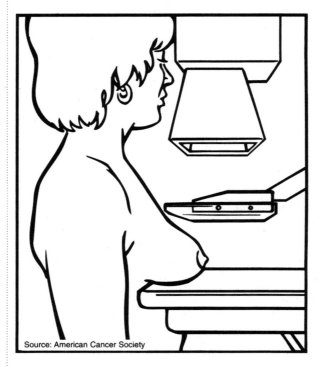

Source: American Cancer Society

2. Compression reduces the superimposition of breast tissue, so it's less likely that a lesion could be obscured by overlying breast tissue.

"But compression should not be painful," Feig emphasizes. If you have tenderness in your breast at certain times of the month, schedule your mammograms shortly after your menstrual period begins, he suggests. This timing has other benefits, as noted in the next section of this chapter. Feig also says the technician is supposed to finish the compression process by hand (the initial compression is done electronically), reaching the final point of compression based on feedback from the patient. The compression is only applied for a couple of seconds, at most, he says.

Timing counts

Researchers at the Fred Hutchinson Cancer Research Center in Seattle, Washington, found that mammography may work better for younger women if the test is done during the first two weeks of the menstrual cycle. The study was published in the *Journal of the National Cancer Institute* (June 1998). The researchers found an association between menstrual phase and breast density, which affects mammogram readings. Here's how: As the menstrual cycle progresses, the breast tissue becomes less fatty, that is, less transparent on a mammogram reading, and more fibrous and dense. The density appears as increased cloudiness in the mammogram, making it more difficult to detect very small malignancies in premenopausal women. The changes are probably due to reproductive hormone fluctuations.

Bottom line? If you're in your forties, get your mammograms during the first two weeks of your menstrual cycle. In addition to a more accurate reading, you'll also feel more comfortable because your breasts will be less tender during this phase of your cycle.

Those who benefit most from this timing are those women who are at or below average body weight because they naturally have denser breasts.

Breast density and its impact on mammography

Breasts are composed of fatty and fibroglandular tissue. Fibroglandular tissue has the same density on the mammogram as a cancer, so it's difficult to tell fibrous tissue from a cancerous mass. Mammograms show fat as black and glandular tissue as white. Cancer, however, also appears white. (See Figure 6.7 to see what normal fatty breast tissue looks like on a mammogram.) The proportions of fatty and fibroglandular tissue

Figure 6.7
It is difficult for
radiologists to
find breast cancer
in dense tissue. It
would be easier
to see it in the
fatty tissue shown
here.

Source: NCI

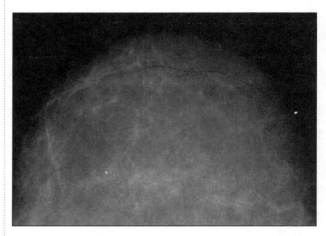

vary from woman to woman, and even in the same woman the proportion varies over time, Feig says. These variations are due to hormonal changes. In general, younger women have denser breasts than older women, he says, explaining that fibroglandular tissue decreases as you age and after you have children, both as a result of changes in hormone levels.

The degree of breast density depends on the amount of glandular and fibrous tissue that make up the breast. Density can only be discerned by mammography and is not related to the size, shape, lumpiness, or texture of a woman's breasts. Breast density is rated on a scale of one to four, one being the least dense and most fatty, four being the most dense, most glandular, and most fibrous.

Who's reading your mammogram?

Mammography has a sensitivity (the ability to find cancer when the woman being screened has the disease) of up to 94 percent, and a specificity (the ability to find the absence of cancer when the woman being screened does not have the disease) of greater than 90 percent, according to the National Cancer

Institute. But not all mammograms are equal, due in large part to the people who read them.

Robert Schmidt, M.D., associate professor of radiology at New York University School of Medicine, has found a weak link in the detection and diagnosis process that may raise considerable concern in women who have been screened for breast cancer. A recent study he led suggests that not all general radiologists are adept at reading mammograms. Among that group of physicians, there's a wide variation in their ability to read mammograms. The study took place at five medical seminar meeting locations in the U.S. during 1997 and 1998, using high-quality copy films of 100 patient cases. These X-rays were shown to more than 250 radiologists and four experts (those with advance mammography reading skill levels), whom Schmidt selected. The radiologists were given about 2 1/2 hours to complete the exercise. The cases were not overly subtle or tricky: 45 contained 50 cancers diagnosed in routine practice, and 55 were normal/benign cases.

In fact, one radiologist, who rated himself as being at an advanced skill level, finished just 80 percent of the mammogram skill reading test and of that, he detected only 30 percent of the breast cancers. This radiologist reportedly reads 5,000 mammograms a year and has been at his job for 10 years. On the other hand, two who said they were beginners did better than the best experts.

The problem? Radiologists spend only two months of their five-year residency learning to read screening mammographies. Moreover, in practice they don't get much, if any, feedback on the accuracy of their readings because they typically don't screen patients recalled for a work-up of the potential abnormality the

Watch Out!
According to published reports, upward of 20 percent of breast cancers may be overlooked on mammograms, and up to 70 percent of them could possibly have been detected sooner.

Unofficially...
Because of low reimbursement, high government regulation, and high lawsuit rates, mammography is often a money loser for radiologists. This may be a factor discouraging radiologists from spending a lot of time reading mammographies.

radiologist questioned on the screening exam. Patients are rarely screened by the same radiologist year after year. Furthermore, there are only minimal government standards for screening ability: (board certification in radiology, 40 hours of continuing medical education credits in mammography, and reading at least 480 mammograms per year, or about two per working day. "A radiologist reading the minimum number of screening exams would only see about two... cancers a year," according to Schmidt. Within the last 10 years, a section on mammography was added to the radiology board exam but this does not test mammography screening ability.

Schmidt emphasizes three points to be learned from this study:

1. Experts are better than general radiologists at reading mammograms because they have both training and experience. Experts know more cancerous patterns because they've seen more. They know where to look for cancerous tumors and they know how to see through the distortions.

2. Radiologists often don't know when they detect a cancerous growth. Patient follow-up is difficult, and few radiologists like to document when they are wrong. The purpose of Schmidt's study was to give radiologists the opportunity to see if they know what breast cancer looks like, give them feedback on their skills, and show them how to improve their technique. Either to protect themselves from lawsuits or due to altruism, a few radiologists who found out their scores gave up reading mammograms.

3. You're more likely to get a radiologist with better abilities if you choose one from the expert group.

How can you tell if you're getting a radiologist who's adept at reading mammograms? You can't be certain. You can ask friends or your doctor for recommendations. The problem is that a typical internist may only come into contact with a few breast cancers a year, so it's hard for her or him to give a good recommendation. Generally, facilities that are dedicated to mammography, that is, that have dedicated mammographers, do better, Schmidt says. University-based facilities often have dedicated mammographers.

If in doubt, ask if the facility can take X-rays with different views. (In the U.S., there are typically two standard screening views per breast. In some states, such as New York, there are three for baseline mammographies. There are also magnification and spot compression views, and other special views, which are part of diagnostic work-ups, supervised by a radiologist.) Ask if they do ultrasound, and if they perform alternative types of breast biopsies, like needle aspirations or core biopsies rather than sending patients directly to surgeons. ("There are certainly excellent facilities which may do screening only, but a facility which also works up the screening abnormalities with special views and does breast ultrasound and needle biopsies will, in general, be one that does higher quality work," Schmidt says.) In addition, ask if the films are sent away to be read. In those cases, the radiologist probably won't have your previous films with which to compare the new ones. Mammography works by looking for changes in the mammograms, so the old films are very important for comparison.

Regardless, don't panic. In many cases where breast cancers are missed, they are often detected on

66

If you don't even use film, you're right in 99.5% of the patients on average.
—Robert Schmidt, M.D., associate professor of radiology at NYU School of Medicine, explaining that only one in 200 screened women will have breast cancer detected on a mammogram.

99

Unofficially...
Misdiagnoses based on failure to detect breast cancer, which almost always includes a mammogram, are the No. 1 cause of medical negligence suits in this country.

Moneysaver
Free mammograms, if not from a center providing longitudinal study data, can end up being costly—because radiologists who do these screenings do not have your prior X-rays to compare with the new ones and detection is more difficult. If the radiologist misses a growing cancer, it can cost you a lot of money in medical bills down the road, and possibly even your life.

subsequent mammograms before the diagnosis is made, because the average breast cancer grows relatively slowly. So there is usually ample opportunity to make the diagnosis.

Bottom line? There's no perfect person around, Schmidt says. But, a radiologist with a certain amount of skill in reading mammograms increases your chances of a more accurate screening, he says.

If you have any doubts about your mammography results, get a second opinion before getting a biopsy, Schmidt advises. A second opinion and additional films can eliminate more than 25 to 40 percent of unnecessary biopsies, according to Schmidt.

Free mammogram screenings—are they safe?

Mother's Day screenings, Breast Cancer Awareness month screenings, and the like may be dangerous, according to Schmidt. Why? First, if you don't have a previous mammogram with which to compare this screening, you may not see changes. Using previous mammogram results for comparison helps radiologists see how structures and tissues have been all along and allow them to more easily find changes. To truly benefit from screenings, you must show up regularly and stick with one place, Schmidt says. If you must go to another place, try to obtain your old films for comparison.

Second, it's not uncommon for women who fear they may have a problem to use free screenings, according to Schmidt. However, he strongly advises that once you have a symptom you should have a diagnostic mammogram, not a screening mammogram. The diagnostic mammogram often has additional mammogram views or involves ultrasound, and must be supervised by a radiologist. Furthermore, these special screenings are usually traveling resources. If you use a mammography center instead, you have the advantage of returning to the same center if you need follow-up imaging.

However, if you are uninsured and cannot afford a mammogram, taking advantage of these free mammograms is a good idea. But try to get a hold of a copy of the X-rays or remember where you had them for later comparisons.

Mistakes you can live with

Most breast cancers grow slowly. They probably grow for five to eight years before they're detectable in a self or clinical exam. Mammograms push that up a couple of years. If the radiologist detects a breast cancer at screening, don't panic.

The slow growth means you have probably detected it early, if you have been screened regularly. Furthermore, the odds are on your side, because there are expert radiologists out there. And if, after you turn 40, you get a routine screening mammogram, you'll increase your chances of detection.

In addition, nearly one third of the women screened during a 10-year period had at least one false positive mammogram or clinical breast examination, according to a study by researchers at the University of Washington and Harvard Medical School who were looking at the cumulative risk of a false positive result of a breast-cancer screening. The study results were published in the *New England Journal of Medicine* (April 1998).

The researchers performed a 10-year retrospective cohort study of breast-cancer screening and diagnostic evaluations of 2,400 women ages 40 to 69 at study entry. The women had a median of four mammograms and five clinical breast examinations during that time. Nearly a quarter of the women had at

Bright Idea
Because oversights occur in readings, be sure to get a mammogram routinely each year after age 40. Something that was missed previously may be found on the next reading.

Bright Idea
You can be more diligent about getting a mammogram each year if you make a set date to remind yourself to make an appointment. If you have e-mail access, the University of Pennsylvania's OncoLink pilot service will e-mail you a reminder. Learn more about this service at www.oncolink.upenn.edu.

least one false positive mammogram, and almost 14 percent had at least one false positive breast examination. The estimated cumulative risk of a false positive result after 10 mammograms was nearly 50 percent. (The estimated cumulative risk of a false positive result after 10 clinical breast examinations was slightly more than 22 percent. The false positive tests led to 539 diagnostic mammograms and 188 biopsies.

The researchers estimate that among women who do not have breast cancer, nearly 19 percent will undergo a biopsy after 10 mammograms, and slightly more than 6 percent will do so after 10 clinical breast examinations.

Overall, the investigators found that during the 10-year study period, one third of the women screened had abnormal test results (false positives), which required them to undergo additional evaluation.

The additional testing can be stressful, not to mention costly and time-consuming.

False positive readings are common. Keep this information in mind if you get a positive result. It may help you to feel less nervous, and, more importantly, to be more assertive about getting a second opinion.

MRI

When it comes to breast cancer, MRIs (magnetic resonance imaging) may help differentiate the number of lesions and determine if a mass is benign or malignant, they are not routinely used. Many physicians consider their use in breast cancer investigational.

MRIs can be an intimidating test to undergo. You are placed in a long tube, usually rather narrow and confining, leading many people to feel panicked. Many patients who have never experienced claustrophobia have difficulty during this test. If you think you may feel uncomfortable, ask your physician for a sedative to take before the test. Many MRI facilities also provide headphones hooked into local radio stations. Using music or talk radio as a distraction may be a great help. MRIs have loud banging and clicking sounds, as well. The headphones can be used to protect your ears. If you don't opt for the headphones, ask for ear plugs to protect your hearing.

There's good news, though. Special techniques and apparatus for breast imaging only are being developed.

More sophisticated screening on the horizon

In the future, computer technology will be used more and more to read mammograms. Research efforts are underway to improve conventional mammography, including the development of digital mammography with computer-assisted interpretation of digitized images. Digital mammography makes it possible for the radiologist to change image contrast and magnify specific areas of an image. Changing contrast allows the radiologist to see into denser areas of the breast. "A digital mammogram lets you get all the parts of the picture into perfect exposure, so you can avoid those ruinous white-outs and black-outs we are all familiar with in taking photographs of our friends and family," Schmidt says. Already computer-aided diagnostic (CAD) systems can detect between 80 to 85 percent of all cancers, which is similar to what you might expect from a very good or expert radiologist. But like people, they send false alarms and may miss occasional obvious cancers. Schmidt thinks that CAD may eventually be used for second opinions, which should increase the radiologist's accuracy about 10 to 15 percent on average, Schmidt says.

On the flip side, in order for digital mammogra-

phy to be more effective, radiologists need more training on these new pictures.

Thermal imaging

Thermal imaging, another technique, has been
around for at least 30 years. This technology, which
uses a heat map of the breasts to detect abnormalities, was first investigated in the 1960s, according to
Yuri Parisky, associate professor of radiology at the
University of Southern California School of
Medicine in Los Angeles. Because the technique was
rather crude at that time, and analysis was subjective,
it was ineffective. But recent technological advances
have renewed interest in thermal imaging. Thanks to
advances in military technology, thermal imaging
cameras are more sensitive now. And there's been
another technological advance: the subtle changes
in temperature are interpreted by computer using an
algorithm, a set of findings or characteristics determined to have a high yield in recognizing the cancer.
"These 'formulas' are then applied to the thermo-
gram of the patient's breast," Parisky explains. Breast
cancer cells have an increased metabolism. The
tumor also grows new blood vessel networks as it
grows. Both of these factors increase the heat the
cancer cells radiate. These improvements have
caught the attention of insurance companies and
physicians, who may move the technology back into
the mainstream of medicine. Since falling into disfa-
vor, thermal imaging had been used outside conventional medicine and therefore not covered under
insurance.

Thermal imaging is still not advanced enough to
use for detection alone. In fact, it will take exceptionally good data to persuade the medical community to reintroduce it because its results were so poor

in the 1960s. However, the goal of using this technology is to eliminate unnecessary biopsies. Only 20 to 25 percent of biopsies are malignant, so most women undergo unnecessary biopsy, according to Parisky.

Parisky and his colleagues conducted a trial on thermal imaging. In the first phase of the trial, which had about 100 women, Parisky and his co-investigators were able to detect 96 percent of the breast cancers. If the technique had been applied in the decision-making process, about 40 percent of the benign biopsies could have been avoided, Parisky says. The results of this study were published in the "Proceedings of the 20th Annual International Conference of the JEEE Engineering in Medicine and Biology Society" in November 1998.

(Note: Digital mammography with computer assisted interpretation and thermography as presented are investigational at present.)

Thermal breast imaging is a simple, noninvasive process. There's no compression or radiation involved. The woman lies on a table and a camera typically takes picture of her breast without contact. (Some technologies do contact the breast.)

Ultrasound imaging

Ultrasound is another type of breast cancer detection tool. It uses sound waves sent through the breast to identify masses. The sound waves are either reflected or transmitted, depending on the tissue characteristics. The physics used in ultrasound are similar to sonar used by submarines. It is not a good screening tool, but it is good for further evaluation of suspected abnormalities.

Ultrasound is a highly reliable tool used to distinguish between cysts (sacs filled with fluid, which usually are not malignant—only 1 to 2 percent of cysts contain cancerous cells) and solid masses, which can be benign or malignant. If the mass is determined to be a cyst, the patient can ignore it because it is not dangerous. But if it's painful, then it can be aspirated, Feig says. That process consists of withdrawing the fluid using a syringe. But there are instances when ultrasound cannot make the distinction between a cyst and a solid tumor. In those cases, a radiologist, using ultrasound guidance, aspirates the mass to determine if it's a cyst. (If the mass is palpable, a surgeon or your gynecologist can aspirate it.)

Ultrasound is not used for screening, although that use is currently under investigation, according to Feig. There's also ongoing research to determine if ultrasound can reliably distinguish between benign and malignant solid masses. (Neither ultrasound nor MRI can detect microcalcifications reliably, however.)

Unlike mammograms, with ultrasound there is no discomfort. Gel is rubbed on the breast and a handheld device containing the detection receiver and sound wave generator is placed on the breast. Sound waves are emitted from the detection device. The radiologist views the sound wave picture of the breast on a computer screen while the study is being performed. Films can then be taken of the images on the screen. The radiologist examines the pictures. If the radiologist thinks a mass might be malignant, a biopsy is performed.

Biopsy methods

A biopsy is a procedure used to get a tissue specimen that is then analyzed under a microscope to determine a precise diagnosis.

Many lumps are caused by hormonal fluctuations, not cancerous growths, so if you have a lump your doctor will consider the findings from your physical exam, mammogram reading, and medical history to determine if it needs to be biopsied or simply monitored for a month or a couple of months. If the lump is not palpable but something questionable is seen on your mammogram, your doctor may tell you to wait a few months and get another mammogram if the area in question does not appear to be cancerous.

If your doctor recommends waiting and you're uncomfortable with that, get a second opinion. If you're still not satisfied, request a biopsy.

There are several biopsy methods used, depending on the characteristics of the growth.

There are several different methods used to perform an image- guided biopsy. Most are based on the mammogram or ultrasound image.

- **Excisional biopsy**—For lesions (masses or calcifications) that cannot be detected by touch, that is, nonpalpable lesions, the radiologist, guided by mammography or ultrasound, places a needle into the breast to mark the affected area. Then the patient goes to the operating room where the surgeon removes the entire lesion. Once removed, the radiologist examines the specimen using X-ray technology to be sure the entire mass has been removed.

- **Core biopsy**—Using this biopsy method, the radiologist typically removes only a sample of the lesion. It is done with either ultrasound or mammogram guidance, and is a less invasive procedure than an incisional biopsy.

- **Fine needle aspiration (FNA)**—Using this biopsy procedure, a thin needle is placed into the lesion. Cells are aspirated and sent to a pathologist who is also a cytopathologist, a pathologist

Unofficially...
Cytology is reliable in determining if a biopsy contains cancer. It cannot determine invasion or infiltration of cancer cells. Histology, in which the pathologist examines the tissues, is used for that. Whereas cytology looks only at cells, histology looks at the surrounding tissues and architecture. Usually, a fine needle aspiration is used for cytology and a core needle biopsy for histology.

trained to interpret the cells in the sample.

- ▪ *Stereotactic biopsy*—Using this biopsy method, tissue samples are removed from the breast using a hollow needle that is guided to the suspicious location via mammography and computer coordinates.

- ▪ *Incisional biopsy*—Used for larger palpable lesions, the surgeon excises a part of the mass for biopsy. This type of biopsy procedure is less common now that mammography screening helps detect growths long before they are large enough to mandate this method. Because such lesions are palpable, image guidance is not necessary.

Once the report of your biopsy is in, ask your doctor to explain it. If the biopsy is positive, keep in mind the following questions when he or she is going over the report:

- ▪ What type of breast cancer is it?

- ▪ What stage is the disease in?

- ▪ Is the pathologist who made the diagnosis experienced in diagnosing breast cancer?

- ▪ Is the tumor estrogen and progesterone receptor positive? (Hormone receptor status determines treatment choices and often indicates the prognosis.)

- ▪ Does the tumor have HER-2/neu antibodies? (Antibodies are used to detect the presence of the over-expression of the HER-2/neu oncogene. Over-expression of HER-2/neu would indicate the tumor may respond well to a new drug called Herceptin currently being tested in clinical trials.)

- ▪ What other tests do I need, if any?

- ▪ What are my treatment choices and where can I

get more information on them?

- What benefit can I expect from each kind of treatment?

- What are the possible side effects that I may experience from the treatments?

- What side effects should prompt me to call you?

- Who takes calls after-hours?

- What are the short- and long-term risks?

- What are the risks of not getting treatment?

- What are the chances of recurrence?

- What are the symptoms of recurrence?

- What is the prognosis?

The role of the pathologist

The pathologist is a behind-the-scenes member of the medical team. The role of the pathologist is to look at the tissue under the microscope and make a diagnosis. The most important thing the pathologist must determine is whether the cells are benign (not cancerous) or malignant (cancerous), says Susan Tannenbaum, M.D., a fellow with the College of American Pathologists and a pathologist at United Pathology Associates, in Port Chester, New York.

If the biopsy is totally benign, nothing further is done. If the growth is suspicious, and the first biopsy was performed by needle aspiration of the tissue, then an additional biopsy, sometimes a surgical biopsy, is done. To make sure the entire cancerous area is removed or treated, the pathologist uses permanent ink to color the outside of the tumor after it is removed. This is referred to as *surgical margins*. The tumor is cut into thin slices and placed under a microscope. If the pathologists sees cancer in the middle of the growth but not on the perimeter, then

Unofficially...
Positive margins are a marker of increased risk of disease recurrence in the breast following lumpectomy for invasive breast cancer. Nearly all surgeons would re-excise and try to have negative margins. Positive margins in the context of mastectomy require irradiation for local control of disease.

he or she can be sure the entire tumor was excised. But if cancer is detected up against the ink, a second surgery must be done to remove the rest of the cancerous tissues.

Under a microscope, the pathologist can identify characteristics of the tumor cells, which determine the diagnosis, the need for treatment, and the prognosis.

Tumor grade

Tumor grade is a classification system used to describe the degree of differentiation—the degree of abnormality of cancer cells in both appearance and function, compared with normal cells of the same type of tissue—which often relates to how the tumor behaves (aggressive versus nonaggressive). Well-differentiated cells look similar to healthy cells. The opposite is also true. Poorly differentiated cells (cancerous cells) look quite different from the healthy cells from which they were created through mutation.

Grades are measured* by four degrees of severity:

1. G1 is well-differentiated and considered low grade, that is (typically) nonaggressive.

2. G2 is moderately well-differentiated and is considered intermediate grade.

3. G3 is poorly differentiated and is high grade, that is (generally) aggressive.

4. G4 is undifferentiated and is high grade, that is (generally) aggressive.

(Note: GX is an undetermined grade and is reserved for those cells that cannot be assessed.)

Aggressive tumors have a lot of mitotic activity. This means that cells are continually multiplying,

Unofficially...
Tumor type, in situ or invasive, vascular or lymphatic invasion, histologic differentiation, and nuclear grade are all important in determining diagnosis and treatment.

*Measurements were established by the American Joint Commission on Cancer.

causing the tumor to grow rapidly (though not overnight).

Note: Grade does not fit atypia, described in the next section, and is just being incorporated into ductal carcinoma in situ (DCIS).

Atypia

Not all growths are cancerous and not all growths are clearly benign. Some waver on the border—a gray area of atypia, or atypical growth. They're not cancerous but could become cancer, Tannenbaum says. These growths serve as markers of increased risk of subsequent breast cancer. This type of cell formation can remain stable or, if hormonal stimulation is reduced, "some of these growth patterns could subside," she says. "[Atypia] gets into the art of medicine as opposed to the science," Tannenbaum explains, so these premalignant growths must be monitored with self and clinical exams, mammography, or ultrasound, especially if you have a personal or family history of breast cancer.

Atypia is important because if detected on biopsy, it increases the risk of a subsequent cancer diagnosis. Atypia plus cellular hyperplasia, although not cancer, further increases the risk of subsequent cancer diagnosis.

Lymph node status

If the biopsy indicates that the tumor is an invasive type of cancer, and the malignant cells are pushing along the edges of the ink, the cancer is no longer classified as in situ. (In situ does not spread—it does not go into the fatty and support tissues of the breast. Invasive does and therefore can spread.) In this case, the lymph nodes must be checked to see if the cancer has spread to the lymphatic system or beyond. When malignant cells break away from the primary tumor, they can travel through the blood vessels or lymphatic system, which is similar to the circulatory system in that it carries a fluid throughout the body. (In fact, sometimes cancerous cells can be seen in breast, blood, and lymph vessels.)

If tumor cells are present in the lymphatic system, the woman has an increased risk of subsequent distant metastases—breast cancer cells found in sites far from the breast such as the liver, bone, lungs or other secondary sites—and an increased risk of a local recurrence for those women treated with breast conservation therapy, such as a lumpectomy. The pathologist must determine if the cancer has spread to the axillary lymph nodes in order to make a prognosis and determine treatment options.

To determine if cancer has spread, that is, if there is axillary lymph node involvement, and to determine the postoperative treatment, typically 10 to 30 lymph nodes must be surgically removed to look for malignant cells. But in an estimated 70 percent of cases, there is no spread of the disease to the lymph nodes. Though sometimes necessary, removing as many as 30 lymph nodes has several, sometimes severe, consequences:

- Numbness in the arm due to the surgery cutting through the nerves to the skin

- Permanent swelling in the upper arm (lymphedema) (This can lead to infection in the affected limb.)

- Decreased shoulder movement

There is hope on the horizon for better lymph diagnosis, however. Another method called sentinel lymph node dissection (SLND) is being employed by more and more surgeons. It is a relatively new diagnostic procedure being used by some highly trained surgeons to detect whether an invasive type of cancer has spread to the lymph nodes. The procedure was developed in 1993 at the John Wayne Cancer Institute in Los Angeles by Armando Giuliano, M.D.

Compared with multiple lymph node removal, SLND is

- Less invasive

- Less painful

- Less tiring, that is, less time is needed for recovery

Unofficially...
There have been no randomized, comparative long-term studies comparing risks and benefits of sentinel node biopsies and complete axillary lymph node biopsy.

While breast cancer diagnosis and treatment have become less radical, more accurate, and more efficient over the years, the same has not been true for lymph node removal. In fact, SLND is the first advancement in lymph node removal since 1900. SLND has fewer long-term side effects compared with complete axillary lymph node removal and does not necessitate an overnight stay in the hospital as does complete axillary lymph node removal. "Less is more here," Tannenbaum says.

In performing SLND, a nuclear mapping system, the surgeon injects a radioactive "tracer" and/or a blue dye into the area around the tumor. This provides the surgeon with both visual (via the dye) and aural (via a hand-held gamma detecting probe similar to a Geiger counter) cues. The added fluids drain into the lymphatic system, and within 10 minutes the surgeon can determine which lymph node the dye enters first (the node the cancer, too, would enter first). This is the sentinel node. Compared with the conventional method of assessing the 10 to 30 nodes, the evaluation of this single node (sometimes two or three) is more thorough and therefore more accurate. It provides more information with less invasion.

There is a high learning curve involved with this

technique and some surgeons are reportedly using SLND without enough training, possibly putting their patients in danger of receiving false negative results. How do you make sure your surgeon is highly trained? Edward Clifford, M.D., chief of the general surgery section at St. Paul Medical Center in Dallas, Texas, and clinical assistant professor of surgery at the University of Texas Southwestern Medical School, says there's no national credentialing process. He suggests asking your surgeon the following questions:

- How many SLNDs have you performed (not assisted in)? (The American College of Surgeons recommends 30 procedures.)

- What is your identification rate? The identification rate, also called a "find rate," (finding the sentinel node) needs to be high. A generally accepted identification rate is anything greater than 90 percent.

- What is your rate of accuracy? More important than the identification rate is the rate of accuracy, the percentage of time the surgeon correctly determines if cancer cells are present and makes an accurate prediction of further node involvement. A generally accepted rate of accuracy is greater than 90 percent.

There are other components in which surgeons must gain skill in order to perform SLNDs with a high degree of accuracy. They must have a thorough understanding of the kinetics of the radiopharmaceuticals or other tracers. They also must be well trained in the use of the detection device used. Furthermore, the nuclear medicine physicians and pathologists the surgeon works with must also have a thorough understanding of tracers and the detection device.

The biggest benefit to this procedure, as noted earlier, is that lymph nodes are not excised unnecessarily. But if cancer is found in the sentinel node, then other nodes must be removed to determine the extent of the spread. The total number of lymph nodes containing tumor cells help to determine treatment options. Stratification is based on the following:

1. No tumor cells are detected in the nodes

2. Between one and three nodes are affected

3. Between four and nine nodes are affected

4. More than 10 nodes are affected

The pathologist also notes whether cancerous cells are present in the fibrous-fatty tissue surrounding the lymph nodes or if multiple lymph nodes are matted together by the cancer.

Back at the lab

Much of the pathologist's role takes place in the laboratory. The surgical margins are marked on the excised mass and the tissue is thinly sliced.

Sections are stained with eosin and hematoxylin, dyes that color the cell's nucleus (the center of the cell) blue and its cytoplasm (the section surrounding the nucleus where most chemical activities take place) pink. Additional staining is used to obtain information on specific cellular elements, like hormone receptor status (discussed in the next section).

Flow cytometry, which detects light absorbing or fluorescing properties of cells or components of cells (chromosomes) passing in a narrow stream through a laser beam, is used to determine the rate of tumor cell growth and the amount of nuclear DNA. This information helps the pathologists make a prognosis

Watch Out!
Sentinel lymph node biopsy is not a choice for women who have had an excisional biopsy for diagnosis. The tumor must be in place to determine the lymphatic drainage pattern.

and determine treatment options.

Receptor and oncogene status

When a biopsy is positive (shows cancer), the pathologist uses molecular biology techniques to determine hormone receptor status. This means that the pathologist looks for markers for estrogen and progesterone, and HER-2/neu antibodies. (Antibodies are used to detect the presence of estrogen receptors and progesterone receptors and overexpression of the HER-2/neu oncogene on and within the cancer cells.) The process, called *immunohistochemical staining*, is achieved by using an antibody, which is hooked in a molecular fashion to a brown dye. Positive receptors will be activated and light up a certain color under the microscope as a result. If no color is present, the cell is negative for hormone receptors. It measures the degree of dependency the cancer cells have on the hormones estrogen and progesterone for growth. Receptor studies are done to individualize therapy, Tannenbaum explains. If there is a receptor present on the cell, the cancer may be susceptible to certain therapies.

Profile summary

If the pathologist has determined that a tumor is indeed cancerous, then a profile of the tumor is developed to determine treatment. A profile includes the following tumor characteristics:

- Invasive/noninvasive

- Aggressive/nonaggressive

- Lymph node involvement/no lymph node involvement

- Markers present/no markers present for estrogen, progesterone, and HER-2/neu.

- Size

66

I would like to encourage women to understand what all these technical terms mean. Don't be afraid to ask questions. The more you know, the more you can take care of yourself, and the better fight you can put up.
—Susan Tannenbaum, M.D., a fellow with the College of American Pathologists and a pathologist at United Pathology Associates, in Port Chester, New York.

99

Tumor size

Part of a properly completed report includes the size of the tumor, which can range from microscopic to several centimeters.

Size is not always the determining factor as to whether a surgeon decides to perform a needle biopsy or excises the area surrounding the tumor. "The technique of fine needle aspiration is used for a variety of reasons—not necessarily because a mass is too small to be biopsied," Tannenbaum explains. Both large and small masses are "needled." For example, a large fibroadenoma, a benign mass, may easily be felt by the patient. A surgeon may perform a needle biopsy to confirm that it's benign to reassure the patient, she says.

But when a mass shows up as calcium flecks on a mammogram, a golf ball size area (or smaller) of tissue containing the calcium is removed by biopsy. Both the surgeon and pathologist, using an X-ray of the removed tissue, make sure that the calcium has been removed from the patient and is present in the biopsied tissue. "Once the calcium has been identified in the specimen, the tissue is then fixed and sectioned into 20 or perhaps even 30 thin pieces [placed on 20 to 30 glass slides]," Tannebaum says. "If the calcified area turns out to be a tumor under the microscope—a microscopic tumor—the pathologist will measure the size of the tumor right from the glass slide, using a ruler, or under the microscope, using a micrometer," Tannenbaum explains. (The size of the specimen on the slide is the size of the cancer.) Such tumors are typically about 1/2 centimeter in size, or possibly less, sometimes more," she says. (A centimeter is about a half inch.)

But some tumors, as noted in Chapter 1, are in

Bright Idea
You can contact the pathologist if you have questions. If you want a second opinion, the pathologist will cut additional sections from the biopsy tissue, place them on slides, and give them to you to take to another pathologist.

situ (noninvasive) and others are a combination of in situ and infiltrating. In these cases, an estimate of the extent of the invasive tumor is measured. Those with small numbers of invasive cells (microinvasive) are described and measured on a glass microscope slide. The size and invasiveness, if any, plays a role in the prognosis and therapy.

Tumor type

There are two main tumor type classifications for breast cancers: ductal and lobular. Ductal carcinoma, found in the cells of the lining of a milk duct, is the most common type of breast cancer. There are several types, some of which can become invasive and some that almost never become invasive.

Lobular cancer begins in the lining of milk lobes or lobules. Lobular carcinoma in situ is not considered an actual breast cancer at this noninvasive stage. But it is considered a warning sign: Women with LCIS have a 25 percent chance of developing breast cancer in either breast over the next 25 years.

Both ductal and lobular cancer can become invasive, spreading beyond the tissue from which it originated. A noninvasive ductal carcinoma is considered to be pre-invasive. Left in place it could spread, so it's surgically removed. Lobular carcinoma in situ, while not considered pre-invasive and therefore not removed, is considered a strong predictor of future new breast cancer in either breast. Sometimes there are overlaps between these two types of cancers.

The two most common types of invasive tumors are *infiltrating mammary duct carcinoma* and *infiltrating lobular carcinoma.*

Most breast cancers are infiltrating ductal carcinomas. These tumors feel like stones (although they are not always palpable) and frequently metastasize

> 66
> To be sure you have a correct diagnosis [of] breast cancer in situ, an experienced pathologist should examine your biopsy slides. You may [also] want to have your slides examined by a second pathologist at a university hospital, cancer center, or breast clinic. This is important because it is sometimes difficult to make an accurate diagnosis.
> —National Cancer Institute, *"Understandng Breast Cancer Treatment"*
> 99

TABLE 6.1 STAGING—SPECIFIC PATTERNS OF BREAST CANCER

Stage 0 Very early breast cancer. This type of cancer has not spread within or outside the breast. It can be DCIS (ductal carcinoma in situ or intraductal carcinoma) or LCIS (lobular carcinoma in situ), though LCIS is not a true cancer, breast cancer in situ, or noninvasive cancer.

Stage I The cancer is no larger than about 1 inch (2 centimeters) in size and has not spread outside the breast. (Also described as early breast cancer.)

Stage II The doctor may find any of the following:

The cancer is no larger than 1 inch, but has spread to the lymph nodes under the arm.

The cancer is between 1 and 2 inches. It may or may not have spread to the lymph nodes under the arm.

The cancer is larger than 2 inches, but has not spread to the lymph nodes under the arm.

Stage III Stage III is divided into stages IIIA and IIIB.

Stage IIIA The doctor may find either of the following:

The cancer is smaller than 2 inches and has spread to the lymph nodes under the arm. The cancer is also spreading to other lymph nodes.

The cancer is larger than 2 inches and has spread to the lymph nodes under the arm.

Stage IIIB The doctor may find either of the following:

The cancer has spread to tissues near the breast (skin or chest wall, including the ribs and the muscles in the chest).

The cancer has spread to lymph nodes inside the chest wall along the breast bone.

Stage IV The cancer has spread to other parts of the body, most often the bones, lungs, liver, or brain. Or, the tumor has spread locally to the skin and lymph nodes inside the neck, near the collarbone.

Inflammatory Breast Cancer Inflammatory breast cancer is a rare, but very serious, aggressive type of breast cancer. The breast may look red and feel warm and swollen. You may see ridges, welts, or hives on your breast; or the skin may look wrinkled. It is sometimes misdiagnosed as a simple infection.

Recurrent Breast Cancer Recurrent disease means that the cancer has come back (recurred) after it has been treated. It may come back in the breast, in the soft tissues of the chest (the chest wall), the lymph nodes in the area, or in another part of the body.

Note: Tumor size is usually reported in metric measurement: 1 centimeter = approximately 1/2 inch.

Source: National Cancer Institute with additions from the Unofficial Guide Panel of Experts

Unofficially...
Cancer confined to the breast is localized. If the cancer cells have spread outside the tumor but are still contained in the area, the cancer is invasive. If the spread is to a distant site, it's metastatic.

(spread to the lymph system and to other parts of the body through the blood or lymph). Infiltrating lobular carcinoma also metastasizes. Tumor types are covered in more detail in Chapter 1.

Stage

The extent to which the disease has progressed, and the extent of lymph node involvement determines the cancer stage. Stage is another diagnostic and prognostic factor used to determine treatment options. (Table 6.1 gives a breakdown of the stages of breast cancer.)

Just the facts

- By far, most breast cancers are detected by women themselves.

- Mammographies and breast exams should be part of your routine.

- Not all radiologists are equally skilled at reading mammographies.

- There many biopsy methods, some that don't require surgery.

- Understanding the role of the pathologist can help you better understand your diagnosis.

Standard Treatment Methods

GET THE SCOOP ON...
How cancer is treated ▪ Why chemotherapy
is given to so many women with breast cancer ▪
Treatment protocols for different stages of
disease ▪ Why there's so much hope for a cure

PART IV

Choosing a Treatment Method

Once diagnosed with breast cancer, you only have about two short weeks before starting treatment, although you can request a couple more. Either way, that's not a lot of time to learn about your diagnosis and treatment options.

In this chapter, we'll give you an overview of treatment options and break them down by stage of disease. We'll also provide you with questions you should ask your physician.

The lowdown on treating breast cancer

There are three primary, conventional treatments breast cancer patients can receive: surgery, radiation therapy, and systemic therapy. (See Table 7.1 to see how they work.) Hormone therapy can use drugs to change the way hormones work (remember, some hormones promote tumor growth) or it can mean surgically removing the ovaries, where the sex hormones are made. (Hormone therapy will be discussed in more detail in Chapter 10.) Still in the experimental stages, and still controversial, is high-

173

TABLE 7.1 TREATMENT METHODS

There are four primary treatments for breast cancer.

Localized treatments

- Surgery
- Radiation therapy

Systemic treatments

- Chemotherapy
- Hormone therapy

Localized treatments remove or destroy the cancer cells in a small area. Systemic treatments destroy cancer cells throughout the body.

dose chemotherapy supported by peripheral blood stem cell transplantation and sometimes bone marrow transplantation, which are discussed in Chapter 9.

There are additional treatments for breast cancer. Scientists are experimenting with boosting the body's immune system, so it can fight off the cancer in a non-toxic way, though the therapy may not always be nontoxic. This is called biological therapy. Biological and other experimental treatments will be discussed in Chapter 10.

Removing tumors

Once you've been diagnosed with a breast tumor, it must come out, which means you have to make a major decision about the type of surgery you want to undergo. There are two primary surgical options: lumpectomy or mastectomy. If you choose a mastectomy, then you must consider which type: a simple mastectomy, modified mastectomy, or radical mastectomy. If you choose any type of mastectomy, you also must consider if you want reconstructive surgery, and, if so, if you want to schedule it at the time of the mastectomy or at a later date.

The diagnosis of breast cancer typically is not an

Unofficially...
Localized breast cancer does not kill. It's the spread of the cancer that has the potential to be fatal. Therefore, surgery, radiation, and systemic therapy are important treatments that reduce the chance of metastases.

emergency situation. Treatments usually begin several weeks after being diagnosed. Many women use this time to explore their options and to deal with the impact of the diagnosis.

Not all patients undergo surgery as their initial therapy. Many patients have preoperative chemotherapy to shrink their tumor prior to surgery.

After the surgery, many women are able to resume most normal activities within two or three weeks. All activities typically can be resumed just six weeks after surgery.

There are several types of breast surgery, as noted earlier. (They will be discussed in more detail later in this chapter.) Which technique is recommended for your situation depends on prognostic indicators, such as the stage of disease and the tumor characteristics (Ultimately, however, the type of surgery is your choice.) More specifically, prognostic indicators include the following:

- *Tumor size*—Generally, the smaller the tumor, the better the prognosis.

- *Hormone receptors*—All breast cells contain receptors for estrogen and progesterone. When there are significant levels of these receptors, tumors are considered estrogen receptor positive (ER+) and/or progesterone receptor positive (PR+). More than half of all breast cancer tumors are ER+ and more than half of those tumors are PR+. Receptor positive tumors tend to be less aggressive, and therefore offer a better prognosis. They also respond better than receptor negative tumors to hormone therapy.

- *Proliferative capacity of the tumor*—This refers to how fast the tumor cells are dividing and correlates with the aggressiveness of the tumor.

Unofficially...
During surgery, drainage tubes are inserted into the wound to drain body fluids that accumulate after surgery. They are removed several weeks after surgery.

- ***Oncogene expression and amplification***—Tumor cells that contain certain oncogenes may have a higher chance of recurrence. Oncogenes are genes that, when activated, cause or promote unchecked cell growth. Tests for oncogenes are experimental and not widely available. However, HER-2/neu testing is being performed more readily now. Metastatic tumors found to have an overexpression of the HER-2/neu gene are often treated with Herceptin.

- ***Lymph node involvement***—If the lymph nodes are found to contain cancer cells (determined through a biopsy)—referred to as lymph node-positive—the cancer has spread to the area around the breast. A positive nodal status is associated with a higher likelihood of recurrence, either locally or distantly (metastases). Lymph node involvement is the most important factor for prognosis because it tells if the cancer has spread.

Unofficially...
Histologic grade looks at the cell as a whole while nuclear grade looks at the nucleus.

- ***Histologic grade***—Grade 1 tumor cells appear very similar to normal cells under the microscope. Grade 4 tumor cells are highly undifferentiated, that is, they grow very rapidly and hence bear little resemblance to the normal cells from which they derived.

- ***Nuclear grade***—Nuclear grading is a cytologic evaluation of the structural features of the cell nucleus; that is, tumor cells are compared with what's normal and graded according to how closely they resemble normal cells. "Nuclear grading is an attempt to semi-quantitate the degree of aggressiveness of a tumor by grading nuclear abnormality on a scale of 1 to 3," explains Susan Tannenbaum, M.D., a fellow with the College of

American Pathologists and a pathologist at United Pathology Associates, in Port Chester, New York. "A grade of 1 means that the nuclei of the cells in a tumor are 'not very abnormal,' or that they appear not too unusual with regard to density, shape, size, irregularity, etc. A grade of 3 means that the features of the nucleus are markedly abnormal, with regard to the appearances [just] listed. Nuclear features in a grade 3 or high grade tumor are often described as 'bizarre,' in that they deviate markedly from normal appearances. A grade of 2 is intermediate. These changes correlate reasonably well with tests used to determine the DNA content of a tumor. That is, if the DNA amount, or the number of chromosomes in a cell—called ploidy—is normal, the cell is most likely to be grade 1. A cell with a very high and random amount of DNA (number of chromosomes) is usually a grade 3. Higher grade nuclear changes correlate with the aggressiveness of a tumor," she explains.

- *Mitotic index*—A third criterion used in grading a tumor. It is an estimate of the number of cells undergoing division in the tumor. With a low score of 1+1+1=3 and a high score of 3+3+3=9, tumors are graded on a scale of 3 to 9—3 is low-grade (least aggressive) and 9 is high grade (most aggressive), Tannenbaum explains.

Lumpectomy

A lumpectomy, which is sometimes called an excisional biopsy or segmental resection, is a breast-conserving surgery. Rather than remove the whole breast, as is done in a mastectomy, only the tumor (the "lump") and the surrounding tissue are removed in a lumpectomy. A lumpectomy leaves much of the breast, the

Watch Out!
One study suggests that women who have breast tumors removed during days three to twelve of their menstrual cycle (the follicular phase) have a poorer prognosis than those operated on during the luteal phase (days zero to two and 13 to 32). Other researchers have questioned the validity of this study, however.

Unofficially...
A scar in the vertical location or through a circumareolar approach may preclude a lumpectomy and make the best surgical choice a mastectomy with reconstruction.

nipple, and areola intact. (Many doctors also remove some of the lymph nodes under the arm, if the cancer is invasive.) This type of surgery is followed by radiation therapy to reduce the risk of recurrence due to the possibility that some cancer cells were not removed by the lumpectomy despite clear margins. Women who don't undergo radiation therapy have up to a 40 percent increased risk of recurrence in the breast.

Typically, radiation therapy takes place a few weeks after the surgery, giving the surgical wound time to heal. Some women also undergo chemotherapy. In that case, chemotherapy is usually started before radiation.

Women in the early stages (stage I and stage II, defined later in this chapter) of breast cancer who have a lumpectomy plus radiation have the same survival rates as those who have had a modified radical mastectomy.

Women who have multiple tumors or are pregnant are not good candidates for a lumpectomy, unless the delivery date is fairly soon, so that radiotherapy (radiation therapy) can be delayed until after delivery.

Mastectomy

Mastectomies are generally recommended when there are multiple tumors in the breast, when the tumor is fairly large in relation to the size of the breast, or when the breast is small or misshapen, making the cosmetic results of a lumpectomy undesirable.

There are three primary types of mastectomy:

Timesaver
Wear clothes that are easy to get in and out of when you go for radiation treatments. This will save you time and energy.

1. *Simple mastectomy*—Removal of the breast only.

2. *Modified radical mastectomy*—Removal of the breast and some axillary lymph nodes. This is the most common type of mastectomy.

3. *Radical mastectomy*—Removal of the breast, chest wall muscle (pectorals), and lymph nodes. This surgery is rarely done now.

Conservation surgery (lumpectomy) has reduced the number of all types of mastectomies.

If you must have a mastectomy, and opt for breast reconstruction, that surgery can often take place at the same time. Breast reconstruction can either be done using an implant or your own tissue. For more information on breast reconstruction, see chapter 15.

Radiation therapy may be used after a mastectomy if the tumor is larger than 2 inches, if cancer cells are found in multiple axillary lymph nodes, or if the tumor is near your rib cage or chest wall muscles.

Modified radical and simple mastectomies have the same survival rate.

Don't just do it

Before agreeing to surgery, consider asking your doctor the following questions:

- Why are you recommending this type of surgery for me?

- What will my breast/chest look like after surgery?

- Where will the scars be?

- What should I do to prepare for surgery?

- How many of these surgeries do you perform per year?

- What type of follow-up care will I need?

Destroying cancer with radiation therapy

We're often told to stay away from radiation because it can cause cancer. For instance, we're told not to sit too close to the television and not to get unnecessary

Watch Out!
There's an increased risk of some surgery-related complications in a small percentage of women who undergo outpatient mastectomies compared with those who have a one-day hospital stay, according to research published in the *Journal of the National Cancer Institute* (June 1998). Complications include wound infection and blood clots.

Unofficially...
Second opinions can be helpful in the decision-making process and should be encouraged by your physician.

X-rays at the dentist's office. Ironically, radiation that comes from high-energy X-rays can be used to kill cancer cells.

Radiation therapy (radiotherapy) can be administered in two ways: externally or internally. Using external radiation, the X-rays are zapped from a machine, through the skin, and into the tumor or the isolated cancer cells. If it is administered internally, radioactive isotopes are placed inside the body through thin plastic tubes to emit radiation into an isolated area.

Moneysaver
Make sure you get a referral for treatment from your primary physician, if necessary, and complete any necessary paperwork for your insurance provider ahead of time. Otherwise, your provider may not cover your treatment.

Radiation may be administered, sometimes along with chemotherapy or hormone therapy, before surgery in cases where the tumor is too large to be surgically removed or when removal is difficult. The goal of radiation therapy and chemotherapy in these circumstances is to shrink the tumor so it can be surgically excised.

Radiation therapy is sometimes used after surgery to destroy cancer cells that may have spread to nearby parts of the body. Radiation therapy is always given after lumpectomy as part of the primary treatment. It is also given for tumors greater than 5 centimeters, matted lymph nodes, and almost always when a woman has four or more positive lymph nodes.

When external radiation therapy is used as adjuvant therapy following breast-sparing surgery, the treatments are given five days a week for five to six weeks. Sometimes an extra "booster" (an additional dose to the tumor bed, the area that remains after the primary tumor is removed) is given at the end of the treatment. The booster can be either external or internal, using an implant. If an implant is used, you will have a short stay in the hospital.

What's the process? Your first appointment will be

used for planning the radiation therapy. Your chest will be marked with a long-lasting ink to mark exactly where the X-rays will be targeted. The exact treatment plan will be based on the following:

- Mammograms
- Pathology and lab reports, including the size of the tumor
- The surgical procedure
- A physical exam
- Your medical history

(During treatment you will undergo regular physical exams and blood tests.)

Before starting the treatment, you may want to consider asking your radiation oncologists the following questions:

- Who will be administering the actual radiation treatment? (The machines are operated by radiation therapy technicians. Make sure he or she is board certified. In the case of an implant(s), a radiation oncologist should deliver the treatment.)

- How long will each treatment take? Will I be able to drive myself home or to work after treatment?

- What can I expect during each treatment?

- What can I expect after each treatment?

- How do I wash and protect the treated area?

- What side effects should I expect? Which ones should I report to you? What phone number should I call?

- How will I know that the treatment is working?

- What will my breast look and feel like after the treatment is completed?

Watch Out!
Radiation treatment may cause fatigue, skin irritation (itchiness, redness, soreness, and peeling) and skin alterations (darkening or shininess of the skin) and decreased sensation in the breast. Down the road, it may cause changes in the shape and color of the breast and leave a feeling of heaviness in the affected breast. Possible long-term adverse effects include rib fractures, lung scarring, and lymphedema.

Destroying cancer with toxic drugs

Even when breast cancer is in its early stages, cancer cells sometimes break away from the primary site. Because the cells are microscopic, there is currently no way for the surgeon or pathologist to determine if this has happened. Chemotherapy, the use of drugs to kill cancer cells, is therefore generally administered after surgery. Unlike surgery and radiation therapy, which work at the site of the tumor, chemotherapy is a systemic treatment—it covers the entire body. It kills cells that have traveled away from the local site.

Watch Out!
Chemotherapy takes a temporary toll on the immune system, so you will be more vulnerable to infections.

Chemotherapy used for breast cancer is generally a combination of drugs. They are given orally or by injection in a series of cycles—a treatment period followed by a period for recovery. Generally healthy patients receive chemotherapy as an outpatient, or even at home.

It works

Adjuvant chemotherapy may be difficult to stomach, so to speak, but it works. Journal article after journal article report promising findings. What follow are a couple of the more recent reports.

Investigators in England found that treating breast cancer with chemotherapy improves long-term survival, even in women whose cancer had not spread to the lymph nodes. Why? Because even after the tumor is successfully removed by surgery, breast cancer cells can remain undetected in the body. The chemotherapy works systemically to kill any microscopic cancer cells that may have traveled from the primary tumor through channels other than the lymph system.

Reporting their findings in *The Lancet* (September 1998), the researchers said after three to six months of adjuvant combination chemotherapy with CMF (cyclophosphamide, methotrexate, and fluorouracil) or an anthracycline-containing regimen, they typically saw an improvement of about 7 to 11 percent in 10-year survival for women under 50 when diagnosed with early breast cancer, and improvement of about 2 to 3 percent for women aged 50 to 69 "unless their prognosis is likely to be extremely good even without such treatment." Longer durations of chemotherapy did not indicate a survival advantage. The researchers also noted a 20 percent reduction in contralateral breast cancer (when the second breast develops a primary tumor). The women in these studies were both node-positive and node-negative.

While 2 to 3 percent may not sound like a big survival advantage, consider this: If 100,000 women have breast cancer and undergo chemotherapy, an additional 200 to 300 women will survive. As the percentage rises, so does the number of saved lives. Furthermore, women at high risk of breast cancer recurrence receive greater benefit statistically. (The increased chance of receiving benefit applies to the population as a whole. It is not possible to predict outcome for individuals.) So for some risk categories 2 to 3 per 100 women will be cured and for others a larger percentage.

The overall decrease in risk of death from breast cancer for all treated populations is about 32 percent +/-9 percent. Thus, for a risk of 5 percent recurrence and death, a 32 percent risk reduction would be a 1.6 percent benefit (32 X .05 = 1.6 percent). For a risk of 90 percent of recurrence and death, this same risk reduction would provide a 28.8 percent benefit (32 X .9 = 28.8 percent).

For some women, therefore, the cure rate is very

Watch Out!
If you don't experience side effects, don't think the chemotherapy isn't working. Some women don't have any. Also, better drugs to control side effects have become available in recent years, so chemotherapy has become easier to tolerate.

high and adjuvant therapy adds little benefit while for others the benefit is substantial.

Controversial role of lymph nodes

Some women who have small tumors, which are typically associated with localized disease, still end up with metastatic cancer, Clifford Hudis, M.D., chief of the Breast Cancer Medicine Service at Memorial Sloan-Kettering in New York, points out. Science does not have an accurate test to determine how an individual's cancer spreads. Does it spread first to the lymph nodes? Or does it spread through other channels? We do not have the tools to answer these questions yet, Hudis says.

Most women with small cancers don't have lymph node involvement. Removal of the lymph nodes increases the risk of other side effects, like lymphedema (severe swelling in the arm caused by the build up of lymph fluid) and cellulitis (an infection in the arm), Hudis points out.

Unofficially...
It is important
to balance risk
reduction and
benefit with
potential
toxicities.

Increasingly, knowing the status of axillary lymph nodes is not very critical in making treatment decisions. In a patient with a clinically negative axilla, one of the main reasons a node dissection is done is that the patient herself wants the prognostic information.

A solution, Hudis says, might be to test the sentinel nodes, those nodes the lymph flows to first, and use them as a guide to see if other nodes are affected. A sentinel node biopsy (also called sentinel lymph node dissection or SLND, discussed in Chapter 6) uses radioactivity or a dye to identify which specific nodes are the first stop from the site of the tumor. These nodes are then analyzed for cancer cells. If the sentinel nodes are negative, the surgeon doesn't have to do axillary dissection, saving the woman from further complications. This approach is now being broadly tested and could become standard in many communities over the next several years.

The procedure is most successful when done by an experienced surgeon. The American College of Surgeons recommends using a surgeon who has successfully completed at least 30 sentinel node biopsies. The surgeon should also have a "find rate," (finding the sentinel node) of greater than 90 percent and a high degree of accuracy, the percentage of time the surgeon correctly determines if cancer cells are present and accurately predicts further node involvement. A generally accepted rate of accuracy is greater than 90 percent.

But lymph node status—whether or not the cancer has spread into the lymph nodes—is not so important anymore in terms of treatment because adjuvant treatment for most breast cancers has become standard practice, Hudis says.

For individual women there is no way to tell whether or not they are in the group that would benefit from chemotherapy or if they have been cured by the surgery because currently there is no way to determine if any cancerous cells have escaped the local site through means other than the lymph.

Better safe than sorry

In comparison to most things in oncology, there are no guideposts for adjuvant chemotherapy. We don't know who's cured by surgery and who needs follow up with adjuvant chemotherapy, or if it's working for an individual woman, Hudis says, adding that it's frustrating for both patients and scientists.

But chemotherapy is not based on guesswork. "What we have is group answers," Hudis explains. It's similar to wearing a seatbelt, he says. We know they save many lives, but we don't know in advance who's

Unofficially...
Chemotherapy kills cancer cells. Hormone therapy, like tamoxifen (Nolvadex), blocks hormone receptors on certain cancer cells (those that are ER+ or PR+), which interferes with their growth. The hormone therapy induces cells to undergo *apoptosis*, programmed cell death, by depriving them of estrogen.

going to get into an accident and thus need a seat-belt. So everyone is required to wear one all of the time to prevent injury in case you do get into an accident.

Decisions about adjuvant chemotherapy and hormone therapy (such as tamoxifen, discussed in Chapter 10) are made on the basis of large studies of groups of patients rather than on a woman's individual case. "The impact of treatment on a percentage basis is typically small...especially for lower risk patients," Hudis says. (Most women with early stage disease are cured by local treatment.)

Unofficially...
Between 60 and 70 percent of women who have node-negative breast cancer are cured with surgery. But 30 to 40 percent suffer recurrences, according to the National Cancer Institute.

As a result, some women at risk look at the percentage of women who will benefit and think it is too small to justify. But when translated into real numbers, it makes more sense why doctors think adjuvant chemotherapy is so important for most women. For example, if chemotherapy only benefits 3 percent of women with breast cancer, it doesn't seem that the benefit will outweigh the risks. But when translated to the large numbers of affected women, if there are 100,000 candidates for chemotherapy, 3,000 would die without it. That's a lot of lives saved. "That's really the thing that drives us," Hudis says.

Women at greatest risk for recurrence are those with positive nodes and those with negative nodes but with tumors greater than 1 cm.

Who gets what chemotherapy and how much? The combinations of chemotherapeutic drugs and dose schedules were developed largely empirically, experimentally, and through observation over the years. "The gold standard is CMF [cyclophosphamide, methotrexate, and fluorouracil]," says Hudis, though other medical oncologists think it is CAF (cyclophosphamide, Adriamycin, and fluorouracil).

More and more studies are determining the advantage of doxorubicin (Adriamycin) in combination with cytoxan in breast cancer, making it a more commonly used combination.

Doxorubicin, in combination with cytoxan may have a small benefit over CMF, but researchers have not yet determined which candidates who would benefit most. Women with excess HER-2 (gene number or receptor) expression probably get a benefit from doxorubicin, Hudis says. (HER-2 over expression also plays a role in determining who may benefit from trastuzumab (Herceptin), discussed in Chapter 10.)

The length of time a woman receives chemotherapy was also arrived at experimentally, according to Hudis. Researchers conducted randomized trials to determine how long treatement was necessary for optimal results. Earlier patients underwent treatments for two years. But study results indicated that a lengthy period was unnecessary. Now the optimal range is three to six months. The dosage is more individualized, based on height and weight and is adjusted for side effects.

Research is ongoing. Current research efforts include fine-tuning the dose and the scheduling of drugs to see if changes will have added benefits.

Hormone therapy, discussed in more detail in Chapter 10, is another systemic therapy some women with breast cancer can benefit from. In the United States, physicians prescribe tamoxifen for women whose tumors have ER+ or PR+ receptors (and on the rare occasion when receptor status is unknown). In addition, combination chemotherapy is prescribed for younger women (who typically have more aggressive cancers and whose hormone levels are higher than those of postmenopausal women) and those generally healthy women of any age with higher risk factors. Hudis notes that these two groups can overlap. So a 50-year-old woman with ER+ receptor status and lymph node involvement may be given combination chemotherapy and a 30-year-old with no node involvement may not be given this treatment, while both would receive the tamoxifen.

Raloxifene (Evista) is FDA approved for the prevention of osteoporosis for postmenopausal women, Hudis says, noting that initial research hints that it may reduce the incidence of breast cancer. But this will be clarified in the Study of Tamoxifen and Raloxifene (STAR), which is looking at women who don't have breast cancer but who are at high risk. There are no data indicating whether this drug will have an effect on those who have already been diagnosed with breast cancer.

Herceptin shrinks HER-2/neu positive cancers in some patients when they have advanced disease and may add further benefit in the adjuvant setting among appropriate patients, Hudis says. But it has side effects, and researchers must determine if the benefits outweigh the risks.

No longer directing therapy

Not too long ago, lymph node status was the determining factor in breast cancer treatment. Removing the axillary lymph nodes, those under the arm, was thought to improve survival by removing the first site that the cancer spread to. But studies showed that this additional surgery wasn't any more effective than nonsurgical options. The procedure was also used to figure out the best adjuvant therapy—chemotherapy, radiation, or both. But times have changed. Doctors treat most breast cancer patients with adjuvant chemotherapy or hormone therapy, regardless of their nodal status.

Axillary lymph node biopsies can still provide prognostic information. Lymph node status indicates if the cancer has spread. Not knowing node status makes informed consent and informed decision-making about risks of the disease and risks and benefits of treatment difficult. Furthermore, for patients with many positive nodes who may be interested in participating in research trials, such as high-dose chemotherapy, the nodal information is important.

In addition to prognostic factors (lymph node involvement, tumor size, grade, hormone receptor status, proliferative capacity of the tumor, oncogene expression and amplification, and lymph node involvement), treatment options depend on the following factors:

- Age
- Menopausal status
- General health
- Location of the tumor
- Whether there are any enlarged lymph nodes under the arm
- The size of the affected breast

The most important factor used to determine treatment is the stage of the disease. Stages and the treatments typically used for each one are as follows:

1. Stage 0

- *Description—Noninvasive carcinoma or lobular carcinoma in situ (LCIS)* consists of abnormal cells that are found in the lining of a lobule that rarely spread. Rather, LCIS is considered a risk factor for breast cancer (in both breasts, not just the breast in which the LCIS is found).

- *Treatment options*—Treatment is not necessary,

but increased surveillance is very important. However, there are preventive treatment options including hormone therapy (tamoxifen) and prophylactic mastectomies (both considered controversial), and promising new preventive treatments available in the STAR trials. (For STAR trial locations call the NCI's Cancer Information Service at 800/4-CANCER.)

■ *Description—Ductal carcinoma in situ (DCIS),* also called intraductal carcinoma, is a diagnosis given when cancer cells are found in an area of abnormal tissue in the lining of a duct. The cells have not spread into the surrounding breast tissue. In contrast to LCIS, cancer cells may break, spread, and eventually develop into an invasive breast cancer. Therefore, treatment is necessary.

■ *Treatment options*—There are three treatment options—conservation (breast-sparing surgery and radiation) or mastectomy (in this case, simple mastectomy). The role of tamoxifen is being tested at this stage. The National Surgical Adjuvant Breast and Bowel Project (NSABP) recently completed a double-blind, randomized, controlled trial to find out whether lumpectomy, radiation therapy, and tamoxifen were of more benefit than lumpectomy and radiation therapy alone for DCIS. Results were published in the *Lancet* (June 1999). The findings were positive.

2. Stage I

■ *Description*—Stage I is considered early stage breast cancer, but unlike stage 0, stage I breast cancer has already spread outside the ducts or lobules of the breast into the nearby tissues surrounding the tumor. In stage I, the cancer cells are contained in the breast and the diameter of the tumor is less than or equal to 2 centimeters (2.5 centimeters equals 1 inch). Stage I breast cancer is considered curable in the vast majority of cases. After 10 to 20 years, only about 21 percent of patients treated with surgery alone had a recurrence (this percentage includes both local and distant recurrences), according to research results by Rosen, et al. published in the *Journal of Clinical Oncology* (September 1989). According to the medical textbook *Diseases of the Breast* (Lippincott-Raven Publishers; January 1996), 75 percent of all node-positive women treated by surgery alone die within 10 years, but only 25 to 30 percent of women with negative nodes die of breast cancer in the first 10 years.

■ *Treatment options*—These include breast-sparing surgery (lumpectomy) followed by radiation therapy, partial or segmental mastectomy, which may be followed by radiation therapy to the remaining breast tissue, or complete mastectomy, with or without reconstruction. Both surgical treatments (lumpectomy and partial or segmental mastectomy) generally include removing the axillary lymph nodes. (However, less than 3 percent of tumors less than or equal to 5 millimeters detected by mammography have spread to the axillary lymph nodes, so lymph node biopsy may not be necessary in these cases.) Studies have demonstrated that these treatments (lumpectomy plus radiation and mastectomy) are all equally effective. However, choosing one over the other is determined by the size and location of the tumor, the size of your breast, specific characteristics of the cancer cells, as well as how important it is to you to preserve your breast. It is uncer-

Bright Idea
It is difficult for pathologists to distinguish between lobular carcinoma in situ and ductal carcinoma in situ. Because treatments differ for these two stage 0 cancers, you may want to consider getting a second opinion from a pathologist at another hospital, specifically, a breast specialist pathologist.

tain, however, whether young women with BRCA1 or BRCA2 mutations are good candidates for breast-conserving therapy. There are no good data yet. Many women will receive adjuvant chemotherapy and/or hormone therapy to destroy any cancer cells remaining in the breast or those that may have traveled beyond the breast after the primary treatment. Other options include clinical trials of adjuvant therapy, no adjuvant therapy, or treatment to block the ovaries from working. The reason for the latter is that ovaries produce estrogen, which makes some tumors grow. Estrogen receptor status, progesterone receptor status, tumor size, and the proliferative capacity of the tumor (i.e., how fast it grows) are strong predictors of the risk of recurrence. Therefore, adjuvant therapy may be necessary for women who have a node-negative status (the cancer was not found in the lymph nodes). Adjuvant therapy may include tamoxifen for women with hormone-positive tumors with negative lymph nodes or combination chemotherapy consisting of cyclophosphamide, methotrexate, and fluorouracil (CMF) for women with negative nodes and aggressive tumors. (There are alternative drug combinations.) Women with negative hormone receptors and a negative nodal status may be treated with combination chemotherapy without tamoxifen. Women with negative nodes and ER+ (estrogen receptor positive) tumors may receive tamoxifen plus chemotherapy. One study showed chemotherapy plus tamoxifen resulted in a 91 percent disease-free survival and a 96 percent overall survival versus an 87 percent disease-free survival and a 94 percent overall survival from tamoxifen alone after five years.

Ovarian ablation, removing the ovaries, in women younger than 50 appears to produce the same survival benefit as chemotherapy in premenopausal women. It may be that systemic chemotherapy works in part through ovarian ablation. The theory is still under investigation. Preoperative chemotherapy (doxorubicin (Adriamycin) and cyclophosphamide) may be beneficial for women who want breast conservation surgery but who do not qualify due to the size of their tumor.

Timesaver
Ask your doctor if treatment appointments run on schedule. If they don't, call in on the day of your appointment to see how backed up the office is, so you don't have to waste time sitting in the waiting room.

3. Stage II

- *Description*—Stage II is also considered an early stage breast cancer. In contrast to stage 0 and similar to Stage I, the cancer has invaded beyond ducts or lobules of the breast into the local tissue. There are three possibilities that qualify a tumor to be categorized as Stage II: 1. The tumor is less than 1 inch across, and the cancer has spread to the axillary lymph nodes (those under the arm); 2. The tumor measures between 1 and 2 inches (with or without spread to the axillary lymph nodes); 3. The tumor is larger than 2 inches but it has not spread to the axillary lymph nodes. There is a fourth possibility; Stage II includes T_3No disease, that is, tumors greater than 5 centimeters but node negative.

- *Treatment options*—Stage II breast cancer is also considered curable in many women. Treatment options are similar to early invasive cancer (Stage I) and always include systemic therapy.

They include breast-sparing surgery followed by

radiation therapy, or mastectomy, which may be followed by radiation therapy to the chest wall. Both surgical treatments generally include removing the axillary lymph nodes. Studies have demonstrated that these two treatment options are equally effective. However, the decision of one over the other is determined by the size and location of the tumor, the size of your breast, specific characteristics of the cancer cells, as well as how important it is to you to preserve your breast. Most women will receive adjuvant chemotherapy and/or hormone therapy to destroy any cancer cells remaining in the breast after the primary treatment and any cancer cells that may have traveled outside of the breast, avoiding removal (or destruction, in the case of radiation therapy) during the primary treatment phase.

There are two additional treatment options: A clinical trial of neoadjuvant therapy (therapy before surgery) or high-dose chemotherapy with a stem cell transplant if the cancer has spread to four to nine lymph nodes.

4. Stage IIIa and IIIb

■ *Description*—Stage IIIa and stage IIIb breast cancer are considered locally advanced cancer. However, they have much different prognoses.

1. A breast cancer qualifies as stage III if it meets one of the following criteria: 1. The tumor is more than 2 inches across with positive axillary nodes; 2. The cancer is found in a large number of axillary lymph nodes, which are matted together or fixed to other structures under the arm; 3. The cancer has spread to internal mammary nodes near the sternum (breast bone); 4. The tumor involves the skin

or extends into the muscles of the rib cage; 5. The cancer is diagnosed as inflammatory breast cancer.

2. A tumor qualifies as stage IIIa if it is more than 5 centimeters and has spread to movable axillary lymph node(s) on the same side, is more than 5 centimeters and has matted lymph nodes (those grown together or stuck to other tissues and fixed in place, not moveable on physical exam) or any tumor with matted lymph nodes. Stage IIIa tumors have a clinically better outcome than stage IIIb tumors, but the approach to treatment is the same or quite similar.

3. A tumor qualifies as stage IIIb if it involves the breast skin, the chest wall, is inflammatory, or has internal mammary nodal metastasis.

■ *Treatment options*—Most oncologists treat Stages IIIa and IIIb with preoperative chemotherapy.

This systemic treatment is most commonly three to four cycles of chemotherapy but may be hormone therapy, or both chemotherapy and hormone therapy. The tumor is then treated with surgery, most commonly with a modified radical mastectomy but sometimes a lumpectomy with axillary lymph node removal followed by three to four rounds of chemotherapy, radiation therapy, and/or tamoxifen for five years if the tumor is ER+/PR+.

Other options may include participating in a clinical trial investigating new chemotherapy drugs, new drug combinations, or new ways of administering old drugs, biological therapy, or high-dose chemotherapy with peripheral stem

Watch Out!
Chemotherapy can deplete your white blood cells, red blood cells, and platelets. As a result, chemotherapy may be delayed until your blood counts return to a near normal level. Your doctor may prescribe medications to try to boost the white blood cell counts.

cell transplantation.

5. Stage IV

- **▪ *Description*—**Stage IV breast cancer is metastatic disease, that is, it has spread to other areas of the body. Stage IV may also include inflammatory breast cancer. (Stage IV also includes women whose cancer has spread above the clavicle or collar bone. There is a subset of women with metastatic disease in this area only who have a better prognosis, with 40 percent survival at 5 years.)

- **▪ *Treatment options*—**Just 10 to 20 percent of women with stage IV disease typically attain long-term, complete remission. A cure is rare but not unheard of. Chemotherapy and/or hormone therapy is used to destroy cancer cells and control the disease. Mastectomy or radiation may be used to control the cancer in the breast, and radiation may be used locally to control tumors in other parts of the body, such as the bone, and to treat any pain they may cause. (Surgery and chemotherapy or hormone therapy are also used sometimes to control pain.) Hormone therapy may be used as a first-line treatment in women with hormone-sensitive tumors whose cancer has spread only minimally to the liver or lung.

Bright Idea
Schedule your chemotherapy sessions on Friday afternoons. That way, if you experience side effects, you'll have two days to recover before returning to work or your daily routine.

If the cancer has spread or the tumor is not sensitive to hormone therapy, combination chemotherapy regimens are used. Doxorubicin-based therapy produces superior results if it has not been previously used. Other options include participating in a clinical trial investigating new chemotherapy drugs, new drug combinations, or new ways of administering old drugs, biological therapy with or without chemotherapy, or high-dose chemotherapy with peripheral stem cell transplantation.

6. Recurrent cancer

■ *Description*—When the same cancer grows back, it is referred to as a recurrence. Sometimes the breast cancer grows back locally in the breast, skin, or lymph nodes. Other times it grows in other places in the body. Although recurrences most often occur within three years after treatment, breast cancer can recur many years later.

■ *Treatment options*—Once there is a recurrence, the surgical oncologist must determine whether it's operable. If the recurrence is located in the breast (post-lumpectomy plus radiation) where the original cancer developed, then you may be a candidate for a mastectomy, which may be followed by adjuvant chemotherapy, according to Lyndsay Harris, M.D., assistant professor in the Multidisciplinary Breast Program at Duke University. The role of adjuvant chemotherapy and hormone therapy has not yet been defined but it is being used. There's a 50-50 chance or better of being cured in this circumstance.

If the tumor is hormone sensitive, you may be given hormone therapy. If the tumor is not hormone sensitive, you may or may not be offered chemotherapy. If you have a slow-growing ER+ tumor, such as those found in the skin, lymph nodes, bone, or fluid surrounding the lungs, a hormone inhibitor such as tamoxifen, or aromatase inhibitors (aromatase inhibitors are drugs that block the conversion of androstenedione to estriol, and as such they reduce circulatory estrogen levels in post menopausal women) if you have already had tamoxifen, are possibilities, Harris says. If the tumor is not hormone sensitive, or you have an aggressive type of recurrence, affecting areas like the liver, lung, or brain, then chemotherapy may be a better option. Your HER-2 status will determine whether Herceptin alone or combined with taxane (paclitaxel or docitaxel, chemotherapeutic drugs) is viable. (Herceptin is used alone on slow-growing tumors.) There are also specialized options for symptom control. Radiation can be used in some situations, such as when there is a painful bone metastasis or when there is a local recurrence in the chest wall or lymph nodes that can be irradiated locally, if radiation to that same area was not given previously. (There is a maximum-tolerated tissue dose for irradiation, so it is not often done.)

Unofficially...
It can be difficult to tell in an intact breast if a tumor is a new primary cancer or a local recurrence. However, it's not impossible.

Radiation can be followed by chemotherapy for more systemic control. Tamoxifen and radiation can be administered at the same time. In addition to Herceptin and tamoxifen, there are other biological therapy options, which are discussed in Chapter 10.

Hope in the headlines

A recent phase III study of 3,000 node-positive women found taking paclitaxel (Taxol) plus standard chemotherapy (doxorubicin plus cyclophosphamide) increased survival rates by 26 percent and reduced the risk of recurrence by 22 percent compared with taking doxorubicin plus cyclophosphamide alone. This news certainly gives more women hope for a cure. The study was headed by the Cancer and Leukemia Group B (CALGB), and findings were presented at a meeting of the American

Society of Clinical Oncology in May 1998. Paclitaxel (Taxol), a chemotherapuetic drug, is rapidly becoming part of the standard chemotherapy regimen used by many oncologists.

Based on preliminary data from a phase II study, an FDA advisory committee has recommended that capecitabine (Xeloda) be made available to women with advanced breast cancer who have not responded to standard treatment. The drug, a pill taken orally, remains inactive in large part until it reaches the tumor site at which time it converts to fluorouracil. As a result of this process, it is expected to have fewer side effects.

Research presented at the annual meeting of the Radiological Society of North America in December 1998 showed a promising alternative for women with small cancers who want to avoid disfiguring surgery. Doctors use interactive magnetic resonance to place a needle in the tumor and then place a fiberoptic wire into the tumor. The wire is used as a conduit to place laser heat there for about 10 minutes. The heat destroys the tumor. This technique is referred to as tumor ablation. The procedure, called laser lumpectomy, doesn't require an incision, so there is no scar. Furthermore, it can be done on an outpatient basis using local anesthesia. The research is being conducted at the University of Arkansas in Little Rock.

Laser lumpectomy is one investigational method of tumor ablation that "cooks" the tissue. It has not been compared to "standard" therapy in randomized trials but may be in the future.

A Canadian study, supported by the National Cancer Institute of Canada Clinical Trials Group, showed that a specific chemotherapy combination— cyclophosphamide, epirubicin (which is chemically

Unofficially...
Docetaxel (Taxotere) is derived from the European yew tree, and paclitaxel (Taxol) is derived from the USA yew tree.

related to Adriamycin), and flourouracil compared with cyclophosphamide, methotrexate, and flourouracil (CMF) can further reduce deaths by 19 percent in premenopausal women whose breast cancer has spread to the lymph nodes. Furthermore, the investigators found that the chemotherapy drugs can reduce the risk of recurrence by 29 percent. This study took place in 36 centers across Canada. Study participants were followed for at least five years. The findings were published in the *Journal of Clinical Oncology* (August 1998).

Just the facts

- Surgery and radiation are local treatments and chemotherapy and hormone therapy are systemic treatments.

- Most women in the early stages of breast cancer are cured by surgery.

- Chemotherapy is given to most women after surgery just in case cancer cells have traveled outside the breast.

- Chemotherapy can be used before surgery to make breast-sparing surgery possible for women with large tumors.

GET THE SCOOP ON...
How to reduce your anxiety during
treatments ▪ How to control side effects through
diet ▪ How to prevent or control lymphedema ▪
What causes cancer pain and what can relieve it

Undergoing Treatment

Chapter 8

Getting through breast cancer treatment and its side effects can be a challenge. Chemotherapy can cause many side effects, including hair loss, nausea and vomiting, loss of appetite, weight loss, mouth sores, and fatigue. Radiation therapy can also cause fatigue as well as tenderness, redness, and dryness in the treated area of the skin. Surgery causes pain and tenderness in the area of the incision and can result in lymphedema, a swelling in the arm and hand as a result of the pooling of lymphatic fluid that sometimes occurs when lymph nodes are removed.

In this chapter, we'll give you tips on how to get through the treatments as well as how to handle the side effects. We'll also give you expert advice on how to get adequate nutrition to keep up your strength during the cycles of treatment.

Preparing for treatment

No matter which treatment or treatments you undergo, it's tough getting through them. The fear can be

Unofficially...
Side effects of cancer treatment differ from woman to woman. They may even differ from one treatment to the next.

so overwhelming, it sometimes produces an anxiety response. For example, a woman may develop nausea before the second round of chemo simply by recalling how unsettled her stomach was following the first treatment. While no doubt a trying experience, there are ways to make your fears more manageable. Anne Coscorelli, Ph.D., director of the Rhonda Fleming Mann Resource Center for Women with Cancer at the Jonsson Comprehensive Cancer Center at UCLA, gives these tips:

■ Let others help you out. Fear uses up a lot of energy. You can preserve some energy by accepting offers from friends and family to drive you to your treatment or run errands. Don't hesitate to ask for help, either.

■ Take action to reduce your anxiety. Doing so may alleviate treatment-related pain. You can reduce your anxiety by using meditation, deep breathing, guided imagery, and progressive relaxation. Learn these skills before the procedure by reading books on the topic, finding groups where they're practiced, or visiting a therapist skilled at teaching these methods.

■ Find people you can talk to. Tell the nurse, technicians, your family, friends, support group, and clergy if you're feeling nervous, upset, or worried about your treatments.

■ Take someone with you to the treatment so you have someone to talk to.

■ Before your first treatment, talk to others who've been through it. They may calm some of your fears and give you tips on how to handle treatment over the long-term.

■ Learn cognitive coping skills. When we talk to ourselves during a frightening situation, we may (understandably) say scary things to ourselves. Take a moment to listen to your thoughts. Then consciously change what you say to yourself. For example, tell yourself "This is a time-limited period," "I only have X number of treatments to go," "I've coped in the past," "At least I don't have to do [fill in the blank]," "I can use my deep breathing skills," and "Other women have gone through this and they're fine now." If you're being treated for a recurrence you may say to yourself, "I'm getting the best care. There's hope." Say positive, reassuring things to yourself, Coscorelli advises.

Sometimes women with a recurrence may be sicker than those who are recently diagnosed for the first time.

Make sure you're comfortable: Wear comfortable clothes, bring your own pillow, and ask for what you need. If you have bony metastases, anything you can do to make yourself more comfortable will help, Coscorelli says.

Plan to distract yourself during treatment. Distraction has "actually been shown to be a very effective tool to get through treatments," Coscorelli says. Here are some ways to distract yourself:

■ Listen to music with headphones.

■ Listen to books on tape.

■ Try needlepoint, crocheting, or knitting.

■ Play video games.

■ Watch videos.

■ Write letters.

■ Write a story about something else.

■ Use relaxation techniques to help reduce pain. There are several different techniques you can use including progressive muscle relaxation, guided imagery, or visualization techniques such as picturing the treatments and your body's own cells like the video game Pac Man, gobbling up the cancer cells. Some physicians claim treatment results may even be better when this technique is used and you are less likely to feel helpless if you are an actual member of the cancer-fighting team. This may help reduce any pain.

Taking control of your health through diet

One way to improve your health to some degree is by eating right. However, the diet that may be best for those trying to prevent breast cancer may be slightly different for those trying to prevent a recurrence.

For example, eating soy has been associated with a lower incidence of breast cancer in some studies. That is, it is thought to help prevent cancer.

As noted in Chapter 5, researchers have noted an association between soy intake and estradiol (a potent estrogen) levels and sex hormone-binding globulin in Japanese women. They believe that the results, if causal, suggest that eating soy lowers breast cancer risk by modifying estrogen metabolism. The report was published in *Nutrition and Cancer* (Volume 20, Issue 3, 1997).

But it's not really the soy your after. It's the isoflavones in soy foods, according to Katrina Claghorn, R.D., Section Editor of OncoLink's "Nutrition During Cancer Treatment" and "Diet and Cancer" menus. The isoflavones, sometimes referred to as phytoestrogens or plant estrogens, have similar properties and chemical shape to human estrogen, but plant estrogens are much weaker. Scientists believe the reason that phytoestrogens may reduce breast cancer incidence is that the weak estrogens fit into the estro-

Watch Out!
Not all women lose weight during breast cancer treatment. Some women actually gain weight, which may be a risk factor for recurrence. It's also an appearance issue, says Laura Kramer, a registered dietitian. In addition to dealing with breast cancer, these women have to deal with the emotional aspects to being overweight.

gen receptor site in breast tissue, preventing the more potent human estrogen from attaching to the receptor site and initiating the cancer-causing process.

How much should you consume on a daily basis to reap the protective effect? The current recommendation is 30 to 50 mg of isoflavones daily, according to Claghorn. "The best sources of isoflavones are soy milk (30 mg/8 oz), tofu (35 mg/1/2 cup), tempeh (35 mg/1/4 cup), roasted soy nuts (60 mg/1/4 cup) and soy protein powder (approximately 60 mg/2 scoops)," she writes at Oncolink (www.onco link.upenn.edu).

Take note: Not all soy products contain isoflavones. For example, "soy foods made from soy protein concentrate may have little if any isoflavones," Claghorn writes.

However, because some soy products have a weak estrogen link, it may be unwise for women who have been diagnosed with an estrogen-positive (ER+) tumor to include it in their diet, Laura Kramer says, a registered dietitian at Massachusetts General Hospital in Boston.

There is considerable concern among some scientists that estrogen may trigger tumor growth in women who have been diagnosed with breast cancer and postmenopausal women.

Eating right during treatment

Chemotherapy can take away your desire for food. "The worst thing a patient can do is not eat," Kramer says. "You want to keep your strength up. Studies have shown that you may be able to handle higher doses of treatment [if you eat well]," according to Kramer. Make sure you eat something.

Loss of appetite is a common problem during treatment. Many factors can affect appetite, including nausea and vomiting, feeling upset or depressed, or feeling fearful about the treatment or disease.

The key to gaining back your appetite is making mealtimes more relaxed. Have healthy food handy when you do feel like eating. Eating several small meals throughout the day may be easier than sitting down to three hearty meals a day. Consider keeping nuts, applesauce, cereal, peanut butter, pudding, muffins, crackers, and juice on hand.

Breast cancer treatment, particularly chemotherapy, has side effects, and these side effects can interfere with good nutrition.

The most common side effects that interfere with good nutrition when it comes to chemotherapy are nausea, vomiting, mouth sores, diarrhea, and constipation. Keep in mind that everyone does not experience these side effects. Furthermore, if you experience side effects during one treatment, it does not mean that you will experience them again after the next one.

Kramer says there are three primary reasons why it's so important to get adequate nutrition while undergoing chemotherapy:

1. Good nutrition may help women deal better with the side effects.

2. Good nutrition may help fight off infection.

3. Good nutrition allows the body to rebuild healthy tissue faster.

A balanced diet consists of food from the following food groups:

- Fruits and vegetables. The National Cancer Center recommends eating five servings a day. The combination doesn't matter, but you should eat a variety of them, and the more colorful, the better. For example, don't eat only green vegeta-

Unofficially...
Medical marijuana is used for appetite stimulation for some patients. It is also used to help control nausea in other patients. In controlled trials, it was not as effective as other anti-emetics, drugs used to control nausea.

bles. Include yellow and orange to get a variety of vitamins and minerals. Fruits and vegetables have antioxidant properties, which may help fight off cancer. They also contain phytochemicals, which may prevent or fend off cancer and may strengthen the immune system.

- Poultry, fish, and lean meat
- Grains, cereals, and breads
- Dairy products

You need to eat enough calories to maintain your body weight, but not so many as to cause weight gain, which puts you at risk for a recurrence, Kramer says. In addition, you need to eat enough protein to help repair your muscles, skin, and hair, she says.

In addition to eating well, Kramer emphasizes the importance of getting enough fluids. Dehydration from vomiting can become a problem. In addition, cytoxan is toxic to the bladder. You need to protect your bladder and kidneys during treatment. In addition to water, you can hydrate yourself by eating flavored gelatin, soup, popsicles, and the like.

Some days during treatment you probably won't feel like eating, Kramer says. She suggests the following:

- Eat small snacks or meals throughout the day.

- Take a walk before meals to stimulate your appetite. This also helps to keep your bones and muscles healthy.

- Distract yourself by eating with friends or family, and if you have to dine alone, eat with relaxing music or candlelight.

- If you live alone, and you find it difficult to cook for one, consider using a service like "Meals on Wheels."

Moneysaver
Shop with coupons. Seeing how much money you save may give you a little pleasure. If possible, put this money aside so you can reward yourself with something special when you finish your treatment.

Try to eat a lot of calories and protein during breakfast because it tends to be a better-tolerated meal, Kramer says.

Coping with side effects

All cancer treatments have side effects you must cope with. But the side effects of chemotherapy—nausea and vomiting, loss of appetite, weight loss, mouth sores, and fatigue—are particularly challenging. However, there are effective ways to deal with them.

Nausea and vomiting

Watch Out!
Don't eat your favorite food before chemotherapy, says Kramer. If you get sick from chemotherapy, chances are you'll never like it again.

"Nausea and vomiting from chemotherapy occur from the drug's effect on the stomach, the area where the brain controls vomiting, or both," Kramer says. Radiation can also cause nausea and vomiting if your gastrointestinal tract is irradiated.

Ginger (ginger ale, ginger snaps, crystallized ginger, and ginger tea) can help reduce the nauseous feelings. You can also use motion sickness bands, acupuncture, and accupressure, she says.

Kramer gives these additional tips for controlling nausea and vomiting:

- Don't eat big meals.

- Don't drink a lot of fluids with your meal. It will fill you up and make you feel bloated. Hydrate yourself after you eat and consistently throughout the day.

- Eat and drink slowly, so your stomach won't fill up too fast.

- Avoid eating greasy, fatty, spicy, or sweet foods.

- Eat foods that can be kept at room temperature. These foods tend to have less odor and are therefore better tolerated.

- Avoid lying flat for at least two hours after you eat.

- Wear loose-fitting clothes so as not to restrict your stomach.

- If you were nauseous during a treatment, avoid eating heavy food for several hours before your next one, but try to eat a little.

- Suck on mints, ice cubes, or tart candy. (But don't suck on tart candy if you have mouth sores.)

To prevent vomiting, your doctor will prescribe a drug called an anti-emetic, a medicine that prevents or alleviates nausea and vomiting. (If you don't think you can keep a pill down, request a suppository.)

Fatigue

Many women experience fatigue as a result of breast cancer treatment. Surgery, radiation therapy, and chemotherapy all cause fatigue. The fatigue resulting from chemotherapy is often a result of anemia, a low red blood cell count, which is caused by the drugs.

Kramer suggests the following tips to deal with fatigue:

- Get plenty of rest. Take naps if necessary.

- Limit your activities. Decide which ones are most important to you.

- Ask for help if you need it.

- Eat well-balanced meals. Snack in between meals.

- Take walks or do light exercise.

Mouth sores

Chemotherapy can cause sores in the mouth as well as in the throat. These sores can become infected from the bacteria and viruses in the mouth, so it's important to have good oral hygiene, Kramer says. She advises brushing your teeth and gums after every meal using a soft toothbrush and seeing a den-

Timesaver
If you are too tired to cook every day, pick one day per week to cook batches large enough to last the whole week. Freeze meals in microwaveable containers.

tist regularly. (You should also see a dentist prior to chemotherapy in order to take care of any existing or potential problems.) She also suggests avoiding mouthwashes that contain alcohol. Alcohol will make mouth sores burn like fire.

What do you eat when your mouth and throat are sore? "Choose soft, soothing foods, like mashed potatoes, chicken pot pie, macaroni and cheese, [and] soft-boiled or scrambled eggs," Kramer says, adding that you can also puree food in a blender. "Eat foods that are at room temperature or cooler," she adds.

You may want to avoid acidic food, such as tomatoes or tomato products, because they can be irritating. In addition, avoid citrus fruits and citrus fruit juices—such as orange juice, grapefruit juice, lemonade—and opt for less-irritating apple or grape juices. Also avoid salty or spicy foods, and rough, dry, or coarse foods, such as raw vegetables, toast, and popcorn.

Dry mouth is common in women undergoing treatment for breast cancer. Both chemotherapy, especially if mouth ulcers develop, and radiation therapy in the head or neck region can reduce the flow of saliva and cause dry mouth. Head and neck irradiation causes the salivary glands to disappear. Having a dry mouth can change the way foods taste.

If your mouth is dry, try some of the following:

- Drink fluids

- Chew gum

- Suck on candy (preferably sugarless because with decreased saliva you're more prone to cavities)

- Dunk foods in gravy, sauce, or salad dressing

- Eat very sweet or tart foods and drink beverages such as lemonade (unless you have mouth sores or a sore throat) to help your mouth produce more saliva. Use soft and pureed foods, which may be easier to swallow.

- Moisten your lips with lip salves.

If you're mouth is still dry, artificial saliva can be purchased at drug stores to increase moisture in the mouth.

Unofficially...
Radiation to the breast does not cause vomiting or diarrhea.

Diarrhea

Chemotherapy targets rapidly dividing cells such as cancer cells. But cancer cells are not the only cells that divide rapidly. The cells that line the digestive tract also divide rapidly.

"If chemotherapy affects the lining of the intestine, the result can be diarrhea," Kramer says. Diarrhea also can be caused by radiation therapy to the abdomen and emotional upset. Severe diarrhea (10 or more stools per day) may cause dehydration and increase the risk of infection if the diarrhea is due to colon or small bowel ulcerations.

If you have sudden, short-term diarrhea attacks, try a clear liquid diet during the first 12 to 14 hours to replace body fluids lost during diarrhea. (If you have severe diarrhea or it lasts for more than a couple of days, contact your physician.)

To control the diarrhea, try some of the following suggestions:

- Drink plenty of liquids to prevent dehydration. (Remember to drink those fluids in between meals.)

- Eat small, frequent meals or snacks.

- Salt and potassium are often lost during diarrhea. Drink fluids that contain sodium (salt)—bouillon or fat-free broth. Eat foods high in potassium— bananas, peaches, and apricot nectar, and boiled or mashed potatoes—and salt.

- Eat low-fiber foods such as yogurt, farina or cream of wheat, grape juice, eggs (not fried), ripe bananas, cottage cheese, cream cheese, smooth peanut butter, white bread, rice or noodles, skinned chicken or turkey, lean beef, or fish (not fried).

- Avoid eating high-fiber foods, including raw fruits and vegetables, beans, whole-grain bread, cereal, nuts, seeds, dried fruit, and popcorn.

- Avoid caffeine (coffee, tea, some sodas, chocolate).

- Avoid eating greasy, fatty, fried, and spicy foods (hot pepper, curry, and cajun spice mix).

- Avoid raw vegetables and fruits and high-fiber vegetables (corn, beans, broccoli cabbage, peas, and cauliflower).

- Avoid dairy products if they make the diarrhea worse. Try replacing milk products with lactose-free or nondairy products.

If these dietary changes don't help, or your can't make the dietary changes, ask your doctor to prescribe a medication such as Imodium or Lomotil to help control the diarrhea.

Constipation

Conversely, some women experience constipation during treatment as the result of pain medication, inactivity, dehydration, or a lack of bulk in their diet. It also can result from being bedridden. To deal with constipation, try some of the following tips:

- Drink plenty of fluids—at least eight 8-ounce glasses a day—to keep your stools soft. Warm and hot drinks can be used to loosen the bowel. Drink something hot about one-half hour before your usual time for a bowel movement.

- Eat high-fiber food, including bran, whole-grain breads and cereals, pastas, vegetables (raw or cooked), fresh or dried fruits, including the skins, nuts, popcorn, dried peas, dried beans, barley, brown rice, and other whole-grain products, and potato skins.

- Do some light exercise, such as walking.

- Sprinkle unprocessed wheat bran into foods such as cereals, meatloaf, casseroles, and homemade breads.

If none of these suggestions works, ask your doctor for medication. Don't take any over-the-counter laxatives or stool softeners without consulting your physician first.

Lymphedema

Lymphedema can occur whenever you have surgery in the armpit. About 30 percent of women who have mastectomies with node biopsies suffer from lymphedema ranging from asymptomatic to severe, according to Caroline Fife, M.D., director of the Hermann Lymphedema Center in Houston, Texas.

The condition can develop right after or within a few months of surgery, or even years or decades later. Lymphedema can also result from radiation due to scarring. (Between 15 to 20 percent of women get lymphedema as a result of radiation therapy within 6 to 12 months after the treatment.)

To understand how lymphedema develops, you first have to understand that lymph (a pale fluid containing white blood cells) moves through lymph nodes via tiny channels called lymphatic vessels.

Watch Out!
Get immediate medical attention with the first symptoms of lymphedema. Symptoms include any swelling in the arm, hand, fingers, or chest wall. If you itch, see a rash, blistering, or redness, or feel an increase in temperature in the arm with lymphedema, or if you develop a fever, contact your physician immediately. An inflammation or infection in that arm could signal the beginning or worsening of lymphedema.

Together, the nodes and lymph vessels make up the lymph (or lymphatic) system. The role of the lymph nodes is to filter out bacteria and other microbes to prevent them from spreading. Cancer cells can pass through and/or grow in the nodes.

When blood cells bring nourishment to the tissues, they carry away some waste products such as carbon dioxide. Other waste products are removed through special cells such as macrophages and through the lymphatic channels. The whole body has an interconnecting system of lymph channels

Lymph channels move a tremendous amount of fluid each day. Removal of lymph nodes and vessels during biopsy results in blockage of lymph flow. Blockage can result in extreme swelling in the hands and arms. The swelling may be both painful and debilitating.

"The swelling makes women more likely to get skin infections," Fife says. "A mosquito bite can put a woman in a hospital [because the immune system doesn't work well in that area]," she explains. If lymph vessels are blocked, the fluid that accumulates can act as a good culture medium. Therefore, relatively minor trauma or infections may become quite serious. Most commonly, this is due to staph or strep bacteria.

Directing the flow

The lymphatic fluid must be moved through alternate routes (venous capillaries, for example) via a mechanical process. This can be accomplished through a technique called Manual Lymphatic Draining (MLD), a type of massage. The therapy uses gentle massage techniques, Fife explains. Afterward, the massaged arm is bandaged in a way that squeezes fluid out of the arm and hand and into the body. There are also mechanical pumps available as well as compression sleeves.

"Unfortunately, the medical community is pretty uninformed about the treatment options for lymphedema," Fife says. "It's not something you learn about in residency," she says. The techniques are new and don't fall into any particular specialist's field. As a result, doctors who become experts in lymphedema come from different backgrounds. Fife's background, for example, is family medicine and chronic nonhealing wounds.

If left untreated, the lymphatic fluid, which is rich in protein, sends out signals to the immune system. The body then reacts as if there is a wound in that area and makes efforts to repair it, resulting in inflammation and scarring. Over months and years a new condition called *hypertrophy* develops, in which enlarged fat and scar tissue form under the skin. That condition can be permanent and extremely painful, and can eventually limit the movement of the arm and hand, Fife says. This condition was common in the era of radical mastectomy, but rarely occurs with modified mastectomy or segmental mastectomy.

Lymphedema is not curable but it is treatable. Following are some of the options available.

Complex decongestive physical therapy

Complex decongestive physical therapy is used to manage lymphedema. This therapy takes place in two phases: Phase I ranges from two weeks for mild lymphedema to eight weeks or more for severe lymphedema. Phase II, which is done at home, must continue for a lifetime. The sooner this therapy is started, the less intensive it will be.

Phase I consists of physical therapy five days a week. Sessions are later reduced to three days a week. Phase I has four components:

Unofficially...
Under the Women's Health and Cancer Rights Act of 1998, if you have coverage under a group health plan or an individual health insurance policy that covers medical and surgical benefits in connection with a mastectomy, your insurance company or HMO must also provide coverage for physical complications of mastectomy, including lymphedema.

1. *Lymph drainage massage*—This is a specialized form of massage used to empty and decompress obstructed lymph vessels. The massage moves fluid to other areas that are able to drain the excess fluid.

2. *Compression bandaging*—This is a multi-layered bandaging technique used to prevent your arm(s) and hand(s) from refilling with lymphatic fluid in between massage therapy sessions. The pressure from the bandages also helps the body's "muscle pump" to move the lymphatic fluid from your arm(s) and hand(s).

3. *Skin care*—You must protect your arm(s) and hand(s) from scratches, wounds, and insect bites, which could become infected. Infection and wound healing can both make the lymphedema worse.

4. *Exercise*—Specially designed exercises are used to stimulate the lymphatic system and aid in dislodging excess lymphatic fluid. These exercises improve muscle strength and minimize the loss of function that often results from lymphedema.

At the end of this phase, you will be fitted with a compression sleeve to wear during the day and you will learn how to bandage your arm(s) at night.

The second phase of complex decongestive physical therapy is the home management program. You must be sure to wear your compression sleeve(s) and bandages routinely. You also must be vigilant about good hygiene, especially keeping your arm(s) and hand(s) clean and dry. In addition, you should periodically see your physical therapist or physiatrist to assess your progress. If your compression sleeve is loose, be sure to get remeasured.

Bright Idea
Visit the National Lymphedema Network at www.lymphnet. org. This Web site has a Net pal registry (pen pals via e-mail), lists support groups, and offers information on legislation and educational material.

How to prevent lymphedema

While lymphedema cannot be cured, it can be prevented. It can also be controlled if you already have it. The National Cancer Institute suggests taking the following precautions.

Do's:

- Protect your hands while doing chores and gardening. Wear gloves. Even minor injuries allow bacteria to enter.

- Practice good hygiene. Keep your skin clean and dry. Be especially careful to dry your skin thoroughly between your fingers and in any creases. Use lotion (Eucerin or Nivea) after bathing to keep your skin supple. Use hypoallergenic soap or deodorant to protect skin from irritation and possible infections.

- Use an electric razor instead of a razor with a sharp blade when shaving under your arms to reduce the chance of cuts and infection.

- When possible, keep your arm(s) elevated above your heart to allow gravity to drain accumulated fluid.

- Keep your arm(s) protected from the sun. Heat increases blood flow, which can increase swelling. Avoid hot tubs, saunas or sunbathing. Avoid washing your hands or dishes in hot water.

- Maintain (or get down to) your ideal body weight. Excess weight will increase swelling.

- Eat a low-salt, high-fiber diet.

- Reduce your intake of sugar to prevent fluid retention.

- With the approval of a physical therapist, walk, swim, do light aerobics, ride a bike, or take specially designed ballet or yoga. Some activities,

Unofficially...
Lymphedema is a high-protein edema. However, cutting back on protein won't reduce the protein content in the lymph fluid. In fact, it will weaken the connective tissue, worsening the condition. If you have lymphedema, your diet should include easily digested proteins, such as those found in chicken and fish.

such as high-impact aerobics, gymnastics, tennis, or golf, may aggravate the condition. (When you choose an exercise, pick one that will not exert the arm at risk. If it begins to ache, lie down and elevate it.)

■ Wear a compression sleeve when traveling by air. You may need to wear additional bandages on a long flight. (Consult your physician.)

■ Wear a light breast prosthesis if you have a large breast. A heavy one may place too much pressure on the lymph nodes above your collarbone. You may also want to consider wearing soft pads under your bra straps. Be sure to wear a well-fitted bra that is not too tight and has no wire support.

■ Wear a well-fitted compression sleeve during waking hours and special bandages at night.

■ Measure the circumference of your arm(s) every month to catch any increased swelling.

Don'ts:

■ Avoid using the arm for lifting heavy objects (over 5 pounds).

■ Avoid carrying a purse, brief case, or duffel bag with a shoulder strap on that arm.

■ Avoid using that arm for rubbing, scrubbing, pushing, or pulling. This type of physical activity causes sudden, rapid blood flow through the muscle and tissue, which will further damage an already compromised lymphatic system.

■ Don't wear tight jewelry such as rings and bracelets on the affected fingers and arm(s). The same goes for rubber bands.

■ Avoid cutting cuticles during manicures to reduce the chances of cuts and infections.

Watch Out!
Better safe than sorry. Never permit a health care worker to draw blood or inject medication into the affected arm. Although there is no data on this, there is concern the needle hole will provide an entryway for infection-causing microbes. If both arms are affected, blood can be drawn from the feet.

- Don't let pets jump on you, and avoid holding cats. Their claws may cut your arm, increasing your risk of infection.

- Avoid insect bites to reduce your chance of infection.

- Don't smoke.

- Get regular check-ups.

The pain of breast cancer

While breast tumors rarely cause pain, many women do experience pain as a result of treatments or when the disease has spread to other parts of the body. Both radiation and chemotherapy cause fluid accumulation and swelling, called edema, which can irritate or destroy healthy tissue. This disturbance of healthy tissue can cause pain and inflammation, and possibly sensitize nerve endings. If the cancer spreads, the pressure of a growing tumor or the infiltration of tumor cells into other organs can cause pain. The good news is that, for the most part, pain can be treated effectively.

The spread of cancer to the bones is the most common cause of pain in women with breast cancer, according to cancer specialist Judith M. Ford, M.D., Ph.D., assistant professor, Department of Radiation Oncology at UCLA and Jonsson Cancer Center. Women feel skeletal pain, not surprisingly, at the site of the metastatic tumor—for example, pain in the hip if that's where the cancer has spread or in the back if that's the site of a new tumor.

Metastatic breast cancer sometimes, though rarely, spreads to the brain rather than the bones. Brain tumors do not cause pain per se, but they can cause headaches due to brain swelling, which causes the covering of the brain to stretch.

If the cancer spreads to the liver, it may cause an aching or irritated feeling, rather than an acute pain. Cancer that spreads to the lung is generally painless, Ford says, with the exception of tumors growing on the surface covering the lung, which may cause pleurisy.

Cancer treatments may also cause pain or discomfort, Ford notes. Surgery causes pain due to the incision and excision of the tumor as well as the stress on the muscles from being moved around. Radiation therapy is usually painless when used to alleviate pain, though in curative treatments the higher doses may cause skin soreness, especially in women with large breasts. Sometimes, during breast surgery, the surgeon hits a nerve. Consequently, the patient suffers from neuropathic pain, which can be treated with low-dose antidepressants because they interfere with the way pain is transmitted down the nerve fiber, says Connie Dahlin, R.N., a nurse practitioner who specializes in palliative care at Massachusetts General in Boston.

Chemotherapy may cause mouth sores. Almost all cancer treatments are associated with fatigue, and fatigue makes it that much harder to deal with the pain, Ford points out.

A world of pain

"Pain isn't just physical. It's multidimensional," Ford says. In addition to physical pain, there is pain from suffering—emotional pain, financial pain, family pain, social pain, and spiritual pain. Each of these can impact the other, she says. For example, anxiety lowers the physical pain threshold, so if you feel anxious, you'll feel physical pain sooner and more acutely than someone without anxiety.

Pain tolerance varies from patient to patient,

Unofficially...
A lot of physicians don't realize that pain *is* controllable. "Good cancer physicians are much less afraid of using opiates than others," according to cancer specialist Judith M. Ford, M.D., Ph.D., assistant professor, Department of Radiation Oncology at UCLA and Jonsson Cancer Center.

Dahlin says. Physical pain disturbs sleep, which in turn compounds other forms of pain and makes everything more difficult for the patient, according to Ford. The longer pain persists, the more likely it is to involve secondary factors—missing work and interfering with personal relationships, for instance. The more that it disrupts, the more it's likely to lead to clinical depression.

Likewise, if having breast cancer interferes with your ability to go to work, the cancer is causing emotional pain. If your family suffers financially as a consequence of your inability to work, you and your family experience financial and family pain.

Emotional pain has several other facets. There's a fear of the loss of control. The doctors are telling you what you must do and thus you must follow their instructions, and you've lost control over your body and your appearance.

Sometimes cancer can impact on your ability to keep up your social schedule. This inability to live a normal life causes social pain.

Some women with breast cancer also suffer from "the sudden realization that it's possible to get a life-threatening disease," Ford says. People think cancer happens to other people. Interestingly, Ford and others note, many women with breast cancer take the opportunity to take stock of their life and feel in the end their life will be better. "So it's a pain you grow through," she says.

All types of pain must be considered and treated, Ford stresses. Doctors must look at many dimensions of pain, not just at what hurts physically.

You don't have to live with pain

Physical pain is the easiest form of pain to deal with, Ford says: "Physical pain is nearly always controllable."

Bright Idea
There's a "hot" candy to soothe painful mouth sores that can result from chemotherapy. The taffy-like candy is made from hot chili peppers, and was created by researchers at Yale University School of Medicine in 1994. The candy contains capsaicin—the active ingredient in chili peppers. It provides pain control after repeated applications. The sugar in the candy prevents the capsaicin from causing burning in the mouth.

The only exception is bone pain. Sometimes bone pain is difficult to control completely if the patient is mobile because the movement causes stress on the bones. But other kinds of pain can be controlled so that you get the right balance between pain relief and functioning without grogginess. "It's not always an instant fix," Ford says. You will only be given small doses of pain medication in the beginning so that your body can get used to the side effects, which will then diminish or go away. The tough part, sometimes, is convincing patients that "the pain control effect will work," she says. Cancer patients resist pain therapy for two main reasons:

1. Some patients think they need to feel the pain. It is true that the pain is telling you something's wrong, but once you're doing something about it it's not necessary to keep feeling it, Ford says. Other times "people feel they should put up with it," she says. "There are no medals for feeling pain," she stresses.

   Note: Caregivers must consider cultural and religious meanings of pain, Dahlin says. Some believe you must endure it, she says.

2. Some patients fear they will become addicted to the pain medication. "It's just not an issue," Ford retorts. This just does not happen when you are using the drug to control cancer pain, she says. "It just isn't the same situation [as a drug addict] at all," she stresses. A drug addict, Ford points out, uses drugs for a completely different reason—a buzz or a high. The pills and patches used for cancer pain control do not have these effects. The most common side effect is constipation, "and that is not addictive," Ford says. (Some people also experience sleepiness or confusion, and that is an

> 66
> Treating the patient and not just the disease is important.
> —Cancer specialist Judith M. Ford, M.D., Ph.D., assistant professor, Department of Radiation Oncology at UCLA and Jonsson Cancer Center
> 99

indication that they are on too high of a dose, Ford says.) Moreover, morphine or other similar opiates are safe drugs when used correctly. They won't damage organs the way aspirin and other pain killers can. If you take too much morphine, you just sleep it off, she says. And, unlike other pain killers, there's no dose threshold where you don't get more effect with more drug. (However, if you've been addicted in the past, there may be a resistance, she says, making pain control harder.) When the cause of your pain is resolved, your doctor can safely wean you off of the morphine, so you won't become an addict, Ford says.

Note: Being put on morphine doesn't mean your cancer is terminal, Ford stresses. It's just to make your life more functional, she says.

Besides medication, there are other techniques, sometimes used in combination, to control pain:

- *Radiation therapy*—Tumors in some areas of the body can cause pain and pressure that can be alleviated with radiation, which works by killing off the cancer cells in the tumor, thus relieving pressure on the nerves, Ford says. An effective method of pain relief, radiation can be used to reduce pain in one or two sites at a time, Ford says. It is particularly effective for bone pain and will often relieve pain due to movement more effectively than medication. Eighty percent of patients with bone pain will obtain some or complete pain relief with external beam irradiation.

- *Surgery*—Surgery is occasionally used to excise tumors causing pain, to stabilize a bone to prevent fracture,or to relieve or prevent spinal cord compression.

Bright Idea
If you're worried about drowsiness, a pain specialist can use implantable pumps, so the morphine is placed in a local area.

▪ *Chemotherapy or hormone therapy*—Both of these treatments are systemic approaches.

In general, the response rate for cancer pain is higher for radiation than chemotherapy, but chemtherapy has the advantage of treating all areas of disease at once. In metastatic breast cancer, however, chemotherapy has one of the highest response rates. Hormone therapy, which is also effective for metastatic disease, has the advantage of having fewer side effects as well as having a systemic effect, but may take about two months to be effective. Chemotherapy and hormone therapy may give the patient prolonged periods of pain control, even though the cancer is metastatic, Ford says. A good response to chemotherapy or hormone therapy may make a woman with breast cancer totally functional and pain free without long-term pain management, she says.

The symptoms of brain tumors, which seldom cause pain, per se, but which may cause headaches due to swelling can be controlled easily with steroids, Ford says. (Note: The tumor itself does not induce pain, but the swelling of the brain and the supporting tissues cause pain.) And there are other ways to control other types of pain—a lesion in the hip, for example, can be treated with a hip replacement to get rid of cancer pain and the tumor.

The list of options to deal with pain is extensive, Ford says, emphasizing that treatment "should be tailored to the patient's need."

In addition to these pain treatments, there are non-drug options, including acupuncture and electrical stimulation. Acupuncture, especially near the point of pain, is thought to work by releasing endorphins, morphine-like peptides that bind to neuron receptors and diminish pain. Electrical methods include transcutaneous electrical nerve stimulation, brief pulses of electricity to nerve endings under the skin, and brain stimulation, which is useful for pain associated with advanced cancer. Brain stimulation, however, involves the risks associated with brain surgery.

Other non-drug treatment for chronic pain includes counseling, relaxation training, meditation, hypnosis, biofeedback, and behavior modification.

The placebo effect can also control pain. Placebos are made from a sugar pill or salt water injection. Patients in some studies are told they may be given a drug or placebo. When administered, they are not told which they received. For years, doctors have attributed the placebo effect to suggestion, distraction, the patient's optimism that something is being done, or the desire to please the doctor (placebo actually means "I will please" in Latin), according to the National Institute of Neurological Disorders and Stroke (NINDS), one of the National Institutes of Health.

However, more recent studies suggest that the placebo effect may be neurochemical. "[P]eople who respond to a placebo for pain relief—a remarkably consistent 35 percent in any experiment using placebos—are able to tap into their brains' endorphin systems," according to NINDS. Endorphins are, as noted earlier, morphine-like peptides that bind to neuron receptors and diminish pain.

To evaluate the placebo effect, investigators asked adults who were scheduled to get their wisdom teeth removed to volunteer in a pain experiment. Following surgery, some patients were given morphine, some naloxone, a drug that prevents endorphins and morphine from working, and some a placebo. About a third of those who took the placebo reported pain relief. These people were then given naloxone. They all reported a return of pain, according to NINDS.

It is not known how people who respond to placebos gain access to pain control systems in the brain. Some scientists think stress may be a factor because people who are very anxious are more likely to respond to a placebo for pain than those who are calmer. However, NINDS says that dental surgery itself may be stressful enough to trigger the release of endorphins.

There are some healthcare providers who are uncomfortable writing prescriptions for pain relief, according to Dahlin and others. If your healthcare provider isn't helping you receive satisfactory relief from any pain you are experiencing, get a second opinion or see a pain specialist. Call a nearby cancer center to get a referral or contact the American Academy of Pain Medicine, 4700 W. Lake Ave., Glenview, IL 60025; 847/375-4731.

Just the facts

- There are many tools, such as distraction and relaxation techniques, that you can use to get through treatments.

- You can alter your diet to reduce or eliminate some side effects.

- Lymphedema can be controlled through massage therapy.

- Cancer pain can be controlled without grogginess.

GET THE SCOOP ON...
What peripheral stem cell support and bone marrow
transplantation are ▪ Why researchers are studying
high-dose chemotherapy supported by peripheral stem cell
or bone marrow transplants ▪ Why the preliminary results of
bone marrow transplant studies are controversial ▪ How
the high-dose chemotherapy trials differed

High-Dose Chemotherapy and Stem Cell or Bone Marrow Transplants

Chapter 9

The use of high-dose chemotherapy supported by autologous peripheral stem cell transplants (stem cell transplant for short) or bone
marrow transplants has been under investigation in
clinical trials for more than a decade. In May 1999,
preliminary results of phase III trials were announced
by the scientific community.

In this chapter, we'll explain what high-dose
chemotherapy supported with stem cell or bone marrow transplant is and why this method of treatment is
thought by some physicians to hold promise. We'll
also summarize and discuss the preliminary results of
these trials.

The lowdown on high-dose chemotherapy

Many women with breast cancer relapse after standard chemotherapy because microscopic cells are

sometimes left behind and grow into metastatic disease. Some of these women enter high-dose chemotherapy trials. High-dose chemotherapy is based on the hypothesis that the high doses will accomplish three things:

1. Kill off any cancer cells remaining in the body after the primary and subsequent treatments;

2. Overcome any drug resistance (cancer cells, like bacteria, can mutate and become resistant to drugs they've already be introduced to);

3. Increase the cure rate.

High-dose chemotherapy is not experimental in leukemia, lymphoma, and some other hematopoietic malignancies. But because its effectiveness in breast cancer remains to be proven, it's considered experimental in breast cancer.

High-dose chemotherapy must be supported by autologous stem cell transplant or, less frequently, bone marrow transplant. The stem cell or bone marrow transplant is used to replenish the blood cells destroyed by such high doses of drugs. Stem cells are the most primitive cells in the bone marrow from which all blood cells are derived. Stem cells, collected from the blood, are used in the vast majority of transplant cases because they regrow faster than marrow cells, which are harvested directly from the bone. (If enough cells from circulation are not harvested then bone marrow cells are used.) Both procedures are delivered by a process similar to a blood transfusion. However, while stem cells can be collected as an outpatient, bone marrow harvest requires an inpatient operation.

As noted earlier, bone marrow transplants are done much less frequently than stem cell transplants,

> "
> We expect that there will be lively discussion, debate, and even disagreement among physicians about the implications of these findings... Some may consider the matter settled, at least for these particular patient groups, and will no longer consider high-dose chemotherapy with transplants worthy of further testing. Others will be more impressed with the limitations of the present trials and will be eager to continue studying different high-dose combinations.
> —Robert Wittes, M.D., director of NCI's Division of Cancer Treatment and Diagnosis.
> "

which work faster and are less invasive. There are four types of bone marrow transplantation:

1. *Autologous*—this form uses the patient's own bone marrow.

2. *Allogeneic*—this uses a closely matched relative's marrow.

3. *Syngeneic*—this uses bone marrow of an identical twin.

4. *Matched unrelated donor*—this uses the marrow of an unrelated donor whose bone marrow closely matches yours. (This BMT method has not been used for breast cancer.)

Prepping the patient

Before entering the hospital, there are a list of things you must do to protect yourself against infection and other complications, including the following:

■ Wash the clothes you plan to wear in the hospital and dry them in a hot dryer. Place them directly from the hot dryer into a clean plastic bag.

■ Do not drink any alcohol for two weeks prior to admission because alcohol can enhance the toxicity of the chemotherapy.

■ Trim your fingernails and toenails prior to admission. You will not been permitted to do so during your hospitalization. That's because a cut may open the door to an infection.

■ To make yourself more comfortable, you may bring a new pillow, one without feathers. It must still be in its original bag to keep it from being contaminated with germs.

■ Plastic and metal items, such as radios and video-cassettes, must be cleaned before being brought

Unofficially...
High-dose chemotherapy is administered to kill cancer cells throughout the body. However, it also kills other cells, such as bone marrow cells. Bone marrow is the spongy tissue inside bones that produces blood and immune system cells, including white blood cells, red blood cells, and platelets. Therefore, the immune system must be replenished with either a stem cell or, rarely, a bone marrow transplant.

into the hospital room. Books, newspapers, posters, and photos require no special treatment.

■ If you're one of the few women not already bald from previous chemotherapy, you may want to cut your hair short before entering the hospital. A short haircut will be easier to manage and be less of an emotional shock if it does begin to fall out after treatment begins. You may bring along a washable turban, hat, or cap, but wigs are not permitted because they may carry germs.

■ Plants are not permitted, nor are floral arrangements, cosmetics, deodorants, lotions, soaps, toothbrush and toothpaste, and razors. Self-care items will be provided at the hospital.

Before entering the hospital you'll undergo a series of tests, including:

■ Blood work

■ CAT scan(s)

■ Bone marrow biopsy(ies)

■ Heart studies

■ Pulmonary function tests

■ Liver and kidney function tests

The last three tests are done to make sure that your organs can tolerate the high-dose chemotherapy.

The actual stem transplant—whether the stem cells were harvested from the blood or bone marrow—is done through an IV, and only takes 5 to 15 minutes. During that time, your blood pressure, heart rate, temperature, and breathing will be monitored by your physician and a nurse, who will be there during the re-infusion process. You'll also be given medication to prevent any minor reactions. The most common side effects of stem cell re-infusion are fever, headache, chills, and flushing.

Bright Idea
If you are considering undergoing high-dose chemotherapy and stem cell transplant, it's important to remember that it remains experimental. Join a trial at an expert center with a proven track record for safety.

Because your immune system will be weakened by the treatment, you'll have your own private room. The door to your room will remain closed most of the time. Your hospital stay will last about two to three weeks. During that time, you should instruct your visitors not to sit on the bed or recliner, use the bathroom, eat in your room, or touch any medical supplies in order to reduce your risk of infection.

(Note: Sometimes follow-up after the stem cell transplant is done on an outpatient basis. This money-saving alternative, when available and appropriate, requires a trained, dedicated team familiar with transplant toxicities and complications to see you on a daily basis. Infection control requires prophylactic broad-spectrum antibiotics.)

It is essential that you wash your hands after going to the bathroom and take a bath every day to decrease the bacteria on your skin. (Bone marrow/stem cell transplant units have baths and showers.) Frequent showers can cause the skin to dry out,so you'll be given lotion to help prevent itching.

Because high doses of chemotherapy can cause mouth sores and a weakened immune system, you'll need to be extra cautious about keeping your mouth and teeth clean. (It's also a good idea to have your teeth cleaned by a dentist before you're hospitalized.) That's because mouth sores serve as entryways for infection-causing bacteria. These infections can be severe because of your low white blood cell counts, granulocytes, and lymphocytes. See Chapter 8 for tips on dealing with mouth sores and other chemotherapy-related side effects.

High-dose chemotherapy can cause a low white blood cell count, referred to as neutropenia. Neutropenia may cause chronic dental infections to flare up. In addition, it can cause mouth sores, mouth

Moneysaver
Your state insurance commissioner's office can often work with your insurance company, healthcare providers, and experts at major cancer centers to get procedures covered that insurance companies might normally refuse, claiming they're experimental, such as bone marrow transplants.

dryness, and yeast infections. Sometimes viral infections are re-activated as a result. To fight infection, you'll receive dental care throughout the treatment and afterward.

You'll also be evaluated by a physical therapist before starting treatment. The physical therapist will provide you with an exercise and ambulation program. It is important to exercise every day and to practice deep breathing and gentle stretches as well as muscle strengthening routines. It is important to keep yourself in good physical condition during and after treatment.

As a result of treatment, your red blood counts, white blood counts, and platelets will dip.

Watch Out!
Salads, fruit, and raw vegetables can have infectious agents on their surface.

To keep close tabs on your blood levels, and to give you intravenous medications (which may include medications for pain, nausea, anxiety, and strep, antibiotics, antifungals, antivirals, and more) one or two central venous catheters will be inserted into your chest. The insertion is done in surgery. You'll have the opportunity to meet with your surgeon before the surgery or, if you choose, just before entering the operating room.

After discharge from the hospital, you'll need to closely follow food preparation guidelines for about two to three weeks. In addition, you will need to avoid certain foods. There are also restaurant concerns that you need to deal with such as avoiding uncooked food. You should also avoid eating food prepared by those unaware of your weakened immune system and who may contaminate food with bacteria by not washing utensils and countertops thoroughly after handling raw meat or poultry.

High-dose chemotherapy trials

High-dose chemotherapy with stem cell support was

evaluated in five trials presented in May 1999 at the annual meeting of the American Society of Clinical Oncology (ASCO). Two of these studies did not show a significant benefit of high-dose chemotherapy in terms of overall survival, and the results of two others were too early to interpret. A study of 100 patients in South Africa did show benefit but used a different high-dose treatment strategy than the others, although the control arm was standard-dose chemotherapy.

There are many as of yet unanswered questions about these transplant studies and their statistical power, including the study size, the power of the dose, and the schedule of drug administration as well as the extent of disease and evaluation prior to high-dose chemotherapy.

The results of these studies have caused controversy among clinicians, especially because of the promising South African study. But others saw the predominantly negative outcomes as a sign that this treatment method offers no benefit to women with breast cancer, except perhaps in a certain subset(s) of patients.

The theory behind high-dose chemotherapy

High-dose chemotherapy followed by stem cell transplant is based on test tube studies and animal models that demonstrate the effectiveness of high-dose regimens on aggressive breast tumors. With lower doses, not all of these cells are likely to be eradicated, and subsequently cancer may grow back as metastatic disease. It is important to understand that breast cancer cells can become resistant to drugs they've already been exposed to.

However, the protective mechanisms that allow cancer cells to survive standard-dose chemotherapy can be overridden, and it is possible to take advantage of an injured cell's natural self sacrifice, a process called programmed cell death (which is also known as *apoptosis*). Since cancer cells are genetically unstable, they are more vulnerable to apoptosis than normal cells. Therefore, researchers use different combinations of drugs to maximize cancer cell death while protecting host tissues and minimizing side effects.

Apoptosis can be achieved using other mechanisms, including immune therapy; however, when a woman has a relatively large tumor, there are a very large number of cancer cells involved. For example, it has been estimated that a 1 centimeter lump of tumor contains up to a billion cancer cells. Thus, locally advanced primary breast tumors have a very high likelihood of spreading outside the breast, even though it can't be obviously demonstrated on scans because the cells are microscopic, and these cells are the most likely of the cancer cells to be resistant to chemotherapy. Such tumors, as well as metastatic disease, are difficult to reduce to a size that can be successfully controlled with other treatments, including hormone and biological therapies. Immune therapy is ineffective in patients with large and small tumors because the number of cancerous cells is so large.

Replenishing the immune system

High-dose chemotherapy with stem cell transplantation attempts to reduce the number of tumor cells so that other treatments can potentially work better. For example, high-dose chemotherapy can be used in young patients for locally advanced, inoperable cancer to make their tumors operable and amenable to radiation therapy.

Because chemotherapy targets rapidly dividing cells, including blood progenitor cells, low blood cell counts make it impossible to administer high doses without protecting the bone marrow. To protect the bonemarrow, a stem cell "transplant" or rescue needs to be done. High-dose chemotherapy supported by autologous stem cell re-infusion allows higher doses of cytotoxic drugs to be administered with more safety. Why stem cells and not bone marrow? Peripheral blood-derived stem cells regrow quicker than bone-marrow derived stem cells because they are more mature.

The stem cells are taken from you before the high-dose chemotherapy and are transplanted afterward to restore your immune system. The stem cell transplant itself is a relatively simple and usually painless process. Here's how it works: You get "plugged" into a special pheresis machine—your blood comes out of one vein, the stem cells are spun out and removed, and your blood is injected back through another vein. The process is called leuko-pheresis and is usually done on an outpatient basis.

The stem cells are processed, "cleaned," and stored at -70°C, a temperature that safely preserves them. Several days after the high-dose chemotherapy, the stem cells are injected back into you in a process similar to a blood transfusion but more quickly in that the re-infusion takes about 15 to 20 minutes. The stem cells circulate back to the bone marrow and repopulate, so red blood cells, white blood cells, and platelets return to normal levels. Bone marrow transplants work the same way.

If you decide to undergo this process, remember that practice makes perfect. Centers that treat fewer patients have higher treatment-related death rates, and as noted in Chapter 16, physicians and hospitals with more experience have better patient survival rates. Nationwide the treatment-related death rate is less than three percent, and in top centers transplant-related mortality is less than one percent.

High-dose chemotherapy on trial

High-dose chemotherapy has been used in the treatment of metastatic and very high-risk primary breast cancer that has spread to multiple lymph nodes, despite a lack of research indicating a benefit in survival. Early phase I and phase II trials showed this strategy may hold promise for increased survival. These results needed to be tested on a large scale and compared with standard dose regimens. To give patients and physicians a better basis for their treatment decisions, preliminary results of phase III trials were presented at the ASCO meeting in May 1999. The trials all differed in their approach—using different drugs, different dosing, different populations, and more. As noted earlier, the results were inconclusive.

Unofficially...
More than 12,000 women with breast cancer in the United States have undergone high-dose chemotherapy with stem cell or bone marrow transplant since the mid-1980s.

Three of the trials presented at the ASCO meeting used high-dose chemotherapy and bone marrow or stem cell transplant in the adjuvant treatment of women with very high-risk primary breast cancer as defined by the investigators as those whose disease had spread into at least 10 lymph nodes. Two trials investigated high-dose chemotherapy treatment of advanced, metastatic breast cancer. (Bone marrow transplants were used more frequently in these trials than they are today because these trials began years ago when the technology was not as advanced.)

The preliminary results of two studies suggest that high-dose chemotherapy with bone marrow or stem cell transplant has similar survival rates to lower doses of chemotherapy but has more toxicity. A third study was inconclusive and a fourth showed more toxicity to the non-transplant arm. (The transplant arms had mortality from the high-dose chemotherapy, but, overall, the lower-dose chemotherapy, because it was of greater duration, gave longer periods of time with chemotherapy symptoms.) The fifth study had positive results.

Take note of the differences

There were many differences among the studies, including:

- Number of study participants (the power to detect benefits and/or harm is dependent on the number of patients)

- Patient characteristics, such as age and menopausal status

- Drugs or combinations of drugs tested

- Dose intensity and number of cycles of drug administration

- Three studies, referred to as the adjuvant trials, looked at women whose cancer had spread to the axillary lymph nodes (those under the arm). These women are at high risk of recurrence.

- Two studies looked at women with metastatic disease.

Take note of the differences—adjuvant trials

The three adjuvant trials (those that enrolled women at high risk of recurrence but without evidence of disease beyond the breast and axillary (underarm) lymph nodes) were based in the United States, Scandinavia, and South Africa. There were differences among these studies, including the following:

- The number of study participants. The more study participants, the better the study can detect small differences between treatments being com-

Watch Out!
The effectiveness of high-dose chemotherapy can depend on the stage of disease, so the adjuvant and metastatic studies should be considered separately.

pared and the less likely that detected differences are due to chance. Large studies have another advantage—they are more likely to have an equal balance of participants sharing the same characteristics (menopausal status, age, number of positive lymph nodes, hormone receptor status, and other medical conditions) in both the experimental and control arms. An imbalance of patient characteristics can lead to inaccurate results referred to as "study bias." (The other two studies didn't have enough participants to draw meaningful conclusions.)

- The U.S. (CALGB-Cancer and Leukemia Group B, a multidisciplinary cooperative cancer treatment group funded by the National Cancer Institute) and Scandinavian trials used several cycles of low-dose chemotherapy prior to administering the high-dose chemotherapy.

- The South African study administered high-dose chemotherapy first.

- The U.S. study was the only one to use the same drugs in both the high- and lower-dose chemotherapy regimens.

Take note of the differences—metastatic disease trials

The metastatic trials were based in the U.S. (ECOG—Eastern Cooperative Oncology Group) and France. They shared both similarities and differences, including the following:

- Both trials were small, but the U.S. trial looked at 184 women while the French study only looked at 61 women.

- All participants in both trials received some initial lower-dose chemotherapy to shrink the

Watch Out!
The findings of the trials only apply to women whose breast cancer had metastasized and those at high risk of relapse because the cancer had spread to many lymph nodes, according to Robert Wittes, M.D., director of NCI's Division of Cancer Treatment and Diagnosis. Furthermore, he cautions, the results may not apply to other high-dose regimens.

metastases. About 25 percent of the women in both studies had a complete disappearance of their cancer due to previous treatment. The rest had a partial response, meaning a partial disappearance. After the responses were noted, the study participants were randomly assigned to the high- or lower-dose treatment arms.

■ The drugs used in the two studies (both high and low dose) were different.

The adjuvant trials—spelling it out

The CALGB intergroup U.S. trial studied 783 women with primary breast cancer that had spread to at least 10 axillary lymph nodes. The women were randomly assigned to two groups: one received high-dose chemotherapy (cyclophosphamide, cisplatin, and BCNU—carmustine) with bone marrow and/or peripheral blood stem cell support and the other received intermediate-dose chemotherapy using the same drugs. All the women received a standard chemotherapy regimen prior to the randomization. In addition, all of the women received radiation therapy to the chest area. Women with positive hormone receptor status or unknown status received tamoxifen.

The preliminary results showed participants in the high-dose chemotherapy group had about a 68 percent chance of surviving without breast cancer for three years and a 78 percent chance of overall survival. Those in the intermediate dose group had a 64 percent chance of being disease free and 80 percent of overall survival after three years. These results showed no significant differences between the two groups.

There were fewer recurrences among the high-dose group, but it is not yet clear how that will impact survival. At a median follow-up of 42 months, an

Bright Idea
If you want to hear the discussion of the trials presented at the American Society of Clinical Oncology meeting, go to www.asco.org. You can listen to the virtual meeting while viewing the slide presentation.

Unofficially...
In earlier trials
bone marrow
transplant was
the only proce-
dure around to
preserve blood
cells. As technol-
ogy advanced,
peripheral stem
cell transplants
were added. Then
peripheral stem
cells were used
alone, with bone
marrow trans-
plants as backup.

updated analysis shows a 67.8 percent relapse-free survival for the lower-dose group versus a 78.4 percent relapse-free survival for the higher-dose arm. But the high-dose group had 29 (7.4 percent) treatment-related deaths, thus the overall survival advantage is likely to be 10 to 15 percent at best. There were no treatment-related deaths among the lower-dose group.

There were no measurable differences in quality of life between the two treatment arms one year following completion of chemotherapy.

The South African trial studied 154 women with primary breast cancer involving 10 or more lymph nodes. The results showed increased survival rates (there was a 17 percent mortality rate in the high-dose arm compared with a 35 percent in the standard dose arm) and lower relapse rates (25 percent in the high-dose group compared with 66 percent in the standard dose arm) after more than five years of follow-up. Women assigned to the standard-dose arm received cyclophosphamide, adriamycin, or epirubicin, and 5-fluorouracil (CAF). Women assigned to the high-dose arm received cyclophosphamide, mitoxantrone, and VP16.

The Scandinavian trial studied 525 women with high-risk breast cancer. The results showed no overall benefit of high-dose chemotherapy versus "tailored" chemotherapy—doses tailored according to the patients' blood counts.

In this trial, women were randomly assigned to a group that received nine cycles of "tailored" FEC (5-flourouracil, epirubicin, cytoxan) or three cycles of standard FEC followed by high-dose chemotherapy supported with stem cell transplant. The women were followed for a median of 20 months. There were 55

Unofficially...
Recurrence rates
are not the same
as survival rates.
The goal of these
studies was to
"cure" the cancer.

recurrences and 15 deaths in the "tailored" group compared with 78 relapses and 25 deaths in the high-dose arm. Two of the deaths were directly related to the high-dose chemotherapy. In addition, eight women in the "tailored" group developed leukemia.

The metastatic trials—spelling it out

The ECOG intergroup U.S. trial, which had results as of March 31, 1999, is the largest metastatic randomized trial of high-dose chemotherapy with stem cell transplant to date—553 women, aged 23 to 60, were enrolled initially. Preliminary results showed no significant difference in overall survival or lethal toxicity compared with prolonged, standard dose, maintenance chemotherapy.

All the women who participated in this trial first completed a standard chemotherapy regimen of six cycles of either cyclophosphamide, doxorubicin (Adriamycin), and fluorouracil (CAF) or cyclophosphamide, methotrexate, and fluorouracil (CMF). Those who had complete or partial responses were randomly assigned to one of the treatment arms: high-dose chemotherapy with stem-cell transplant or conventional-dose maintenance chemotherapy for another 18 months. Those treated in the high-dose arm completed treatment in approximately six months, whereas those in the lower-dose arm were treated for up to two years. Of the initial 553 women, 199 women (median age of 46) were eligible and agreed to continue participating in the trial. Of the 199 patients, 184 were able to be analyzed (101 women in the high-dose chemotherapy/stem cell transplant group and 83 in the maintenance chemotherapy group). The women were followed for a median of 37 months.

Of the metastatic trials, the results of the U.S.

Unofficially...
In the adjuvant trials, neither the U.S. nor the Scandinavian trial demonstrated a difference in survival rates between the high- and lower-dose groups. There were, however, fewer recurrences among women in the high-dose chemotherapy group in the U.S. trial.

Unofficially...
The South African study demonstrated a significantly increased survival rate. The challenge is whether they can apply these findings to American patients.

Unofficially...
What is the difference between CAF and CMF? Adriamycin is substituted for methotrexate. Randomized trials have shown CAF (or FAC) is more effective than CMF in metastatic breast cancer.

study do not suggest an advantage of high-dose chemotherapy with stem cell support exists for women who had only partial responses to induction chemotherapy, the first phase of standard treatment. But the study did not include enough women who had a complete response to induction chemotherapy to draw a conclusion of whether that group would benefit from high-dose chemotherapy supported by stem cell transplant. Many researchers would like to see continued investigation of high-dose chemotherapy in women with complete response to induction chemotherapy. Furthermore, high-dose chemotherapy may prove useful for women with partial responses to induction chemotherapy if a different regimen than the one tested is used or if the high-dose regimen is used up front, as it was in the South African study, rather than after repeated cycles of standard-dose chemotherapy. There was no significant difference in toxicity between the two treatments. One woman died during the stem cell transplant from liver disease, which was likely caused by the high-dose chemotherapy plus the initial standard chemotherapy.

In France, 61 women with metastatic breast cancer who had responded to chemotherapy were randomly assigned to either high-dose chemotherapy—cyclophosphamide, mitoxantrone, and melphalan supported by stem cell transplant—or standard doses of chemotherapy (anthracycline-based) treatment arm.

Preliminary results showed no statistically significant difference in progression-free survival or overall survival after five years, but progression-free survival (cases in which the breast cancer does not progress) was noted at three years as well as a quality-of-life advantage among the high-dose arm.

The overall survival rate was 18.5 percent in the standard-dose arm compared with 29.8 percent in the high-dose arm. The rate of recurrence was 50.8 percent in the high-dose arm and 79.3 percent in the standard-dose arm at three years. But at five years, the recurrence rates were nearly the same: 90.7 percent and 90.8 percent, respectively. The delay in relapse for women who received the high-dose chemotherapy could mean a longer treatment-free period, increasing quality of life. There were no therapy-related deaths or unusual toxicities.

Analyzing the data

There were several experts who analyzed the data presented at the May 1999 ASCO meeting. Robert Livingston, M.D., a well-recognized researcher at the University of Washington and one of the experts who analyzed the data, said the U.S. ECOG (PBT-1) study suffers from attrition (women leaving the study). "You have heard that PBT-1 was a negative study. One question we must ask is, 'What is our confidence in a negative result?'" he asked.

For 184 patients in the metastatic trial, "the absolute degree of difference in three-year survival which could be detected with 90 percent power was 25 percent," Livingston said. "On the other hand, for the 45 complete responders, even had the randomization resulted in an equal distribution between the two arms, we have the power only to detect a 50 percent absolute improvement in three-year survival with reasonable confidence," he noted. Bottom line? There is uncertainty about study results due to some inadequacies in the study's design.

It is also difficult to interpret it as a negative trial, Livingston said, because the patient group studied would be expected to show little improvement from

Unofficially...
A national trial testing high-dose chemotherapy in women with four to nine positive nodes is currently in progress as is a trial testing higher doses of another drug in women with 10 or more positive lymph nodes, according to the National Cancer Institute.

the application of high-dose chemotherapy. The three patient groups not expected to do well include those with the following:

1. Drug-resistant disease

2. Three or more metastatic sites or CNS (central nervous system) metastases

3. Prior adjuvant chemotherapy

(Note: These three groups generally do not respond as well to chemotherapy as their opposites. Opposites would be patients with drug-sensitive disease, limited metastatic disease sites (that is, one or two), and no central nervous system disease. Opposites also would not have had prior adjuvant therapy. All of these opposite groups have been shown to have better results with chemotherapy.)

Patients with chemotherapy-resistant disease were excluded in this study as were those with known central nervous system disease, and it's unknown how many people had three or more cancer sites. But 55 percent in the transplant arm had received prior chemotherapy, and today that portion could be even higher, Livingston said. Again, these factors show weaknesses in the study design.

Livingston said that in women who had some response (partial responders to the initial standard chemotherapy) to high-dose chemotherapy is not justified as a standard policy after induction (standard) chemotherapy. However, for women whose tumors were completely eradicated (complete responders) the design of the PBT-1 "trial is inadequate to detect even a large difference in response to the high-dose chemotherapy, if one exists," he said. Earlier studies showed promise in complete responders. So, if you have a complete response to the initial chemotherapy, high-dose chemotherapy may still be helpful.

"
Now is not the end. It is not even the beginning of the end. But it is, perhaps, the end of the beginning.
—Winston Churchill
"

Livingston summarized his analysis of the role of high-dose chemotherapy plus autologous stem transplant for metastatic breast cancer in 1999 by stating that trials up to this point do not support the use of high-dose chemotherapy supported by stem cell or bone marrow transplant on a routine basis. But, he said, it is unclear if there is a subset of women—those who have had a complete response to the initial standard chemotherapy—who may benefit from this treatment method because of the study design weaknesses "and the possible contribution of non-treatment related factors in a comparison across studies."

Livingston theorized that a delayed transplant—when the high-dose chemotherapy takes place well after the standard regimen—might fail because conventional chemotherapy may result in visual shrinkage of the tumor, but "may at the same time promote the survival, multiplication, and further mutation of multi-drug resistant cells initially present as a relatively small population [those that weren't killed by the standard chemotherapy but were too small to detect on a scan]." This in turn may produce resistance by the cancerous cells to the high-dose chemotherapy.

He noted that the South African study used high-dose chemotherapy with stem cell support first, that is, there the patients did not undergo standard chemotherapy before undergoing high-dose chemotherapy. Twenty percent of the women had a long-term, disease-free period. Livingston thought that up-front, high-dose chemotherapy may work by eliminating the postulated microscopic cancer cells that may remain after standard chemotherapy. Because these cancer cells develop a resistance to the drugs, it is thought that they therefore cannot be eradicated by standard chemotherapy and will ultimately account for failure of subsequent high-dose chemotherapy.

Even if the results of the South African trial are reproduced, there is still an 80 percent failure rate. Why? It may be that the high-dose drug regimens and autologous stem cell transplants, which are limited to one or two cycles (rounds), only kill a percentage of the cancer cells, Livingston says. For patients with a large tumor burden, this might not be enough.

(Note: The cycles to which Livingston refers are from another trial, using CNV, by the same South African investigators.)

For the future Livingston made two suggestions:

1. High-dose chemotherapy supported by stem cell transplant clinical trials should be considered for women whose cancer has spread but who have had a complete response (that is, their tumors are gone on scans) to standard chemotherapy. (Long-term remission can be achieved in up to 35 percent of women whose cancer has spread and who have a complete response to standard chemotherapy. In contrast, prior studies suggest that only 5-10 percent of women with complete responses to initial therapy but who do not get high-dose chemotherapy stay disease-free long-term.)

2. A new paradigm of high-dose chemotherapy with autologous stem cell support followed by conventional or novel therapy should be considered in clinical trials.

Gabriel N. Hortobagyi, M.D, from the University of Texas M.D. Anderson Cancer Center also discussed the data presented at the ASCO meeting. He gave the following possible explanations for the lack of major therapeutic benefit seen in most of these trials:

1. Chemotherapy drugs have, at best, modest therapeutic effects.

2. There's a limit to how much a dose can be intensified.

3. Rapid tumor recovery begins after incomplete eradication.

4. Re-infusion of contaminated stem cells may contribute to relapse. (In metastatic disease, tumor cells circulate in the blood.)

Hortobagyi stated that high-dose chemotherapy as the first or only treatment done in the South African study should be tested, as should multiple cycles of intermediate-dose chemotherapy.

But Hortobagyi concluded that high-dose chemotherapy adds little or no benefit to standard adjuvant programs and the toxicity is higher. However, he said, we need to see more mature data. In addition, high-dose treatments must continue to be done in controlled trials and not as standard treatment. (Many women have received high-dose chemotherapy outside of the trial setting. Based on these data, it is no longer ethically acceptable.)

One must distinguish between strategies and tactics (methodologies) in deciding what information you get out of a study, says John Durant, M.D., executive vice-president of ASCO. The strategy in these studies is using extremely high doses of chemotherapy (supported by stem cell transplant and/or BMT), which the investigators hypothesized would improve outcomes for some breast cancer patients. But there were a variety of patient groups (patients with certain shared characteristics) that were not the subjects of these trials and who are most likely to benefit. Those who were included in the study were at the highest risk for poor outcome without the high-dose chemotherapy. (The "good" patients left the trial.)

You must design trials to test the strategy, and there was only one trial that did that—the South African trial, Durant points out. It tested whether high-dose chemotherapy used as the initial chemotherapy treatment worked more effectively than the same drugs used at standard doses. There was no attempt to produce a tumor response with standard-dose chemotherapy before they attempted the high-dose chemotherapy. Whether that tactic made it a positive study is a different question, he says. But if the methodologies used by the other study investigators weren't correct, then this could be the reason for their failure to illicit a positive response. Furthermore, the Swedish and CALGB trials used very high doses for the standard regimen, so those studies didn't have a real comparison of high-dose to standard chemotherapy, he notes.

Another problem? These trials are antiques, Durant says. (They used older drugs and older technologies.) Many were started a long time ago and they suffer from slow accession (accumulation of participants).

Meanwhile, better and new drugs of different kinds are appearing. We don't know what paclitaxel (Taxol) or trastuzumab (Herceptin) would have added to the outcome and where they fit into this strategy. These drugs must be added before conclusions on the effectiveness of high-dose chemotherapy can be drawn, he says. In addition, it must be determined who might benefit from this strategy.

Durant, like others, points out that the results in some cases are premature, so outcomes may change. He doubts this is the case for the metastatic cases. For women with metastatic disease these trials were

Unofficially...
The only consensus among oncologists is that further research on high-dose chemotherapy and bone marrow transplants is necessary, according to the American Society of Clinical Oncology.

not encouraging with regard to the use of high-dose chemotherapy as a strategy, even though the tactics, the way the trials were set up, may have been poor, he says.

This is really just the beginning, Durant adds. It took 25 years to get the right monoclonal antibody to develop Herceptin, he points out. The monocolonal antibody strategy had been all but abandoned before it hit paydirt. There will be new trials testing this high-dose strategy, Durant says. If the South African study is right, it taught us something very important about developing chemotherapeutic resistance, he says.

Bottom line? The jury is therefore still out, and the question of the role of high-dose chemotherapy in breast cancer remains open.

The jury is out

Although many members of the jury voiced strong opinions based on the preliminary data presented at the ASCO meeting, the final verdict won't be in for several years. Much work remains to be done to determine the true results of most of these studies and, if possible, to replicate the South African study.

The positive results of the small South African study should not be disregarded, according to Richard Klausner, M.D., director of the National Cancer Institute (NCI), which sponsored the two U.S. trials. "The chemotherapy agents used in this trial were different from those in the other trials and the particular approach employed by the South Africans may be responsible for the positive results," he explains.

Klausner stressed the overall importance of participating in trials. "These five trials took nine years to yield preliminary data because it took so long to enroll the required number of patients," he said. "Greater participation by physicians and patients in

Bright Idea
If you have advanced or an aggressive form of breast cancer and you or your doctor has ruled out high-dose chemotherapy supported by a stem cell transplant, there are alternative treatments available, including standard chemotherapy regimens, hormonal therapy, and other investigational treatments.

clinical trials would speed answers, not only to crucial questions concerning high-dose chemotherapy with transplants, but other cancer treatments as well."

Other researchers believe that high-dose chemotherapy is a modality that may be beneficial for a subset of patients. It may also provide a platform for other treatments, such as hormone or immune therapy, to work more effectively. In their view, this is a field in evolution and represents a continuum of incremental progress.

Future directions include novel combinations of high-dose chemotherapy, approaches targeting minimal residual tumor with immunotherapy, modulation of drug resistance, stem cell selection, integration of biotherapeutics such as Herceptin, and manipulation of tumor micro-environment with regard to angiogenesis.

Just the facts

- Most of the phase III clinical trials on high-dose chemotherapy did not support the positive findings of earlier trials.

- The findings of all these trials are preliminary, meaning it will take several years for the results to be final.

- The one study with positive findings used high-dose chemotherapy as the first line of treatment versus the other three studies that used it as a follow-up treatment.

- All the studies used different drugs, so they cannot be accurately compared with each other.

GET THE SCOOP ON...
Drugs that block tumor hormone receptors to stop tumor
growth ▪ How the body's own defenses are being enlisted in
the war on cancer ▪ How vaccines are boosting the body's
immune response to prevent recurrence ▪ Drugs that cut off
the tumor's blood supply to halt tumor growth

The Advancement of New Treatments

Chapter 10

The war on cancer continues to gain ground. For many years, the standard artillery included surgery, chemotherapy, and radiation. Now investigators are looking at the body's own mechanisms and resources to halt cancer growth and, in some cases, send it into retreat. There are also new, promising treatments, called angiogenesis inhibitors, that cut off the tumor's blood supply. On the horizon is gene therapy, which also holds promise for future victories.

In this chapter, we'll tell you about hormone treatments, immune therapy, angiogenesis inhibitors, and other biologically based treatments being used to fight cancer.

Digging into the arsenal: Hormone therapy

Some hormones, namely estrogen, cause cancer cells to grow. To keep cancer cell growth at bay, hormone therapy keeps malignant cells from getting the hormones they need to grow. There are two methods used to prevent the growth, spread, or recurrence of these tumors:

1. Systemic drugs, which deprive the cancer cells of hormones by blocking the hormones from the cell's hormone receptors.

2. Surgery, typically to remove the ovaries (oophorectomy), which make estrogen. The ovaries can also be made nonfunctional by irradiation. Both of these procedures are referred to as *ovarian ablation*. New methods of ovarian ablation have promoted new research in this area. Ovarian ablation is a treatment option for premenopausal women with ER+ metastatic breast cancer.

Hormone therapy is generally given to women whose tumors have estrogen and/or progesterone receptors, regardless of axillary node status (whether the cancer has traveled into the lymph nodes under the arm) and menopausal status. Sometimes it is given alone after surgery; other times it is administered after surgery and a regimen of chemotherapy—or in combination with the chemotherapy. It is also given to some women who are at high risk of developing breast cancer.

Unofficially...
Tamoxifen has been used for 20 years to treat women with advanced stage breast cancer.

Tamoxifen

Tamoxifen(Nolvadex), a selective estrogen receptor modulator (SERM), is the most common hormone therapy used for women with breast cancer. Not only does it help prevent cancerous growth in the affected breast, it also reduces the chances of a tumor developing in the other breast. Tamoxifen works by combining with estrogen receptors on the cancer cells, out-competing estrogen for the spot. By binding to these receptors, it blocks the stimulatory effects of estrogen and inhibits the growth and metabolism of breast cancer cells.

Tamoxifen is a pill usually taken one to three months after breast cancer surgery and continued for up to five years. Women at high risk of developing breast cancer may be prescribed tamoxifen in an attempt to prevent the disease from developing.

Prophylactic use of tamoxifen stems, in large part, from the results of the National Surgical Adjuvant Breast and Bowel Project (NSABP), which found that the drug reduced the rates of invasive and non-invasive breast cancer in healthy women. This co-operative study group looked at 13,388 healthy women who had an increased risk of breast cancer because they were either age 60 or older or age 35 to 59 with an increased risk greater than or equal to that of a 60-year-old woman. (At age 60, an estimated 17 out of every 1,000 women are expected to develop breast cancer within five years.) Of the women who were followed for almost four years, 89 women taking tamoxifen developed invasive breast cancer compared with 175 women who were in the placebo group. This demonstrated a 49 percent reduction. In this study, women on tamoxifen had 50 percent fewer diagnoses of noninvasive breast cancer—35 women taking the drug developed localized breast cancer compared with 69 women who were taking a placebo.

Tamoxifen works not only as an anti-estrogen, blocking estrogen receptors on cancer cells, but it also works as an estrogen in other parts of the body, including the bones. In the NSABP study, tamoxifen reduced the risk of hip, spine, and wrist fractures by almost 20 percent. However, tamoxifen increased the risk of endometrial cancer (36 women in taking tamoxifen developed endometrial cancer compared with 15 women in the placebo group), but this increased risk was seen predominantly in women aged 50 or older. All endometrial cancers in this group were localized (stage I), and the risk was similar to or less than that of postmenopausal women taking (single agent) estrogen replacement therapy.

To give you some perspective, in general, 0.7 per 1,000 healthy women in the general population develop endometrial cancer. About one in every 1,000 women with breast cancer develop endometrial cancer. In contrast, between 2 and 3 per 1,000 women with breast cancer who are treated with tamoxifen develop endometrial cancer. Because of this increased risk, you must not skip your annual pelvic exams.

Tamoxifen, particularly in women who are receiving chemotherapy, can cause blood clots in the inner thigh or leg (deep vein thrombosis) or lung (pulmonary embolism). In the NSABP trial, 53 women in the tamoxifen arm versus 28 women in the placebo arm developed pulmonary embolisms or deep-vein thrombosis. Both of these side effects are uncommon, but dangerous, and the consensus in the medical field seems to be that the benefits of taking tamoxifen far outweigh the risks. However, because these risks are present, you will undergo frequent blood tests and physical exams.

In addition, other side effects can result from taking tamoxifen, including the following:

- Nausea

- Hot flashes

- Irregular menstrual periods

- Vaginal spotting

- Increased fertility in younger women

Less common side effects caused by tamoxifen include the following:

- Vaginal itching, skin irritation, bleeding, drying

Watch Out!
Tamoxifen is associated with an increased risk of developing endometrial cancer. Symptoms of endometrial cancesr include pain and unusual vaginal bleeding.

of vaginal mucosa, or discharge

■ Depression

■ Loss of appetite

■ Headache

■ Eye problems

■ Weight gain

Anastrozole (Arimidex)/Letrozole (Femara)

Anastrozole (Arimidex) as well as letrozole (Femara)—the same class of drug with a similar mechanism of action—is a very effective drug in some patients with metastatic breast cancer, specifically those with breast cancer that has progressed despite using tamoxifen. It works by limiting the amount of estrogen a woman produces.

In postmenopausal women, the principle source of natural estrogen comes from the conversion of adrenally-generated androstenedione (an androgenic steroid produced by the ovaries and adrenal cortex) to estrone (a metabolite of estradiol, a potent estrogen) by aromatase (an enzyme that converts androgens to estrogens). Many breast cancers contain aromatase. Arimidex is a non-steroidal aromatase inhibitor that works by lowering estradiol (estrogen) concentrations in the blood.

Arimidex, a tablet, was approved by the FDA in late 1995 for treating stage IV breast cancer.

Arimidex's possible side effects include:

■ Nausea and vomiting (for which your doctor may prescribe medicine to prevent or treat)

■ Abdominal pain

■ Constipation

■ Diarrhea

■ Loss of appetite

- Hot flashes
- Night sweats
- Menstrual irregularity
- Bone or tumor pain
- Blood clot (pulmonary embolism—a blood clot in the lung)
- Shortness of breath
- Cough
- Inflammation of the pharynx
- Edema (swelling caused by the accumulation of large amounts of fluid)
- Dizziness
- Headaches
- Depression
- Rash
- Generalized weakness

Raloxifene

Raloxifene (Evista), like tamoxifen, is a selective estrogen receptor modulator approved by the FDA for the prevention of osteoporosis in post menopausal women. It is currently under investigation for its effect on breast cancer. STAR (Study of Tamoxifen and Raloxifene) is a multicenter clinical trial comparing the effectiveness of the two drugs in reducing the incidence of breast cancer in postmenopausal women who are at increased risk of developing the disease. A separate study on raloxifene and premenopausal women at increased risk of developing breast cancer is underway at NCI. For more information on entering the STAR trial, call NCI's Cancer Information Service at 800/4-CANCER or visit their Web site at http://cancertrials.nci. nih. gov.

Raloxifene acts like estrogen in some parts of the body, such as the bones, but it blocks the effects of estrogen in other parts of the body: In addition to strengthening bones, raloxifene, like tamoxifen, appears to reduce the risk of breast cancer.

But unlike tamoxifen, raloxifene does not appear to increase the risk of endometrial cancer. There are no data indicating whether this drug will benefit women who have already been diagnosed with breast cancer.

The Multiple Outcomes of Raloxifene Evaluation (MORE) trial of women taking raloxifene showed a 54 percent reduction in the incidence of newly diagnosed breast cancers when compared with their counterparts who were taking placebo, according to information pooled from nine separate, randomized, placebo-controlled, double-blind osteoporosis treatment and prevention trials.

The MORE trial was designed to assess the ability of raloxifene to reduce the risk of bone fractures in postmenopausal women, not to assess its effect on breast cancer incidence rates. But a decrease in breast cancer incidence was observed, and it is noteworthy that there was no increased risk of endometrial cancer in raloxifene-treated women.

More than 10,000 postmenopausal women, aged 41 to 80, participated. The mean period for follow-up was 33 months.

Raloxifene has rare but serious side effects: blood clots in the veins, which occurred in clinical trials at a rate similar to that reported for estrogen replacement therapy. More common side effects included hot flashes (18 percent incidence in the placebo group and 25 percent incidence in the raloxifene group) and leg cramps (2 percent incidence in the

Watch Out!
Osteoporosis is associated with a lower incidence of breast cancer. The initial raloxifene trials examined the drug's effect on women with osteoporosis, so the raloxifene trial outcomes and tamoxifen trial outcomes cannot be compared. The University of California-San Francisco MORE (Multiple Outcomes of Raloxifene Evaluation) trial looked at ralox-ifene and older women. The NSABP tamoxifen trial looked at mostly younger women who were at high risk of developing breast cancer.

placebo group and 6 percent in the raloxifene group). Raloxifene is not considered safe for women who are pregnant or who may become pregnant because preclinical data suggest the drug can cause fetal harm.

Biological warfare

Biological therapy uses the body to fight cancer. Its arsenal of weapons includes materials made by the body or made in a laboratory to repair, enhance, stimulate, direct, or restore the body's natural defenses against cancer. Biological therapy is sometimes called *biological response modifier (BRM) therapy* or *immunotherapy*. These treatments, which can be used alone or in conjunction with conventional treatments, are currently under investigation in clinical trials.

A quick immune defense primer

To understand how biological response modifiers work, you must understand the body's immune system. The immune system and how it relates to cancer is discussed in detail in Chapter 2. What follows are the basics:

Immune cells fight off non-self molecules, such as bacteria, viruses, and in many cases, cancer. There are many different types of immune cells and they each have special roles.

The immune cell "role" call is as follows:

- *Lymphocytes (white blood cells)*—B cells, T cells, and NK (natural killer) cells. B cells mature into plasma cells. These cells secrete antibodies, proteins called immunoglobulins, that recognize and attach to antigens (non-self molecules) in a perfect puzzle piece fit. T cells attack foreign invaders and call other immune system defenders to the scene. T cells and B cells produce proteins called lymphokines, a type of cytokine. Cytokines bind to receptors on target cells and recruit many other cells and substances to the battlefield. NK cells produce chemicals that bind to and kill foreign invaders. Unlike T cells, NK cells don't need to recognize an antigen to destroy it.

■ *Monocytes (white blood cells)*—These cells travel into tissues and transform into macrophages when needed to fight foreign invaders. Monocytes and macrophages essentially eat old or broken cells and foreign invaders.

Biological response modifiers can stop tumors in their tracks or help healthy cells to do so. Some biological response modifiers, such as antibodies and cytokines, occur naturally in the body while others can be made in the lab to imitate or influence antibodies and cytokines.

Biological response modifiers used to treat cancer include the following:

■ Cancer vaccines

■ Monoclonal antibodies

■ Interferons, interleukins, and tumor necrosis factor

Currently, only monoclonal antibodies, specifically trastuzumab (Herceptin), and cancer vaccines are being used to treat breast cancer.

Monoclonal antibodies are made in the laboratory in large quantities to target specific cancer antigens. Herceptin is a monoclonal antibody. Cancer vaccines help the immune system recognize and destroy cancer cells. These vaccines may help the body prevent cancer from recurring.

Herceptin

HER-2 (human epidermal growth factor receptor2) is a gene that everyone has but about 20 to 30 percent

Unofficially...
Scientists believe that the immune system sometimes recognizes cancer cells and destroys them. But sometimes some slip by the body's natural defenses, perhaps because they are so similar to the healthy cells from which they are derived and the similarities serve as a camouflage. In other cases, it appears that the immune system may break down or be overwhelmed.

of women with breast cancer have extra copies of it. Those extra copies usually lead to extra copies of the receptor. The HER-2/neu gene produces a protein on the cell's surface. This protein receives biological signals to grow. An overabundance of the gene translates to out-of-control growth, which means an aggressive cancer that spreads rapidly.

Herceptin is an antibody developed to target breast cancer cells that are over expressing HER-2. Herceptin binds to the protein, halting the out-of-control growth by preventing the cells from receiving and/or transmitting a growth signal.

Tumors that over express HER-2 respond to Herceptin because they are more sensitive to chemotherapy treatment, says John Glaspy, M.D., a researcher and oncologist at UCLA's Jonsson Cancer Center. In addition, Herceptin alone can sometimes shrink these tumors, he reports.

On May 15, 1999, at the annual meeting of the American Society of Clinical Oncology (ASCO), Larry Norton, M.D., head of the Division of Solid Tumor Oncology at Memorial Sloan-Kettering Cancer Center in New York, announced updated results from a phase III trial. The results (shown in Table 10.1) showed that at a median follow-up of 29 months, overall survival in women with metastatic tumors that over expressed the HER-2 protein treated with Herceptin plus chemotherapy (anthracycline and cyclophosphamide or paclitaxel) was 25.4 months compared with 20.3 months, an improvement of 25 percent, in patients treated with chemotherapy alone. For women treated with Herceptin plus anthracycline and cyclophosphamide, the median survival was 26.8 months. In contrast, in women treated with anthracycline and cyclophosphamide alone the median survival rate was 22.8 months. The median survival for women treated

> " There's a whole new area of biological therapies.
> —Lyndsay Harris, M.D., assistant professor in the Multidisciplinary Breast Program at Duke University. "

TABLE 10.1 MEDIAN SURVIVAL IN WOMEN WITH METASTATIC TUMORS THAT OVER EXPRESSED THE HER-2 PROTEIN

Treatment	Median survival time
Herceptin plus anthracycline and cyclophosphamide	26.8 months
Anthracycline and cyclophosphamide	22.8 months
Herceptin plus paclitaxel	22.1 months
Paclitaxel	18.4 months

with Herceptin plus paclitaxel was 22.1 months compared with 18.4 months for women receiving paclitaxel alone.

The major value of Herceptin is that "it is a paradigm for a different way of doing cancer research," Glaspy says, that is, if scientists can figure what's broken in the cell, they can work on fixing it. With modern molecular tools, it is possible to understand what's different between cancer versus normal cells. That information can be used to find drugs that attack cancer and ignore normal cells. This more targeted approach is expected to eliminate many of the side effects associated with chemotherapy.

It is likely that there are drugs better than this that have yet to be discovered, but this drug is leading the way in setting the tone for how it is done, Glaspy says, comparing it to the Wright brothers who set the tone for flight.

Herceptin, like cancer vaccines and other biological therapies, is administered once a week intravenously for 30 to 60 minutes. Unlike chemotherapeutic drugs, Herceptin does not cause side effects such as nausea and vomiting, hair loss, fatigue, and a drop in blood counts. But it does cause fever and chills, primarily after the initial administration in about 40 percent of women. In addition, some women who take Herceptin either alone or along with certain chemotherapeutic drugs (anthracyclines) experience cardiac abnormalities, which can be fatal. Often these side effects are controllable with medication.

Herceptin can be used as a first-line therapy in combination with paclitaxel and alone in second- and third-line therapy.

Herceptin does not work for all women whose breast tumors have an overabundance of the HER-2/neu gene.

Cancer vaccines

Vaccines work by exposing the body to a foreign agent, an antigen, that stimulates an immune response. T cells and B cells are activated, and some become memory cells. The result is an acquired immunity—the immune cells remember that specific antigen and attack at any subsequent sighting. Cancer vaccines work in a similar way. (See Chapter 2 for more details on the immune system and cancer vaccines.)

Scientists are developing tumor vaccines that are expected to help the immune system recognize, remember, and destroy specific cancer cells to help prevent recurrences.

One such vaccine under investigation targets the HER-2 protein. As noted earlier, the HER-2 protein is a tumor antigen, and some women have an immune response to it—the response just isn't strong enough to generate a complete remission. Effective cancer vaccines are expected to boost this immunity, potentially to therapeutic levels.

Cutting off supplies

There is a vast network of capillary blood vessels throughout the body. Each of these vessels is thinner than a hair and structured throughout the body so

> "
> Never go to a doctor whose office plants have died.
> —Erma Bombeck
> "

that nearly every healthy cell can live on the surface of one of these vessels.

Under normal conditions, the formation of new blood vessels (called *angiogenesis*) occurs during three processes:

- Tissue growth and repair
- The female reproductive cycle
- The development of the fetus during pregnancy

In abnormal circumstances, blood vessels grow in cancer tissue, allowing the tumor to grow or spread. Angiogenesis in tumor growth is called *neovascularization*.

Tumors also need blood vessels to grow beyond the size of a pinpoint. Therefore, they must form new capillary blood vessels. These new blood vessels bring in an ongoing supply of oxygen, nutrients, and proteins, known as growth factors, and take out waste products.

Angiogenesis inhibitors are drugs that block the development of new blood vessels. In doing so, researchers are hoping to cut off the tumor's supply of oxygen and nutrients and therefore block its continued growth and spread to other parts of the body.

In breast cancer, as the cells multiply and grow into a few millions cells—a microscopic, in situ tumor —they are distanced from their blood supply. Hence, the tumor stops increasing in size. At that point of stabilization, the number of growing cells and dying cells counterbalance each other. This cycle in breast cancer can go on for many years. At this point the tumor is too small to be detected in a clinical examination. By the time a tumor is detectable on a mammogram, the tumor has already become vascularized.

After several years of being in limbo, tumor cells may attempt to trigger angiogenesis, starting the

Bright Idea
Lyndsay Harris, M.D., assistant professor in the Multidisciplinary Breast Program at Duke University, usually tells her patients to consider a clinical trial using a biological agent *after* starting standard treatments to put the tumor in remission, a stable state.

invasion of surrounding tissue, using the following strategies:

■ Tumor cells may produce high levels of proteins that trigger the growth of new blood cells.

■ Tumor cells may activate naturally occurring proteins that trigger angiogenesis.

■ Tumor cells may call into action angiogenic proteins in nearby healthy tissue.

■ Tumor cells may trigger immune response cells (macrophages, for example) to release proteins that will induce angiogenesis.

Once angiogenesis is initiated, the tumor grows rapidly. And once a tumor develops blood vessels, it tends to continue to grow and develop more vessels, continuing its spread. Some of the cancer cells that break off and travel to distant sites are angiogenic, that is, able to produce new blood vessels. In those cases, the spread and growth of new cancer is rapid. In contrast, other cancerous cells that have traveled to distant sites may not have angiogenic cells. They can lie dormant for years after the primary tumor has been surgically removed and treated with chemotherapy or radiation therapy. Suddenly, the metastatic tumor will go through the process of stimulating angiogenesis, and will grow and spread rapidly.

Angiogenesis permits metastasis

Angiogenesis plays a large role in metastasis. Consider the following:

1. Tumors cannot grow beyond the size of a pinhead without becoming vascularized (forming new blood vessels).

2. Tumors with dense networks of blood vessels are often more aggressive and tend to have poorer clinical outcomes.

3. Tumor cells may not break away from the primary tumor until a network of blood vessels has formed.

4. Both angiogenesis and metastasis require enzymes that break down surrounding tissue (called the extracellular matrix) during blood vessel formation and tumor invasion.

Inhibiting angiogenesis

Currently, investigators are using four strategies to design angiogenesis inhibitors:

1. They are trying to block the ability of endothelial cells, which are responsible for forming new capillary blood vessel networks, to break down the surrounding extracellular matrix. (Once the endothelial cells break the matrix, they begin dividing. Strings of new endothelial cells form into hollow tubes, creating new blood vessel networks, making tissue growth and repair possible in normal circumstances.)

2. They are trying to directly inhibit normal endothelial cells.

3. They are trying to block certain factors that simulate blood vessel growth.

4. They are trying to block the action of a specific molecule on the endothelial cell surface.

There are five categories of angiogenesis drugs being tested in clinical trials, including those that:

- Block the ability of the endothelial cells to break down the surrounding matrix

- Inhibit normal endothelial cells directly

- Block factors that activate angiogenesis

- Block the action of integrin, a molecule on the endothelial cell surface

Unofficially...
About 20 angiogenesis inhibitors are currently being studied in early clinical trials, according to the National Institutes of Health.

- Have nonspecific mechanisms of action (These are not currently being tested on breast cancer.)

Angiogenesis inhibitors versus chemotherapy

There are several differences between standard chemotherapy and anti-angiogenesis drugs. The most notable: Angiogenesis inhibitors target dividing endothelial cells and standard chemotherapy targets tumor cells themselves. In addition to having different targets:

- Angiogenesis inhibitors are less likely than chemotherapy to cause hair loss, nausea, or vomiting, and destruction of bone marrow.

- Angiogenesis inhibitors can slow down wound healing and stop menstruation. (No clinically relevant changes in wound healing have been shown to be associated with standard dose chemotherapy.)

- Angiogenesis inhibitors shrink a tumor and hold its growth at bay, while standard chemotherapy drugs are used to kill the tumor itself.

- Angiogenesis inhibitors work by limiting the tumor's blood supply by stopping the formation of new blood vessels around the tumor and by reducing the existing network of capillaries surrounding the tumor; chemotherapy works by killing tumor cells.

- Most cancer cells are genetically unstable, that is, they are prone to mutating. This change in genetic structure allows them to develop a resistance against chemotherapy. In contrast, endothelial cells, which anti-angiogenesis drugs target, are genetically stable, making drug resistance unlikely.

- Because angiogenesis inhibitors stop the growth

of new blood vessels but do not attack healthy blood vessels, in theory they should not harm blood vessels serving healthy tissues. Chemotherapy attacks rapidly dividing cells, including healthy cells, such as bone marrow cells (causing increased susceptibility to infections) and hair cells (causing hair loss).

Because anti-angiogenesis and chemotherapy drugs have different targets, they may have more of an impact on tumor growth when used together—one drug attacks the tumor and the other its source of nutrients. Or it may be that they just appear to work better together because new tumor cells require new endothelial cells at about a ratio of between 10:1 to 100:1 to grow. As a result, for every endothelial cell whose growth is halted, up to 100 cancer cells cannot grow.

Back at the lab

Other angiogensis inhibitors that show promise are still in the early stages of research. In animal studies, a protein called angiostatin appears to be a potent angiogenesis inhibitor. Angiostatin targets endothelial cells associated with the tumor only. As a result, there are no toxic side effects, at least in the animals studied. In addition, drug resistance doesn't develop; again, at least not in animal studies.

Endostatin also seems to be a promising angiogenesis inhibitor in animal studies. The National Cancer Institute is planning an initial testing (phase I trial) of human endostatin in people. The trial will be open to people with solid tumors (cancer of body tissues other than blood, bone marrow, or the lymphatic system), including breast cancer.

More than 20 angiogenesis inhibitors are being tested in clinical trials sponsored by drug companies and the NCI. If you are interested in finding out more about these trials, contact NCI's Cancer Information Service at 800/4-CANCER or visit their Web site at http://cancertrials.nci.nih.gov.

Gearing up the troops

Scientists are turning to the body's own defense mechanisms to help ward off breast cancer as well as other cancers. Cancer results from broken (mutated) genes. The damaged genes either cause or permit uncontrolled cell growth. Genes become damaged as the result of the following:

- Environmental carcinogens

- Viruses (viruses are not thought to be associated with the development of breast cancer, but they are associated with other cancers)

- The aging process

- Heredity

The resulting genetic mutations occur in at least one of the following three gene categories:

1. *Oncogenes*—These are cancer genes that result from carcinogens (as well as viruses).

2. *Suppressor genes*—These genes suppress cell growth.

3. *DNA repair genes*—When genes that help repair damaged DNA are not functioning, that cell may become cancerous.

Gene therapy is based on the idea that if you can fix the gene by providing cells with healthy copies of missing (deleted) or broken genes, you can prevent or treat cancer.

Here's how it works: healthy cells are taken from the blood or bone marrow and grown in the laboratory. (Remember, each cell contains a copy of all of

Watch Out!
Unforeseen side effects from angiogenesis inhibitors may occur in clinical trials.

your genes; they are not just activated in each cell.) The healthy copy of the gene is then reintroduced into the unhealthy cells by way of an inactivated virus. The healthy cells are grown and returned to the body. Another method uses inactivated viruses or fatty particles to deliver the healthy gene directly to cells in the body.

Gene therapy, like other biological treatments discussed in this chapter, is experimental and still in phase I and phase II trials.

Just the facts

- Hormone therapy blocks the hormone receptors on the cells, so the hormone can not longer promote cell growth.

- About 20 to 30 percent of women with breast cancer have extra copies of the HER-2/neu gene

- Cancer vaccines are being used to boost the body's own immune system to recognize and fight cancer.

- Angiogenesis inhibitors limit the tumor's blood supply, controlling its growth.

Experimental and Alternative Treatment Methods

PART V

Experimental Treatment Methods

Chapter 11

N ew treatments go through a rigorous evaluation process to make sure they're safe and effective and better than currently available treatments.

A large part of that process involves volunteers. People choose to volunteer to be subjects in scientific studies for many reasons. Some have exhausted all conventional treatment and turn toward experimental therapies for new hope. Others may want the extra care they receive as a participant or the comfort of knowing they're being treated by some of the best and brightest clinicians. Some people with limited finances may find that, in a trial, certain medications may be provided free of charge. No matter what the reason, society benefits from those who participate.

In this chapter, we'll tell you how scientific studies are set up, what types of studies there are, the benefits and drawbacks to participating in one, and what protection you receive as a participant. We'll also tell you what it's like to be part of a study.

Why participate in a clinical trial?

If you decide to take part in a clinical trial, you will be helping researchers evaluate the treatment's effectiveness as well as possibly benefiting from it yourself. In addition, your participation may help scientists find better ways of preventing, detecting, or treating breast cancer.

Trial participants are usually assigned to a doctor who wants to take the time to get to know them and who must rigidly follow the study's protocol, a specific treatment given in a specific way at specific time intervals. There are some doctors in the community who base their methods on what they *think* works—mixing and matching chemotherapies—not what has been shown to work, says Lee Rosen, M.D., assistant professor of medicine and director of the Cancer Therapy Development Program at UCLA's Jonsson Cancer Center, a clearinghouse for clinical trials for patients who have failed conventional therapies. While they are probably well-intentioned, it isn't good science, he says. As a participant in a clinical trial, you'll be given a very specific treatment regimen, as noted earlier, and you'll be watched more closely by the physicians because they must gather data.

Not everyone will agree, but Rosen thinks every cancer patient should participate in some sort of clinical trial "because there's so much room for improvement in what we know." Physicians should be treating patients based on scientific evidence, not because one patient did well on something, he says. But Rosen doesn't think you need to put your life or health on the line to participate. A clinical trial can be anything from using a new drug or sequence of drugs to just providing information on how cancer has affected you, he says. Studies provide scientists a way of gath-

Unofficially...
You don't have to have breast cancer to participate in a trial. You may qualify for a trial that is studying women at high-risk of developing breast cancer. In addition, it's not necessary to have gone through prior treatment for your breast cancer. Some women choose to enter cancer trials as a first line of defense.

ering information so they can learn from it.

"Every patient should seek out what clinical trials are available," he says. Local cancer centers will tell you what's available in treatment trials and supportive care trials, as well as questionnaires or family interviews.

But there are drawbacks to consider. You may have to make extra doctor visits and undergo extra lab tests. You may not benefit from the treatment, or you may receive the standard conventional treatment you would have received outside of the trial. The trial may take place in another city or at a center that is less convenient than your doctor's office. Researchers may ask you to give up something, such as a particular food, or ask you to add something to your daily routine, such as exercise. In addition, you may be asked a lot of questions about your health or be asked to fill out questionnaires from time to time over several years. If you've already been diagnosed with cancer, you may not want to dwell on it once the treatment ends.

How trials are set up

Once a treatment has reached the stage of being tested in a clinical trial, it has been through rigorous testing in both laboratory and animal studies.

As described in chapter 3, most clinical research is done in steps. Phase I trials, which enroll only a small number of participants, evaluate how a drug should be given—orally, by injection, or intravenously—and how often without eliciting unbearable side effects or toxicity. It can also explore how other treatment methods should be optimally performed, such as the timing of surgery, for example. At this stage, not much is known about the benefits and risks of the treatment.

66

You can leave [a trial] at any time—
Lee Rosen, M.D., assistant professor of medicine and director of the Cancer Therapy Development Program at UCLA's Jonsson Cancer Center, a clearinghouse for clinical trials for patients who have failed conventional therapies.

99

Watch Out!
New treatments have unknown risks.

Phase I drugs come out of the lab to be tested in animals and human cancer cells and are deemed to be promising enough to try in humans, Rosen says. The researchers go to the FDA for permission to use these drugs in a trial. The purpose of a phase I trial is to determine the optimal dose schedule and side effects. Phase I trials begin at what is thought to be a nontoxic dose, which may be too low to be effective.

In a typical design, the researchers observe three patients for a period of days or weeks. If there are no adverse effects, then three more patients at the next dose level are observed. This process is repeated again and again until side effects are seen. Some trials test one drug, others test combinations. There may be more than one study testing these drugs. The treatment may be tested on different populations or at different schedules. In the end, scientists have identified the dose and side effects of a single drug, a combination of drugs, or a specific schedule.

Phase II trials find out more information about safety and effectiveness of the drug or other treatments being studied. A phase II trial tries to determine if the treatment shrinks the tumor or has other anticancer effects. These trials are also limited to a small number of people. They typically involve about 20 patients with the same disease and same stage of disease, Rosen says. All these patients have had the same amount of prior therapy and all of them get the same drug at the same dose. Researchers observe what percentage of the population has a response or other clinical benefit.

Phase III trials examine hundreds or thousands of people and compare conventional therapy to a treatment that holds more hope in terms of effectiveness or fewer side effects. Trial participants are

Watch Out!
While many treatments studied in clinical trials will benefit patients, some treatments that show promise in animal studies aren't effective in humans.

randomly divided into two groups—one group is given the standard treatment and the other is given the experimental treatment. Sometimes these studies are *single-blinded*—the patient does not know if she is receiving the standard therapy or the experimental one. Sometimes these studies are *double-blinded*—neither the doctor nor patient know which treatment the patient is receiving (though a behind-the-scenes administrator does know who is receiving the experimental treatment and who is receiving the standard therapy.) Phase III trials compare the side effects and survival rates between the two treatment groups, referred to as the *study arms*. A phase III trial is the definitive study that goes to the FDA for its approval of the drug.

Note: If you are placed in the experimental arm and the treatment doesn't work, you'll often get the opportunity to cross over at the end of the study and receive the conventional drug. The same is true if the experimental treatment is much more effective than the conventional treatment. If the experimental drug causes an unexpected or dangerous side effect, the investigators are required by law to notify patients and doctors expeditiously.

Phase IV trials use drugs that have already received FDA approval. These trials are conducted because the FDA wants to see how well the treatment works in other stages of the disease or other diseases.

Clinical trials involving treatment often provide the same amount of physical exams and other care, but they can include additional tests. In most good clinical trials conducted at major cancer centers, the experimental drug and extra tests are free, Rosen says.

But you must check with your insurance to make sure that the basic care is covered. NCI has a useful

Unofficially...
Trials don't always test only new drugs. Sometimes a combination of a conventional drug and a new drug is tested and sometimes an old drug is tested for a new use.

page titled Clinical Trials and Insurance Coverage: A Resource Guide at http://207.121.187.155/NCI _CANCER_TRIALS/zones/TrialInfo/Deciding/ insurance.html. It lists strategies that may help you obtain coverage and deal with the costs associated with clinical trials.

Note that you don't have to be at a cancer center to participate in a trial. There are clinical trials at universities and private practices. Make sure the protocol of the study you are considering is approved by the Institutional Review Board at the study site. Note the study's sponsorship, which is disclosed in the informed consent document. Valid sponsorships include NCI and pharmaceutical firms. Check with 800/4-CANCER or the PDQ at www.nih.nci.gov.

No whim nor fancy

There is no room for creativity in a study protocol. Clinical trials follow strict guidelines that specify who can participate, how many people can participate, and what they must be told before entering the study. The protocol also specifies what information scientists will gather.

In addition, the study protocol includes the following:

Unofficially...
NCI doesn't fund most of the clinical studies. Many clinical trials are sponsored by pharmaceutical companies. Some are sponsored by cooperative research groups such as the Southwest Oncology Group and the Eastern Cooperative Oncology Group.

- The eligibility requirements for the study. Eligibility criteria help ensure that results of the study are reliable. Those who are enrolled must share common characteristics, called eligibility criteria. Examples of eligibility criteria include stage of disease, menopausal status, node-negative or node-positive status, age, geographic location, age at first live birth, and general health. These criteria help researchers to determine whom the new treatment might help most. For instance, the drug Herceptin was found to help women whose breast tumors produced excessive HER-2 proteins. In addition, the eligibility requirements help protect patients from drugs that would otherwise harm them. For instance, some drugs are excreted by the kidneys. Women with renal (kidney) dysfunction would be excluded from the study in the eligibility criteria because the drug may have an adverse effect on them. In this instance, the treatment for one disease could worsen another disease. Eligibility criteria may also include whether or not the patient has had prior cancer treatment.

■ What will be studied, whether it's a single drug or new combination of drug treatments, new approaches to surgery or radiation therapy, new methods such as gene therapy, or food supplements, dietary regimen, vitamins, minerals, herbs, lifestyle changes, etc., or a combination of any of these. In phase I and phase II trials, all the participants receive the same treatment. In phase III trials, patients are randomly separated into two groups. One group will take the best drug available for conventional use and the other group will take the experimental drug that scientists hold hope in.

Study stages and designs

There are two main types of trials: intervention and prevention. Intervention trials attempt to learn how and why a treatment might work. If you enter one of these trials, you may or may not receive a benefit, depending on the phase and on the effectiveness of the treatment and dose level and scheduling if the treatment being tested is a drug. A prevention trial is set up to prevent the disease from occurring.

There are three categories of intervention trials:

Bright Idea
If you don't have
breast cancer but
are consumed
with worry about
developing it,
consider entering
a prevention trial.
Taking action
to protect
yourself might
alleviate some of
your anxiety.

1. *Early detection*—The goal of these trials is to detect cancer in its earliest stages.

2. *Quality of life*—These studies look at ways to improve the quality of life for people living with cancer.

3. *Prevention trials*—These studies evaluate methods of reducing risk.

There are two types of primary prevention trials:

1. Those designed to prevent cancer from developing in those who do not have it.

2. Those designed to prevent a new type of cancer from developing in those who been previously diagnosed with the disease.

Prevention studies are set up in one of two ways:

1. *Action study:* This study design is used to try to determine if cancer can be avoided if people take certain actions, such as exercising regularly.

2. *Chemoprevention study:* This set-up is used to try to determine if taking something—a specific drug, vitamin, food supplement, herb, mineral, or a combination of them—can prevent cancer. Researchers use this type of study to learn about the safety and mechanism of action of the agent being studied. As with other clinical trials, each phase tries to answer different questions about the agent being studied.

Being a guinea pig

If you participate in a clinical trial, you receive treatment at a cancer center, hospital, or doctor's office. Your medical team will follow your progress closely. Part of being watched closely means you'll probably undergo more tests and visit the doctor more often than you would if you were being treated outside a study. The number of treatments, tests, and doctor's visits will depend on the treatment plan that you're to follow. In addition, you may be required to keep notes on your health. Furthermore, for years after your participation in the study, you may be asked to provide information to members of the research team.

The study protocol explains the details—what will be done and why. It notes the number of participants, the kind of medical tests involved and how often participants will receive them, and the treatment plan. Whether you participate in a cancer center, hospital, clinic, or doctor's office, you'll be receiving the same treatment—as well as the same tests and the same number of doctor's appointments—as all other study participants, regardless of location.

Unofficially...
While there are risks inherent in participating in a clinical trial, steps are taken to protect patients.

Armor and other protection

To protect patients, clinical research is carried out in accordance with scientific and ethical guidelines. Each study protocol must be approved by the study's sponsor, often the National Cancer Institute, as well as the Institutional Review Board at each hospital or other study site. The board is made up of health professionals, clergy, and consumers who review the protocol to ensure that the research won't expose patients to extreme risks or unethical practices. Phase III trials are scrutinized by the Data Safety and Monitoring Committee that reviews test results, monitors patient safety, and ultimately decides if the study should continue as planned. The Data Safety and Monitoring Committee is composed of external, nonparticipating scientists appointed by the principal investigator. Furthermore, each participating doctor agrees to provide the same exact treatment to all study participants. Doctors are not permitted to vary from the protocol.

Patients are also protected by eligibility require-ments, which, as noted earlier, protect patients from being exposed to treatments that are likely to cause them harm.

Should you participate?

The decision to participate in a study may be diffi-cult for some women and easier for others. Before deciding, you might want to discuss the possibility of entering a study with your family, your doctor, the staff of any clinical trial you consider entering, and your support group, if you belong to one.

There are several benefits to consider, including:

▪ You may benefit from a new treatment.

▪ If you end up being a member of the control arm of the study, you'll receive the best conven-tional treatment available. This may turn out to be better than the new approach.

▪ You'll be contributing to science.

But there are drawbacks to consider as well, including:

▪ If you receive the new treatment, it may not work as well as a standard therapy.

▪ There may be unknown side effects that are worse than those of the standard treatment.

▪ If you receive the standard treatment, it may not help you.

▪ If you receive the standard treatment, it may not be as effective as the experimental therapy.

▪ Your insurance may not cover all of the costs involved if you participate in a clinical trial.

As a patient in a clinical trial, you're also protect-ed by a "Patient Bill of Rights." These rights include:

▪ Your right not to participate in the study after

going through the initial appointments.

■ Your right to drop out of the study at any time.

■ Most importantly, your right to informed consent. You must be given all the facts about the study before deciding to participate. You should be given details on the treatment you may receive and the possible risks and potential benefits. All the information should be detailed in writing in the consent form, which you must sign if you want to participate. Informed consent continues throughout the trial. If the researchers learn about risks, they must tell you. At that point, you may be asked to sign a new consent form to continue participating. But remember, even though you sign a consent form, you can still drop out of the study whenever you like. It is not like signing a legally binding contract to purchase an item or membership.

■ Your right to ask as many questions as you have. This is your health and well-being at stake.

■ Your right to be taken seriously by the team and to get answers to all your questions.

You also have the right to expect quality care. You should expect your health care team to follow your response to treatment carefully, and if the treatment is causing you harm, you have the right to expect them to take you out of the study immediately. (You should consider returning to your referring doctor for treatment at that point.)

If you're thinking about joining a study, Table 11.1 has some important questions you can ask the study's investigative team—the doctors, nurses, and administrative staff.

Your decision may also depend on how participating in the study will affect your daily life and your family. To find out about the possible social or emotional impact, ask to speak with other study participants and

TABLE 11.1 QUESTIONS YOU SHOULD ASK BEFORE ENTERING A TRIAL

■ What's the purpose of the study?

■ Is the study in phase I, phase II, or phase III?

■ Why do researchers believe the new treatment being tested may be effective?

■ Has it been tested before? If so, what are the prior results of the treatment in women with the same type of breast cancer and the same stage of disease and menopausal status? How do these results compare with those of standard treatment for the same group of women? Have these results been confirmed in other trials? Were there enough participants in those trials to make the results meaningful and generalizable? (If you are entering a phase I or phase II trial, or an early phase III trial, there will not be a large amount of generalizable data. You must carefully consider whether you want to take on the risk of the unknown and you must determine what other treatment alternatives are available.)

■ How does the experimental treatment differ from conventional treatment?

■ Who are the researchers? What are their qualifications? What university, institution, or corporation are they affiliated with?

■ Who is sponsoring the study? Who has reviewed and approved it? What are their qualifications?

■ How will the study data be checked and verified?

■ How will patient safety be monitored?

■ When and where will study results and information be published?

■ Will my identity be protected?

■ Will I have to pay for any medical expenses?

■ Will all the drugs I receive be free of charge? (If not, check with your insurance company to see if it will cover that expense.)

■ Will I receive financial compensation for participating in the trial?

■ What side effects have been associated with this experimental treatment in earlier studies or trials?

■ What measures will be taken for relief of any side effects and any pain?

find out if there is support available for you and your family. There are also groups that can help such as NABCO (www.nabco.org), the Susan G. Komen Breast Cancer Foundation (www.komen.org, 800/462-9273), and Anderson Networks (www..mdanderson.org/centers/pathway/andnet/index.html, 800/345-6324).

In addition, be sure to weigh the risks against the benefits. To help you do that, Table 11.2 lists some questions you may want to ask the team of investigators.

TABLE 11.2   QUESTIONS ABOUT RISKS AND BENEFITS

■ What standard treatments are available for my type of breast cancer and my stage of disease?

■ What are the short- and long-term risks, benefits, and side effects of that type of treatment?

■ What are the known possible short- and long-term risks, side effects, and benefits of the experimental treatment?

■ What are the expected survival rates for each?

You should also expect top-notch care from experts in the field of breast cancer. You may want to consider asking the questions like those listed in Table 11.3, although many of them should be answered in the informed consent form.

How to find a clinical trial

There are many ways to find out about clinical trials. You can ask your physician, call the NCI's Cancer Information Service toll free at 800/422-6237, or call cancer centers and medical schools.

There are also many Web sites that list trials. Some even talk about the pros and cons of entering a trial. Here are some that are especially helpful:

■ **http://cancertrials.nci.nih.gov**—Cancer Trials is NCI's comprehensive clinical trials information

Watch Out!
Sometimes physicians only tell patients about clinical trials that they themselves or local hospitals are involved in. There are a multitude of trials in the United States, internationally, and even locally that your doctor may not be aware of. That doesn't mean you can't investigate other trials. Some of them may offer you more promising results.

center. It includes information on finding specific trials and research news.

- **http://cancernet.nci.nih.gov**—CancerNet contains information from PDQ® (NCI's comprehensive cancer database), which has a registry of about 1,700 open and 10,300 closed cancer clinical trials around the world and CANCERLIT,

TABLE 11.3   FINDING OUT ABOUT THE CARE YOU'LL RECEIVE

- What treatments, medical tests, or procedures will I have during the study?
- Do they cause pain?
- How often will I receive the treatment(s)?
- How long will appointments last? How often will they be scheduled? Will I need someone to drive me to appointments?
- How long is the study expected to last?
- Will follow-up care be provided?
- Will the study have a follow-up phase? If so, what role will I be expected to play?
- Where will the treatment take place? (If outside of your city, you may want to ask if they've arranged for special rates at nearby hotels.)
- Will the treatment require a hospital stay? If so, for how long? How frequently?
- Who will be overseeing my care? What are his or her qualifications? If our personalities clash, will there be someone else to oversee my care?
- Whom should I contact in the event of an emergency?
- What constitutes an emergency? What symptoms are expected and not harmful?
- Have there been deaths associated with this experimental treatment? If so, what percentage of the patients and what were the causes? What is the mortality rate of the experimental treatment compared with the conventional treatment?
- At this point in the research, is the experimental treatment thought to be as safe as the standard treatment?
- If there's an impressive result or the drug causes an unexpected and dangerous side effect, how quickly are patients and doctors notified? If either of these events occur, what are my options?

where you can search literature.

- **www.oncolink.upenn.edu/clinical_trials**—The University of Pennsylvania's OncoLink lists cooperative cancer research group trials as well as those open at the University of Pennsylvania. In addition, it has clinical trial news updates. You can also sign up for a moderated newsgroup and e-mail alerts to new trials.

- **http://bcc-ct.his.ucsf.edu**—The University of California at San Francisco Breast Care Center Clinical Trials list.

- **http://www.ca-coalition.org/**—The Coalition of National Cancer Cooperative Group represents six cancer cooperative groups (large networks of researchers, doctors, and healthcare professionals at both public and private institutions nationwide that participate in cancer clinical trials) funded primarily by the National Cancer Institute, including the Cancer and Leukemia Group B (CALGB); Eastern Cooperative Oncology Group (ECOG); North Central Cancer Treatment Group (NCCTG); National Surgical Adjuvant Breast and Bowel Project (NSABP); Pediatric Oncology Group (POG); and Radiation Therapy Oncology Group (RTOG). Their trial page is currently under construction.

- **www.canceranswers.org/treat.htm**—The Breast Cancer Answers California Clinical Trials Matching System does a little more than just list trials—it searches for breast cancer clinical trials in California to see if there are any that are recruiting women with your medical history. You can also review the list of trials at the site.

- **www.centerwatch.com**—CenterWatch is a clinical

trials listing service. It also lists new FDA approvals and has an e-mail service that will notify you by e-mail when additional breast cancer trials are added to the site. In addition, it contains profiles of the centers conducting the research.

- **www.cto.mrc.ac.uk/ukcccr**—A database of randomized clinical trials taking place in Great Britain.

- **http://cancerguide.org/clinical_trials.html**—Cancer-Guide's information on clinical trials may be particularly useful because it is written from the perspective of a person with cancer.

Another way to find a trial: Research the scientific literature and call the authors of the papers. There's always contact information on the study's lead investigator. The other authors are described by their affiliation with an institution. You can find contact information (an e-mail address and phone number) for the researcher fairly easily by searching for faculty at the Center's Web site or by calling the main phone number to the school, cancer center, or pharmaceutical company. Many researchers are willing to provide information through brief e-mail correspondence or phone calls, or their support staff may be willing to send you information. There's often information on the institution's Web site on preliminary findings. Check at the bottom of the Web page, though, to see when the information was updated to ensure that it's current.

Bright Idea
At www.fda.gov/cder/ob, part of the Food and Drug Administration's Web site, you can access the FDA Electronic Orange Book, which lists newly approved drugs.

Joining the ranks

Thinking of joining a trial? Get a buddy. The pilot Buddy Program for Breast Cancer Clinical Trials pairs women who have breast cancer and are eligible for a clinical trial with a buddy who already has been through a study. The program is run by researchers at New England Research Institutes and funded by the National Cancer Institute and the National Action Plan on Breast Cancer.

The goal of this program is to determine if having a buddy helps women decide whether or not to participate in a clinical trial. You can find more information at http://www.gis.net/~allisonm/gfx/buddies.html or contact Allison C. Morrill, Ph.D., New England Research Institutes, 9 Galen Street, Watertown, MA 02172; Phone: 800/775-6374 x547; Fax: 617/ 926-8246; E-Mail:AllisonM@neri.org.

You can also contact members of the Institution Review Board to ask questions, as well.

Sold out shows

Not everyone will qualify for every trial, and some trials will be closed to new participants. Even so, there is good news. If you don't qualify for one trial, you may qualify for another. For example, treatments are sometimes tested on different populations and variations of treatments are studied, opening up spaces for new participants. (Sometimes variations of conventional or experimental treatments have added benefit, sometimes they don't.)

Take note that timing could be everything. You typically only have 30 to 90 days (depending on the trial's protocol) after surgery to enter an adjuvant treatment trial. If you're considering entering a phase I or phase II trial, you generally must not have had any treatment for four to eight weeks (depending on the trial's protocol).

All is not lost if you don't qualify for a trial or you want the treatment but don't want to be a trial participant. In some circumstances, the investigators are testing combinations of FDA-approved drugs. If that's

Timesaver
Read review papers in peer-reviewed journals, such as the *Journal of the National Cancer Institute*, to find out quickly what trials are being conducted and where. Review papers summarize all the current work in a specific area of research. Look for one that's hot off the press to get the most updated information.

the case, your oncologist can prescribe that same drug combination and scheduling.

But what if the drugs being investigated are not FDA approved? There's still a chance your doctor will be able to prescribe them, depending on your circumstances. There are three possible approaches:

1. Ask the FDA to grant "compassionate care" use. Compassionate care may be granted when the drug isn't fully approved and patient is very ill. The FDA may allow a patient to use a drug even if it's not appropriate or has side effects or risks that they normally wouldn't want someone to have.

Unofficially...
If you find a list of trials testing the same treatment, you can be pretty sure that treatment holds promise.

2. Check with the FDA to see if the drug is nearing approval. If it is, it may be available with special permission for use outside the trial setting. The drug manufacturer, however, would have to agree.

3. Look overseas or to Canada. Some drugs and other treatments are approved in other countries before they are available here. (Make sure the treatment is backed by solid scientific research.) You may have to go overseas for treatment, though sometimes it is possible to legally import the drug. Contact a lawyer who specializes in pharmaceuticals or palliative treatments.

Drugs are expensive. If affordability is a problem, contact the Institute at Capitol Hill Office, 611 Pennsylvania Ave., S.E., Suite 1010, Washington, D.C. 20003-4303 or visit their Web site at http://www.institute-dc.org. You can download free of charge or order a paper version (for a $5 fee) of *Free and Low Cost Prescription Drugs*. They also offer *Free and Low Cost Hospital Care, Free and Low Cost Nursing Home Care*, and *Free and Low Cost Outpatient Care*.

Just the facts

- You don't have to have a disease or a condition to participate in a trial.

- You can leave a trial whenever you want.

- You may receive an experimental treatment or a conventional treatment.

- You may not know which treatment you are getting.

- The experimental treatment may have added benefits and dangerous, unknown side effects.

- Study participants may receive more attentive care than non-participants.

Bright Idea
The same or similar treatment may be under investigation in different phases at different institutions. So you may be able to join a phase III trial at one institution rather than a phase II trial at another.

Alternative/Adjuvant Methods of Treatment

Chapter 12

No doubt about it, American consumers are setting the agenda for researchers. Noting that some cancer treatments are toxic, many cancer patients and others have turned to alternative medicine practices, some which view the body as a whole rather than parts (holistic medicine) and treat disease and symptoms in that light through mostly nontoxic modalities, such as mind-body therapy, acupuncture, music, nutrition, and more. Some consumers are turning toward herbal remedies, some of which may have medical validity. However, some herbal remedies have been found to be contaminated with heavy metals and valium. In contrast to mainstream drugs, the Food and Drug Administration (FDA) does not regulate the production of herbal remedies.

In this chapter, we'll tell you why scientists are taking another look at Eastern medicine techniques, why there has been a delay implementing some of these practices, as well as what's available. We'll also warn you about some unsafe alternative treatments and some of those that remain unproven in terms of measurable effectiveness. And we'll tell you how to conduct your own research of peer-reviewed journal articles to find out what alternative treatments are being studied and which may hold promise.

Proceed with caution

First, a warning: There is an important difference between alternative and complementary therapies, says Barrie Cassilleth, Ph.D., chief of integrative medicine at Memorial Sloan-Kettering Cancer Center in New York. "Alternative therapies are often promoted for use instead of mainstream care and as a cure for cancer. They are biologically active, expensive, and by definition unproved," in Cassilleth's view.

"If they were proven they wouldn't be alternative. They'd be used everywhere," Cassilleth points out. "Complementary therapies, in contrast, are used in an adjunctive fashion along with mainstream care or as wellness approaches for people who are healthy. They don't claim to cure diseases. They deal with enhancing quality of life, managing symptoms [nausea, fatigue, pain, stress, anxiety, and depression], and they work effectively to improve well-being both for patients and for people who are healthy," Cassilleth says.

Complementary and alternative medicine (CAM) is a broad label for many treatments that seek to balance forces within the body that practitioners believe is the cause of disease or of symptoms. These treatments are broadly defined as those not widely taught in medical schools in the United States.

CAM treatments are tailored to the individual, so two people with the same symptoms may not receive the same treatment. The term "integrative medicine," which is preferred by Andrew Weil, M.D., a well-known author and director of the Program in

Timesaver
If you want a
quick primer on
integrative medi-
cine, visit the
University of
Texas Center for
Alternative
Medicine Research
at www.sph.uth.
tmc.edu/utcam
and Dr. Andrew
Weil's Web site at
www.drweil.com.

Integrative Medicine at the College of Medicine of
the University of Arizona, is reflective of his desire to
see the best of both conventional and alternative medicine integrated.

If you are under treatment for any serious illness,
it's essential to discuss your use of unconventional
(complementary) therapies with your physician,
Cassilleth stresses.

"People should be aware of the fact that over-the-
counter remedies, including herbal products, home-
opathic remedies, [and] vitamin and mineral collec-
tions that are promoted as improving health at one
level or another, are not regulated by the FDA,"
Cassilleth warns.

The FDA has *some* authority over these products,
but it's *very* restricted. The FDA regulates these products through the Dietary Supplement Health Education Act of 1994. The question of purity is not in the
Act.

There are different rules for drugs and dietary
supplements. These products are not regulated and
tested like drugs are by the FDA. "This means that
the products are not reviewed or controlled for safety and efficacy, and we have to exercise great caution
in using them," she says. They don't undergo the rigorous scrutiny drugs do pre- and post-marketing.

"These products often are found to be contaminated with chemicals that can be harmful," Cassilleth
says. Other times you simply don't get what you're
paying for. In the vast majority of test cases, particularly herbal remedies, "they are found to contain less
[than] the promised active ingredient," she says.

The collection of herbal products in Asian food
markets are probably the most likely to be contaminated, Cassilleth says. Those that are packaged in

Unofficially...
Alternative medi-
cine refers to
using treatments
outside of stan-
dard, Western
medical practices.
Complementary
and integrative
medicine refer to
combining con-
ventional Western
medicine and
ancient Eastern
medicine prac-
tices.

Watch Out!
High levels of vitamin C have been associated with boosting the immune system, but a researcher at Memorial Sloan-Kettering found excessive amounts of vitamin C, the type offered in alternative medicine clinics, which give high-dose vitamin C intravenously, help a tumor to grow.

protected ways and manufactured by companies with which the consumer is familiar are most likely to be safe, she says. "However, with few exceptions, these products have not been studied, and we do not know whether they work, whether they can block other medications, or whether they contain harmful ingredients."

Many of the herbal products are promoted as treatments for cancer or as immune enhancers. Currently, she says, there is no evidence that they are effective. However, as scientists investigate these products they may very well find evidence of efficacy.

In addition, dietary supplements cannot claim on the label to "cure, treat, mitigate, or prevent diseases" under the Act. The intent of the Act was to make products widely available without a lot of restriction. The FDA does, however, take reports of adverse events. (For more information on the Act, go to www.fda.gov, click "Foods" and read the section on dietary supplements.)

Where Western medicine has failed

"Because we are focused on scientific truth and objective data, we do not as physicians always adequately meet the needs of human beings...for a sense of empowerment,...a sense of comfort and being in control of the random forces that threaten their lives," says John Glaspy, M.D., a researcher and oncologist at UCLA's Jonsson Comprehensive Cancer Center. In the past, tribal civilizations always had a person in the community—a healer called a shaman—to provide that service, he explains. In simple language and stories, the shaman explained an illness to the person suffering from it, and told that person how he or she could make himself or herself well. This need is not extinguished because we have medicine, and is not addressed in the modern medical system, Glaspy says.

In modern medicine, there are no stories to help people with cancer understand their disease, nor are they told what they can do to alter the outcome of the disease. Because this human need is not being met by Western medicine, other practitioners and so-called practitioners have entered the scene to fill that gap, he says. It's easier to deal with the powerlessness and terror with a simple story and remedy— the immune system failed, so take this vitamin, for example, he says. There are many remedies and many stories to go along with them, but they can't all be true, and they may all be wrong, but at the heart is the need for simple story, he says.

Certainly that is true for those practicing quackery, and might well be true for other practices. But the same argument can be made against psychoanalysis and certain practices in psychiatry and psychology, yet Western medicine accepts those theories without solid scientific evidence. Certainly, as discussed later, other factors have played a strong role in keeping promising alternative practices out of the lab.

Digging up the problem

According to Glaspy, Western doctors haven't done a good job educating people about the process of discovering how drugs work. Doctors don't teach patients about trial methodology, he says. As a result, people think researchers and the FDA are rigid, noncreative bureaucrats that demand impossible levels of proof, Glaspy says. But, he points out, a false conclusion in a scientific study impedes medical progress and inflicts untold suffering on the human population. The answer? Scientists must explain the concept and importance of experimental methods, he says. It is important to understand the process of scientific discovery so you don't get tricked into believing unsophisticated, forceful investigators, those touting alternative practices that have not been rigorously tested by scientific standards, he says.

The difference between Western medical practices and many alternative therapies is that Western practices have been studied, the benefits measured, and the rational reasons behind the discoveries explained. Alternative medicine does not have that level of evidence supporting it, he points out. When considering alternative complementary approaches, you should consider asking, "What percentage of the time does it work?" and "Does this treatment conflict with other treatments?" There are so many unknowns with these treatments, Glaspy points out. It is difficult, if not impossible, to get answers to these questions for many alternative and complementary practices because funding hasn't historically been provided to back research on unconventional practices.

Why the cold shoulder?

Although research would answer some questions about the efficacy of alternative treatments, many of these therapies haven't been studied. One reason, as noted earlier, is a shortage of research money.

There's no lack of scientists looking hard for cancer remedies, but they can only study a certain number of things at a certain time, according to Glaspy. Science approaches treatments by first understanding how they work and then testing them, not the other way around, he says.

But others would disagree, at least in part. Observing a result shows promise. Just like aspirin, the mechanism can be studied later.

To many patients and alternative and complementary medicine practitioners, an observation of an apparent cause and effect is critical. It shows a strong possibility of a causal effect that should be recognized and validated through scientific study. To dismiss these observations as insignificant or unlikely or even the placebo effect seems nothing less than arrogant and closeminded by those who have witnessed changes or believe strongly that cause and effect in practices not currently accepted in Western medicine are not just possible but likely.

But there are practical difficulties in studying alternative medicine, according to Jeffrey White, M.D., director of the Office of Cancer Complementary and Alternative Medicine at the National Cancer Institute. "There are logistical and scientific problems involved in comparing the efficacy and toxicity of whole natural products [such as herbs] or their extracts to single, isolated, purified components of these whole products," White explains. For example, if you look at herbal remedies as whole products, it requires different resources than looking at an isolated compound.

Some effects may be interactions of compounds rather than several single compounds having their own effect on tumors. The same principle may exist for taking single vitamins rather than eating a fruit or vegetable that contains several vitamins and eating soy versus some of the elements that make up soy. That is, it might be the combination at certain ratios rather than the single vitamins themselves having an effect.

The question remains is it the whole product or single agent? The answer is difficult to determine because you can't put these products under a microscope to determine what the "active" ingredients are and how they work—alone or in combination with

Unofficially...
Like alternative and complementary practices, the placebo effect, a powerful response by the body's own healing mechanisms, has been ignored by Western medicine in general.

other ingredients. You have to know what you're look-ing for to detect it.

Furthermore, with herbal products, in order to do a cohort study, one that compares a group using the herbs to one that is not, you need to make sure that there is no variability among the batches of the product given to the study participants. "What is it that you're going to look at to say the product is the same?" White asks. Without knowing what's in the herb, the investigator cannot easily identify it.

The problem is further complicated because nature is so intricate. Plants can vary by the soil and climate. Processing can also affect the product. The answer does not lie in growing the plant at the lab. If scientists did so, they might not be able to replicate growing conditions that would guarantee the plant's effectiveness in treating illness. How would they know if the active ingredient was present in it? For example, mistletoe, used in Europe, is a semi-parasitic plant; it grows attached to a tree, and its composition varies according to the tree it grows on. "Those differences may be clinically significant," White points out.

You need to know something about the product before a clinical trial will give you answers, White says. However, scientists, pushed by public demand, have begun to take a closer look at what alternative approaches may have to offer conventional medicine.

The answers to these problems may take some time to get, "but research into the therapeutic use of herbs [such as St. John's wort] and extracts of other natural products [such as shark cartilage extract] is beginning," White says.

But it may be a long row to hoe. "Without a clear understanding of the complexity of these compounds and the potentially intricate ways that they might act on the body, it will be easy to misinterpret the results of these trials," White says.

White believes that it is likely that herbal research will evolve over time, addressing more and more of these issues. "However, since this research is so complex, I think it will only evolve if we can find examples of a whole herb being more useful—more clinically effective or less toxic and equally effective—than the single most active ingredient within it," he says.

Responding to the critics

The difficulty doesn't just lie in the challenges in the laboratory. It lies in the attitude of investigative researchers and conventional clinical practitioners.

Many physicians are traditionalists—hard-core scientists who base their beliefs on proven facts. Their ideas start in the laboratory based on solid theory. In contrast, some alternative methods are based on folklore and other belief systems. The challenge for the field of integrative medicine, a field that combines conventional with alternative practices, is twofold.

First, science studies medicine at the molecular level, an approach that has provided Western medicine with a wealth of important advances in the understanding of diseases and treatment methods. This same approach, however, may be missing important information on other therapies because, as noted earlier, alternative therapies are based on practices that have been handed down through the centuries.

A traditional scientist waits for verifiable and reproducible concrete data before accepting a therapeutic approach to a disease. While it would be generally unwise, and in many cases downright dangerous, to take any other approach due to toxicity or the possibility of just wasting time, in some areas of practice it may prove beneficial to make exceptions.

When the therapeutic method complements that of acceptable protocols and where it causes no harm is one of those exceptions, according to Samuel D. Benjamin, M.D., director of the University Center for Complementary and Alternative Medicine at SUNY Stony Brook School of Medicine, Stony Brook, New York.

The second challenge is for researchers to look at the "big picture." Western medicine is based on reductionism, that is, "Everything can be broken down to a molecular level," Benjamin says. "I agree with that, however, that approach makes us miss the woods from the trees. We have not spent enough time looking for things from a broader perspective. I think you need both [approaches]," he says. Benjamin wants more focus on population trends—looking at how people are faring and determining why. "Sometimes when you look at things from a broader perspective you see more," he notes.

One population-based trend that has been explored and reported in peer-reviewed scientific journals is the Japanese diet and its apparent correlation to low rates of breast cancer among Japanese women living in Japan. (Japanese women living in the United States have a higher rate of breast cancer.) The Japanese diet places a heavy emphasis on soy, a plant product that contains both isoflavinoids and phytoestrogens. Phytoestrogens, most importantly, genestein (as noted in Chapter 1), compete with estrogen receptors and may have a protective effect on breast cancer development. The Japanese diet also includes green tea, which has catechins. Green tea appears to inhibit tumor growth. This ingredient may be an important factor in the lower numbers of diagnosed breast cancers in Japan. Incidentally, indole-3

Watch Out!
The toxicity of high levels of indole-3-carbinol, a substance found in lower levels in cruciferous vegetables such as broccoli, is not known and is being considered for investigation by the National Institute of Environmental Health Sciences.

carbinols, Benjamin notes, can also contribute to decreasing cancer in general, breast cancer specifically, and can be found in vegetarian diets.

Even though these nutritional elements have been the focus of population-based studies, you don't hear of many doctors recommending them because the science behind them is not well understood. However, there is a considerable amount of published research on soy and on green tea.

By eating a diet high in soy or by drinking green tea as a preventive method, "What have you got to lose? These are not things that will cause you any harm," Benjamin says. We may not be able to prevent breast cancer, but we can take measures to prevent it, he adds. This is one approach.

Benjamin comments, though, that "the critics are absolutely right. [Complementary medicine] has not been adequately studied. A lot of what you hear is mumbo jumbo." That doesn't mean the techniques are not useful or scientific, he says. Aspirin was used for decades before scientists understood how it worked. "Because something hasn't been explained yet doesn't mean that it doesn't have validity," Benjamin stresses. "The key is that it [should do no] harm."

Benjamin, like others in his field, points out that the practice of dismissing an observed change because its mechanism of action is not understood has devalued probably the most important tool a person has against disease: the placebo effect. Because it has yet to be rigorously explored and explained, the placebo effect, the healing of the body due to the strong belief that the body is being healed by a drug, although it's not, hasn't gotten much attention from scientific investigators as a healing mechanism. Yet it

Unofficially...
Green tea is thought to have numerous biological activities, including antimutagenic, antibacterial, hypocholesterolemic, antioxidant, antitumor and cancer preventive properties (*Anticancer Drugs*, June 1996).

is the body at its peak state of remedying what has gone awry. The placebo effect is something that scientists need to master, not ignore. Since it is elicited by an expectation (a sugar pill replaces an actual drug without the patient knowing which he or she received), it is not only powerful, it is nontoxic.

Pushed into action

Four out of 10 Americans used alternative therapies in 1997. The total number of visits for alternative treatments increased by 47 percent from an estimated 427 million visits in 1990 to 629 million visits in 1997. This exceeded the total number of visits to all primary care physicians in the United States (386 million) in 1997, according to an article in the November 11, 1998, issue of *The Journal of the American Medical Association* (JAMA*).*

The authors of the JAMA study suggest "that federal agencies, private corporations, and foundations and academic institutions adopt a more proactive posture concerning the implementation of clinical and basic science research,...credentialing and referral guidelines, improved quality control of dietary supplements, and the establishment of post-market surveillance of drug-herb (and drug-supplement) interactions."

In fact, the Office of Cancer Complementary and Alternative Medicine was formed in 1998 to help determine which alternative medicine approaches should be examined by the National Cancer Institute (NCI).

Tools of the complementary medicine trade

If you do develop breast cancer, or have already been diagnosed with it, there are complementary

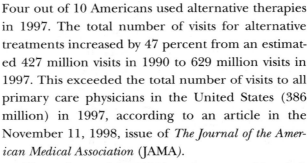

Watch Out!
Due to rising consumer interest and demand, there has been a tremendous growth of unconventional and unproven medical treatments in the United States. Some of these therapies may pose a risk to your health (such as herbal remedies with heavy metal contaminants or herbs that conflict with conventional medications) as well as your pocketbook.

approaches to Western medicine that may provide you with some relief. These include diet, acupuncture, mind-body medicine, physical medicine, some herbal medicines, guided imagery, and spirituality.

"There are many techniques that may be helpful in surviving the symptoms and improving the quality of life of the women who have been afflicted," Benjamin says. The key is, they should do no harm.

Diet

There is scientific evidence that poor nutrition can contribute to the development of breast cancer and other diseases. Conventional medicine recognizes that eating fruits and vegetables, especially those with antioxidants (beta carotene is found in squash, cantaloupe, carrots, and yams; vitamin C is found in citrus fruits, broccoli, green pepper, and spinach; vitamin E is found in wheat germ, oils, nuts, avocado, fish, and oil) and phytoestrogens (found in soybeans, soy flour, flax seed oil, and red clover sprouts), fiber (found in bran cereal, oatmeal, whole grain breads, prunes), soy (found in tofu, soy milk, soybeans, soy flour), and genestein, a plant product that is a good source of estrogen (found in soy beans and other soy proteins) can reduce your risk of developing cancer.

Nutrition is key, says Karen Koffler, M.D, a fellow at the University of Arizona program in integrative medicine. Koffler, who is also an internist and who worked as a hospitalist (a relatively new type of specialist who sees hospitalized patients) prior to starting her fellowship suggests the following:

- **Fruits and vegetables**—A high fruit and vegetable intake (five or more fruits and vegetables a day) lowers the incidence of recurrence in women who have had breast cancer. Furthermore, Koffler

Watch Out!
Beta carotene
supplements
increase the risk
of lung cancer
in smokers.

says that earlier scientific studies have demonstrated that people who eat vegetarian diets have a lower overall incidence of cancer. Fruits and vegetables contain antioxidants and carotenoids, both of which help protect healthy cells from damage caused by free radicals. Free radicals are substances produced by normal body functions such as breathing and physical activity and not-so-normal activities such as smoking. Free radicals attack healthy cells. When healthy cells are weakened, they are more susceptible to mutations. Antioxidants include both vitamins C and E. Fruits and vegetables rich in vitamin C include citrus fruits (oranges and grapefruits), strawberries, broccoli, and potatoes. Foods rich in vitamin E include nuts, peanut butter, and seeds as well as whole grain products, seeds, vegetable oils and salad dressings, margarine, and wheat germ. Carotenoids, which include beta carotene, lycopene, and lutein, are found in red (tomatoes), orange (carrots), deep-yellow (sweet potatoes), and some dark-green leafy vegetables (broccoli).

■ **Soy**—Like many other physicians, Koffler encourages premenopausal women to eat soy and soy products. However, she cautions that while soy and other phytoestrogens seem to have a protective effect against the development of breast cancer in premenopausal women, it is unclear if they will help or harm postmenopausal women and women who have been diagnosed with breast cancer. The concern centers on the theory that soy and other phytoestrogens have a weak estrogen link. It is thought they may trigger tumor growth in these two groups of women. Koffler says there is no scientific evidence to support this belief and adds that while soy may land on the cell's estrogen receptor, it does not lead to the same cascade of events as when estrogen binds with the receptor. Soy can be found in many forms in many food products including tofu and tofu-based products such as tofu ice cream and tofu cream cheese, soy nuts, soybean vegetable oil, soy milk, and soy flour.

Watch Out!
Eating soy may interfere with tomoxifen's protective effect.

- **Antioxidants**—Koffler recommends adding more antioxidants to your diet, such as grape seed extract and green tea. Additional antioxidants are noted earlier under "Fruits and Vegetables." She advises avoiding selenium because there is a possibility that it may increase a woman's risk of developing breast cancer. Selenium is found in meats, fish, grains, and Brazil nuts.

- **Water**—Water detoxifies your body, so drink lots of it, she says. Dehydration is a strain to the immune system, and the immune system plays an important role in combating cancer. Take note that we only sense thirst when we've already been dehydrated by 10 percent. So drink water even when you're not thirsty. To be well-hydrated, the average sedentary adult woman needs at least nine cups of non-caffeinated, nonalcoholic fluid per day, according to research published in the *Journal of the American Dietetic Association* (February 1999).

- **CoQ10**—For metastatic breast cancer, Koffler suggests vitamin Q10 (Coenzyme Q10; CoQ10), a substance involved in energy production within all the cells. Found in high levels in organ meats such as heart, liver, and kidney, as well as beef, soy oil, sardines, mackerel, and peanuts, it also protects cell membranes against oxidation.

Two small studies showed that women with metastatic breast cancer who took CoQ10 along with conventional therapy had complete remissions of the metastatic tumors (*Biochemical and Biophysical Research Communications;* July 1995). Koffler says it is especially helpful for women with shortness of breath or fatigue because it improves the uptake of oxygen into the cell. It is also an antioxidant.

In addition, Koffler suggests eating hormone-free meat and organic fruit to stay away from pesticides, some of which are carcinogenic. When storing and microwaving food, don't use soft plastic containers or plastic wrap. They have a hormone-like substance that can be leached into food. Use glass or hard plastic.

Although most mainstream dietitians believe you can get all of the nutrients necessary through a balanced diet, Benjamin, a physician who practices integrative medicine, and others disagree. He believes you need supplements, specifically, mixed carotenoids, natural vitamin E, and CoQ10. Benjamin also cited the *Biochemical and Biophysical Research Communications* study that reportedly showed five complete remissions among women who took CoQ10 along with the standard treatment for breast cancer. "The studies were not controlled or methodologically significant, and while intriguing, could not lead to any conclusions. However, no undesirable side effects were noted," Benjamin says.

The effects of administering CoQ10 combined with standard chemotherapy is being investigated in laboratory studies by researchers at the Center for Alternative Medicine at the University of Texas.

In an article in the journal *Cancer* (March 1996), Cassilleth, chief of integrative medicine at Memorial

Bright Idea
Make sure you use a good water filtration system, as tap water and some bottled waters may contain carcinogens. Not all filtering systems are equal. Use a carbon filtering system.

Sloan-Kettering Cancer Center in New York, notes that anticancer diets and nutritional supplements are some of the oldest alternative cancer treatments. "Today's most popular anticancer diet is probably macrobiotics," she writes. "The diet...promotes soybean consumption," Cassileth says in the article.

The philosophy underlying this ancient Japanese diet is yin and yang, two antagonistic but complementary forces that operate in the universe: extremes find their opposites for balance.

From a yin/yang perspective, foods range from dense (red meats) to less dense (fish). Root vegetables, whole grains, and cereals, followed by the stalks and leaves of vegetables, fall in the center of this continuum. More expansive foods include fruits followed by refined sugars and alcohol. Eating too much on one end of the spectrum, according to this yin/yang philosophy, creates a craving for food at the opposite end. Eating beef would create the desire for drinking alcohol, for example. Constant cravings can disrupt metabolism, leaving you vulnerable to stress and disease, according to the philosophy. So the diet is centered on whole grains and cereals.

However, the contemporary macrobiotic diet is less restrictive. Only 50 to 60 percent of the diet needs to be from whole cereals and grains. The rest can come from vegetables and beans, fermented soy products, and sea vegetables as well as tea and soups. The diet can also include small amounts of white-meat fish and fresh organic fruits. Occasionally, you can eat lightly roasted nuts and seeds.

The NIH Office of Alternative Medicine is funding studies on the macrobiotic diet.

Acupuncture

Acupuncture is an ancient Chinese practice that has

Watch Out!
Using high-dose vitamins may benefit some people, depending on the vitamins, dose, scheduling, and disease. But vitamins can be toxic, and some can interfere with conventional treatments. Ask your doctor before taking any vitamins.

been practiced for at least 2,500 years. It's based on the belief that energy (qi) flows in patterns through the body. These energy channels, called meridians, are essential for good health. In Eastern philosophy, it is believed that disease is caused by a disruption of the energy flow. The obstruction is similar to a dam obstructing the flow of a river, which backs up the other rivers that nourish the body. Acupuncture is believed to correct the flow, and qi plays an important role in evaluating patients and determining treatment. Asian acupuncturists use different acupuncture points for different applications.

American acupuncture is an adaptation of the Asian method, which uses fine needles that are manipulated manually or by electrical stimulation. These are the most studied mechanisms of stimulation of acupuncture points. Other techniques used to stimulate acupuncture points, which are close to the skin, include lasers, pressure, and heat.

The scientific data supporting acupuncture is as strong as that for many Western medical therapies accepted by the medical community. According to the NIH Consensus Statement on acupuncture (November 1997), the result of a 2 1/2-day conference to evaluate the data on acupuncture procedures for a variety of conditions, acupuncture is useful for several side effects associated with cancer treatments:

- ■ *Nausea associated with chemotherapy.* Though scientists aren't sure how it works, it may have an effect on the central nervous system and the part of the brain that deals with nausea.

- ■ *Post-surgical pain.* By stimulating an endorphin response, it helps reduce pain.

Some doctors believe acupunture also helps with the following:

- ▪ *Fatigue associated with breast cancer.* Acupuncture has a temporary, cumulative effect. If the effects last for a week after the first treatment, for example, they will last more than a week after the next treatment.

- ▪ *Improved immune response.* The science behind this effect is not understood, nor it is known how long the effect lasts.

Scientific studies have demonstrated that acupuncture can cause specific biological responses, both at the needle site and areas distant from the site, mediated mainly by sensory nerves to the spinal cord and brain.

There is considerable scientific evidence that opioid peptides, which have morphine-like activity, are released during acupuncture and that analgesic effects are at least partially explained by their actions. Endorphins, released from the body by rigorous exercise such as long-distance running, is at least in part responsible for "runner's high." Endorphins are one class of opiate peptides.

Acupuncture may also stimulate the hypothalamus and the pituitary gland, resulting in systemic effects. Alterations of neurotransmitters and neurohormone secretions and changes in blood flow also have been documented, and there is evidence that the immune function changes as a result of acupuncture, though it is not understood which of these changes among others mediate the effects.

However, there are questions that remain unanswered. Some of the same biological effects have been observed when "sham" acupuncture points, those considered false, are stimulated, and similar effects, including changes in blood pressure and the release of endogenous opioids are seen after exer-

Unofficially...
The effects of both conventional and alternative medicine rely on several factors, including: the quality of the relationship between the health care giver and the patient; how compatible their belief systems are; the degree of trust the patient has in the health care worker and the therapy; and the patient's expectations.

cise, relaxation, and pain, according to the consensus report, which notes that at this point it is "unclear to what extent acupuncture shares similar biological mechanisms."

In the wrong hands, acupuncture can be dangerous. Dirty needles are a problem with some backroom practitioners. And some "acupuncturists" don't know where to place the needle, Benjamin says. If a needle is inserted too deep into your chest, you run the risk of puncturing your lung, for example. You must place the needle in the right places to get the energy flowing in the right way.

To locate a physician who is trained in acupuncture, contact the American Academy of Medical Acupuncture at 800/521-AAMA or visit their Web site at www.medicalacupuncture.org or check the International Association of Healthcare Practitioners Directory, http://www.iahp.com/pract.htm, which lists over 40,000 complementary therapy physicians. (For more information or to purchase a copy of the directory for $15, contact IAHP, 11211 Prosperity Farms Road, D-325, Palm Beach Gardens, Fl 33410-3487; fax: 561/622-4771; e-mail: iahp@iahp.com.) To locate a nonphysician practitioner, contact the National Certification Commission for Acupuncture and Oriental Medicine at www.nccaom.org or at 703/548-9004. Be sure the specialist you choose is licensed or registered in your state, Benjamin says. Enhancing the Accountability of Alternative Medicine at www.milbank.org/mraltmed.html is a good site to learn about states' regulation of health professionals.

Mind-body medicine

The placebo effect is a good example of how strongly the mind can affect the body. Mind-body medicine is accomplished by altering the state of consciousness so patients can "harvest their own body's ability to heal themselves," Benjamin explains. He added that these altered states of consciousness can help with all the side effects of breast cancer, and perhaps the cancer itself, but more research is needed.

Benjamin illustrates his point by citing a study done by David Spiegel, M.D., who runs the alternative medicine program at Stanford University. He divided a group of women diagnosed with breast cancer and given traditional treatments into a control group that didn't attend a support group, and a case group that did. Those who attended the group lived 50 percent longer. If Spiegel showed that the camaraderie of a support group can increase survival by 50 percent, why aren't doctors pointing this out to their patients, Benjamin asks. It does no harm and will take years for scientists to replicate the study findings, he notes.

"What it shows you is that mind-body medicine can really make a difference," Benjamin says. He theorizes that the case group may have become more optimistic in their prognosis. Another of Benjamin's concerns is the impact of a doctor's attitude. Giving a poor prognosis may be a death warrant in some cases, he says. Doctors need to balance honesty with admitting they can't predict the future. "We don't realize the incredible transcendence that those statements have on people's lives," Benjamin says.

There are many different ways of eliciting the mind-body response:

- Guided visual imagery
- Meditation and yoga
- Mindfulness
- Biofeedback
- Hypnosis

"Good documentation exists for the effectiveness of meditation, biofeedback, and yoga in stress reduction and the control of particular physiologic reactions," Cassilleth writes in the journal *Cancer*. She also says, "Learn to appreciate how good it feels to walk around in the body you have. It will help you develop gratitude, and it's through gratitude that you gain hope."

Information on mind-body research can be found at the National Institute of Health's National Center for Complementary and Alternative Medicine at www.nccam.nih.gov.

Hope, which connects the mind and body, is the biggest healing mechanism, both physically and in terms of quality of life, Koffler says.

Women who express themselves do better than those who accept their diagnosis and pain stoically, Koffler says. You have a more stressed system when you don't express who you are—when you keep silent about your most profound experiences. It takes a lot of energy to hide an experience, she points out. Self-expression can come in many forms—writing, talking, painting, and dancing.

Researchers at the Center for Alternative Medicine Research at the University of Texas-Houston School of Public Health and M.D. Anderson Cancer Center in Houston confirmed Spiegel's findings about the importance of group support. Investigators studied three groups of women with primary breast cancer (excluding those with Stage IV) who were not previously treated with tamoxifen (which can affect the immune system). The focus of the study was to determine the effects of imagery and group support on these women's coping skills, their life attitudes, immune function, perceived quality of life, and their perceived emotional well-being after breast cancer

Unofficially...
Giving a poor prognosis can impact patient attitude, which may affect how aggressively they fight their disease.

diagnosis and treatment.

Forty-seven women participated. They were randomly assigned to three groups: one group received six weekly imagery sessions, one got six weekly support sessions, and one got nothing but standard therapy, that is, they were the control group. Afterwards, their immune function was assessed and psychosocial measures were used to assess their emotional well-being, quality of life, social support, and coping strategies.

The imagery group fared best, with the support group coming in a close second, according to Blair Justice, Ph.D., professor of psychology at The University of Texas Health Science Center School of Public Health and one of the study's authors. It appears there also is some benefit for women to attend support groups, he says. (The imagery group had support implied in it because they met in a group. The added imagery may be why they had a small advantage over the next group, Justice says. The trend was in the right direction though the numbers were not statistically significant because the number of women studied was too low.)

Several years later, Justice interviewed some of the women who participated in the study. He was struck by his findings—so much so he wrote the book, *A Different Kind of Health: Finding Well-Being Despite Illness.* Asked if they considered themselves healthy, these women gave the same kind of answers as healthy, cancer-free adults who respond to epidemiological surveys, Justice says. Twelve of the 13 women he interviewed believed they were healthy, even though they had cancer. Most interesting, Justice points out, is that this belief that they are healthy is more predictive of length and quality of life than a physician's predictions. This, he says, is a good

Bright Idea
Not only does the doctor's attitude have an impact, so does the attitude of those with whom you surround yourself. Surrounding yourself with supportive, caring people can drastically change your outlook.

example of the mind-body effect.

Justice took this opportunity to explore how someone can acknowledge her disease and yet still feel healthy. He found that these women see themselves as having other parts—mental, emotional, and spiritual, and if all these parts are healthy, they view themselves on the whole as healthy.

The basis on which women came to say, "I'm healthy," says Justice, boiled down to two themes:

1. They found something of value as a result of having breast cancer. Some examples include:

   ■ They considered it a blessing because it forced them to reprioritize their life.

   ■ It deepened their faith. (Some women lost their faith but came back to it.)

   ■ They created better relationships.

   ■ They repaired old relationships. "Many learned the importance of forgiveness," Justice says. By learning to forgive and to ask for forgiveness, they were able to renew old friendships, he says.

2. They found they felt better when they focused on positive things outside their illness. The philosophy is based on Fordyce's Law—named after Willard Fordyce, a pain researcher at the University of Wisconsin's medical school—people suffer less when they find something good to do. The degree of suffering is altered when you get outside yourself, Justice explains. Some women he interviewed found a driving purpose. He notes that many cancer survivors become volunteers as a result of that driving force to do good for others. The drive and subsequent behavior helps alleviate the pain. "[The mind-body connection

is] not going to cure you," according to Justice. But healing is something else, he says. It's internal. You can repair what's broken in the non-physical parts, the emotions and attitudes, and that has an effect on the physical parts, the body, he says. There's a lot of research supporting this, he notes.

However, the mind doesn't cause cancer, and cancer patients don't "need" their cancer for the secondary gains it brings such as attention from family and friends, as was theorized by one physician and popular author. "Bernie Siegel, M.D., former surgeon and author of *Love, Medicine, and Miracles* and other best-sellers, is a leading and popular proponent of the link between mind and cancer," Cassilleth wrote in the journal *Cancer.* "Siegel organized groups of 'exceptional cancer patients' based on his observation as a cancer surgeon that attitude influenced survival time. He encourages patients to maintain positive attitudes and to assume responsibility for their own health. He asks them to consider why they might 'need' their cancer. The implication is that cancer results from unhealthy emotional patterns," she explained.

But a study co-authored by Siegel of the "exceptional attitude" patients compared with the controls found no difference in length of survival. The follow-up study was published in the journal *Clinical Oncology* (January 1993). The conclusion stated in the abstract said, "While the program may have beneficial effects on quality of life, this study does not indicate a significant favorable impact on survival with breast cancer or that the program is serving as a social locus for the gathering of exceptional survivors." The earlier positive results were due largely to

Unofficially...
One can be cured but not healed, healed but not cured, or healed and cured!

selection bias, according to the authors of an article published in the *Journal of Chronic Diseases* (Volume 37, Issue 4; 1984). (The authors of that study, however, did not rule out a possible positive effect on survival because of the lack of statistical power and a statistically nonsignificant benefit observed for women who entered the program shortly after diagnosis.) This study, Cassilleth notes, got no press.

Using your head to heal your body

"Guided imagery is a phenomenon," Koffler says. She starts her patients with a relaxation exercise and then moves into imagery, the theme of which the patient must choose. Patients often choose to focus on the tumor or an image of themselves being healthy. Imagery has three possible benefits:

1. It can reduce anxiety and enhance the quality of life.

2. It can boost the immune system.

3. It can affect how the body works by tapping into the molecules where the mind and body connect. (Daydreaming is another way to connect with the body.) In a relaxed state, you are more in tune with those images. You are to some degree directing molecules.

Imagery gives you more control over the situation or provides insight into what you need to do to get a desirable outcome. It gives hope, Koffler says, which is not something to be overlooked. Imagery can also be used for pain relief and to control nausea. With imagery, you can go away from where you are to another place or another time.

Breathing exercises are mostly used to control anxiety, which helps to ease the mind. Controlled breathing also serves as a connection between the mind and body. It is an automatic bodily function that you can take control over. Slow, deep breathing changes your body's biology and brings you into a deep, relaxed state. In many languages, "breath" is the same word as "spirit."

When going through chemotherapy, many women lose their hair and experience other side effects that alter their looks and hence the way they feel about their bodies. One effective way to deal with this is through exercise, Koffler says. She suggests paying attention to how the sun feels on your face and body and how the ground feels underneath your feet.

Spirituality

We don't understand the nature of prayer, says Benjamin. But the power of prayer and spirituality is apparent. A well-known, unreplicated example is the San Francisco intercessory prayer study, a prospective, randomized, double-blind study of 393 patients, one-half of whom were randomly selected to be prayed for by people at a distance. Results were significant ($P < 0.0001$), suggesting that intercessory prayer had beneficial therapeutic effects.

In an article titled "A randomized double-blind study of the effect of distant healing in a population with advanced AIDS. Report of a small scale study," researchers at Geraldine Brush Cancer Research Institute, California Pacific Medical Center in San Francisco reported on a double-blind, randomized trial of 10 weeks of distant healing in 40 patients with advanced AIDS in the *Western Journal of Medicine* (December 1998). Distant healing treatment was performed by self-identified healers who represented different healing and spiritual traditions. Healers were located throughout the United States. The subjects and healers did not meet. At six months, the

> **"**
> It's those subtle influences in life that medicine hasn't paid any attention to that have an enormous impact.
> —Karen Koffler, M.D, a fellow at the University of Arizona program in integrative medicine.
> **"**

researchers found that treatment subjects acquired fewer new AIDS-defining illnesses, had lower illness severity, and required fewer doctor visits, fewer hospitalizations, and fewer days of hospitalization when they were hospitalized. The treated patients had improved mood compared with controls who didn't receive the distant healing.

There have been several studies of the effects of prayer in curing disease, including some that looked at intercessory prayer. Unfortunately, there are no definitive results.

"Stories of individuals who successfully prayed to be healed or who experienced miraculous cures from cancer and other illnesses are frequently reported," Cassilleth writes in the journal *Cancer*.

66
Prayer indeed is good, but while calling on the gods a man should himself lend a hand.
—Hippocrates
99

Whereas religious people may attribute it to prayer, science takes a different view. Spiritual healing may be an example of the placebo effect, where expecting a positive result actually produces one. These two views, however, are not incompatible.

The danger, Benjamin says, is in denying standard medical care because of faith in prayer alone. Another problem is "I'm praying, why isn't it working?"

Even if prayer doesn't cure a person's cancer, it can help create a positive outlook, reduce stress, and strengthen her will to live with the cancer. Religious beliefs also can add purpose and meaning to life, as well as hope.

Because faith plays such an important role for patients, hospitals have chapels and most have ministers and rabbis on call.

Physical medicine
Physical medicine includes the following:

- Osteopathy
- Chiropractic

- Tai chi

- Yoga

(Note: Tai chi and yoga are crossovers of the mind-body connection.)

Watch Out!
Be sure to have your physician and alternative medicine health practitioners work together. Everyone on your medical team should be aware of and in agreement on all your treatments to ensure the best and safest outcome.

During breast surgery, the patient is moved around a lot on the operating table, especially if she is undergoing TRAM-flap surgery taking muscles from the back, so afterwards there is skeletal pain, Benjamin says. He believes that osteopathic medicine (which is based on the philosophy that all body systems are interrelated and dependent upon each other and today treats illness within the context of the whole body with conventional medicine and osteopathic manipulative treatment, a set of manual techniques) or chiropractic therapy is helpful. Chiropractic is a century-old health practice that focuses on the relationship between structure (primarily the spine) and function (as coordinated by the nervous system), and the impact structure and function have on the preservation and restoration of health. Benjamin recommends gentle cranial manipulations, which he says should do the least amount of harm. The theory is that the movement stimulates certain parts of the nervous system. Although many people do not think the skull bones move, real time MRI imaging shows the skull moves around, he says.

Traditional Chinese medicine relies on exercise techniques such as Qi Gong and Tai Chi to strengthen and balance chi, the life force, which flows through postulated energy channels known as meridians, Cassilleth says in the *Cancer* article.

Herbal medicine

Herbal medicine is an area of alternative and complementary medicine with some similarities to chemotherapy in that they are both medicinal but which demands great caution for two reasons:

1. These herbs can interact with chemotherapy and other medications.

2. Herbal products are sometimes poorly produced, not containing what they claim are the ingredients, and the FDA doesn't have stringent control over them as it does with drugs. Herbal products may contain contaminants such as heavy lead, steroids, harmful bacteria, and diazepam (Valium). These contents are not disclosed to the buyer.

"The field is rife with irresponsible people making products that are potentially dangerous," Benjamin warns.

These impurities also make it difficult if not impossible to determine if research outcomes are accurate for pure herbal products.

If you're doing well, you may not want to take herbal remedies. If you're not responding at all to traditional treatments, you may want to join a study that's investigating herbs. But before taking any herbs, consult your physician.

Do your homework

Before integrating an alternative therapy into your medical treatment, explore several important areas to be sure the cure is not worse than the disease. Consider the following:

- Is the treatment considered safe and effective by the conventional medical community? Have study results been published in reputable peer-reviewed journals? Positive findings from published scientific studies would indicate that this treatment may, in fact, be potentially beneficial.

- Is the treatment promoted in the mass media

through advertisements in magazines or through books and TV talk shows? If the treatment is promoted through paid advertisements (except from recognizable pharmaceutical companies), especially advertorials (magazine and newspaper advertisements that look like editorial content but have a disclaimer at the top of the page such as "Advertising Supplement") and 30 to 60 minute paid TV or radio advertisements that are formatted like talk shows, then you may want to view the treatment with skepticism. The same goes for books, unless the author is well-recognized in the field of medicine and the treatment is backed by scientifically sound studies that have been published in reputable peer-reviewed medical journals.

- Is the health practitioner you've chosen well qualified and licensed by the state?

- Do the treatment's promoters dispute the value of conventional therapies? Do they attack the scientific/medical community?

- What are the risks, side effects, expected results, and length of treatment?

- How does the treatment compare with conventional therapy? What percentage of people using it show benefits? Is the benefit measurable?

These are all areas you can research. Check with your state to see if the practitioner is registered with and/or licensed to practice that particular therapy and read peer-reviewed journal articles for safety and outcomes research. Credible information can be found through online searches and at public, medical (hospital), and university libraries. Even after starting therapy, continue to look for updates in the literature.

Here's where you can search on the Internet:

- **MEDLINE (National Library of Medicine)** is accessible through the Internet Grateful Med at http://igm.nlm.nih.gov. It contains more than 11 million journal article abstracts and records dating back to 1966 that can be searched electronically through the Internet. (Full-text articles can be ordered through Loansome Doc or found in many public and medical libraries, which are located in both medical schools and local hospitals. Typically these libraries have hours when the public can access their stacks.)

- **The National Center for Complementary and Alternative Methods at the National Institutes of Health** has a Web site at http://nccam.nih.gov that lists research grants and information resources.

- **The National Center for Complementary and Alternative Medicine at the National Institutes of Health** has an overview of seven alternative medicine fields at http://altmed.od.nih.gov/nccam/what-is-cam. The topics include diet, nutrition, lifestyle changes, herbal medicine, mind-body control, bioelectromagnetic applications, alternative systems of medical practice, manual healing, and pharmacological and biological treatments.

- **The University of Texas Center for Alternative Medicine Research** (UT-CAM) at The University of Texas-Houston Health Science Center at www.sph.uth.tmc.edu:8052/utcam has research on some complementary therapies, a list of studies at the center, and links to other complementary and alternative medicine sites.

- **The Agricultural Research Service** maintains a

Timesaver
Don't understand all the technical jargon? CancerWEB at www.graylab.ac.uk/omd/online has an extensive medical dictionary.

database of herbal properties at www.ars-grin. gov/duke. You can search for the chemical and activities in a certain plant, plants with certain chemicals, or activities of a chosen chemical. It also has a botanical dictionary.

- **The FDA Guide to Choosing Medical Treatments** at www.fda.gov/oashi/aids/fdaguide.html summarizes the criteria that it uses to evaluate the safety and effectiveness of new treatments, lists some clinical trials testing alternative treatments, and gives explicit warnings about fraud and alternative medicine.

- **Quackwatch** at www.quackwatch.com alerts consumers to fraudulent practices and alternative medicine.

Picking a practitioner

Good integrative practitioners are hard to find. Columbia University in New York has a Web site at http://cpmcnet.columbia.edu/dept/rosenthal devoted to helping patients understand complementary and alternative medicine. It contains lists of academic and research centers in the United States, residency programs, and medical schools that have courses in complementary medicine. You can use these listings to locate a practitioner.

It also has links to resources for cancer research on the Internet.

Investigate

In the unlikely event that your physician practices poor medicine or acts unethically, you have a few places you can turn. You can contact the medical board in your state, the American Medical Association, a specialists' professional association (if your doctor has a specialty such as oncology) and Public

Watch Out!
The National Cancer Institute and other scientific organizations have not been able to find any evidence that the following unconventional therapies are useful in treating cancer: Laetrile, Cancell, Gerson Therapy, Livingston-Wheeler Vaccines, Krebiozen, Koch Synthetic Antitoxins, the Greek Cancer Cure, and various dietary regimens.

Citizen, a consumer advocate group. But what about alternative/complementary health practitioners?

When you choose an alternative/integrative health practitioner, shop around:

- Ask friends and other cancer survivors who they recommend.

- Ask your doctor who he or she recommends and why.

- Contact the Cancer Information Service at 800/4-CANCER or the American Cancer Society at 800/ACS-2345.

- Read peer-reviewed journals and contact the investigators to see whom in the field they recommend. Or, if the investigator is a clinician in your area or you are willing to travel, ask if you can see him or her.

- Go to an integrative medicine center with a good reputation.

Then do your homework on the individual practitioner you're considering:

- Contact your state regulatory agency that has authority over the type of practitioner you're seeking.

- Find out if the practitioner is licensed or registered (if licensure is not required) with the state, what his or her educational background is and what accreditation he or she holds, and whether complaints have been filed against the practitioner. You can get this information from local and state medical boards, other health regulatory boards or agencies, and local consumer affairs departments. You can also check with national organizations representing practitioners in specific specialty practices.

Watch Out!
If you get a referral to a complementary medicine practitioner from a professional organization, remember that the organization exists, in large part, to promote its members. They are not regulators.

- Talk to your doctor to find out if his or her colleagues have teamed up with this practitioner before.

- Talk to the practitioner. See if you like his or her approach and demeanor.

- Ask the practitioner about possible side effects and potential problems.

Make sure the practitioner you choose is licensed by the state and has a solid educational background as well as experience in the field of practice.

Just the facts

- The study of complementary treatments has been impeded, in part, by politics.

- More and more investigators are studying ancient healing techniques.

- Not enough is known about alternative treatment methods—it's buyer beware.

- There are many complementary treatments that are nontoxic, such as mind-body techniques.

Watch Out!
Complementary and alternative health practitioners usually are not as thoroughly regulated as those who practice conventional medicine.

Relationships and Emotional Impact

GET THE SCOOP ON...
Cancer myths in the workplace ▪ Dating again
▪ How to deal with your children if you have
breast cancer ▪ Sex after surgery ▪ Why it may
not be safe to get pregnant after being
diagnosed with breast cancer

PART VI

Dealing With the Aftermath: Life Post-Diagnosis

Chapter 13

Women who have been diagnosed with breast cancer often experience a range of physical and emotional difficulties. In addition to fear and anxiety, there are other less predictable situations that you may encounter. For instance, working women may have to deal with the emotional anxiety of going back to work in addition to the physical results of surgery and treatment, such as fatigue or hot flashes. Those in the work force may also find themselves getting a few cold shoulders from co-workers who don't understand what cancer is or just feel awkward and unsure of how to deal with someone who has cancer.

Most women of all ages will have to deal with sexual issues. In addition, single women, who already have to deal with the regular travails of dating, now have to worry about how the breast cancer and its ramifications will affect their ability to attract Mr. Right. Mothers, especially those in single-parent households,

331

Bright Idea
Join a workplace
support group for
cancer survivors.
If one doesn't
exist, start one.

have their fair share to handle, such as telling the children about the diagnosis and treatment. Younger women who are diagnosed have to come to heart-breaking terms with fertility issues and others may have to decide whether or not to risk pregnancy.

These are all big challenges. In this chapter, each of these topics is addressed and top experts share their knowledge and advice from psychological and biological perspectives.

Breast cancer and your job

Eighty percent of cancer survivors choose to return to work, according to the NCI. Some end up benefiting from supportive employers; others just slip back into their routine without much assistance. But there are those who return to co-workers who have misconceptions and false fears about cancer that cause job-related problems. In these cases, unjustified co-worker fear is another hurdle breast cancer survivors must jump.

Research has found that some people believe three myths about cancer that affect their attitude toward cancer survivors. The myths are as follows:

1. Cancer is a death sentence.

2. Cancer is contagious.

3. Cancer makes workers less productive.

There are more than eight million cancer survivors alive today in the United States, according to the NCI. Cancer survivors are just as productive and don't miss work any more often than other workers. However, about one in four cancer survivors experience some form of employment discrimination, according to the NCI.

Working women who have been treated for breast cancer may have to deal with physical hurdles, as well as emotional ones. Physical symptoms such as fatigue, nausea, and hot flashes during the workday are common. Normally, estrogen is prescribed to help ease hot flashes in post-menopausal women, but it's not usually recommended for women with breast cancer, because estrogen plays a large role in the development of the disease. Nausea can be treated with diet (ginger, saltines—see Chapter 8 for more information on diet and controlling treatment side effects) and acupuncture (see Chapter 12 for more information on integrative medicine) as well as medication. You can deal with fatigue by getting enough rest and eating a healthy diet.

If you have a supportive employer, you may want to ask for flex time, job sharing, or a telecommuting arrangement if it would make it easier for you to keep your job. But if your employer refuses to help you out, keep in mind that the federal government and many private companies, under the Americans with Disabilities Act, are now required by law to make "reasonable accommodations" to meet the needs of "disabled" employees if it does not cause the employer "undue hardship." As a cancer survivor, you may qualify for protection. To find out more about your legal rights, contact:

- The Job Accommodation Network at (800/526-7234). This agency can help you and your employer find out about accommodations that have worked for other companies.

- Contact the organizations that enforce anti-discrimination laws: your state commission on discrimination and state affirmative action offices, for example. If your company contracts with the federal government, contact the U.S. Department of Health and Human Services, Office for Civil Rights and U.S. Department of Labor, Office of

Bright Idea
If you're fatigued as a result of your treatments but still want to work, ask your employer if you can telecommute at least part-time to give yourself some extra time each day to rest. Or consider asking your employer if you can share your job with a co-worker.

Federal Contract Compliance.

- The National Coalition of Cancer Survivorship offers limited referrals to attorneys with experience solving on-the-job discrimination problems. Call them toll-free at 888/YES-NCCS (888/937-6227), or visit their Web site at www.cansearch.org.

- The Cancer Legal Resource Center, a joint program of the Western Law Center for Disability Rights and Loyola Law School, can provide some legal direction. They can be reached at 919 South Albany St., Los Angeles CA 90015; 213/736-1455; www.lls.edu;barbara.schwerin@lls.edu

You can also contact your congressman or senator, or file a discrimination complaint under state or federal laws. (Remember that the Family and Medical Leave Act requires employers with 50 or more employees to provide up to 12 weeks of unpaid leave for you or your family if you need help.)

If, however, you feel that the stress is too much, or you just don't want to waste your time fighting your company, you may want to consider finding another job. Of course, you'll probably want to find one at a large company whose health insurance carrier doesn't screen the health of new employees in order to get immediate health insurance coverage. And, you might want to consider taking your current health coverage with you through COBRA for 18 months, just in case the new job doesn't work out. You don't want to be left without health insurance. That said, you'll probably want to organize your resume by skills rather than by dates of employment.

Keeping your health coverage through COBRA

The Consolidated Omnibus Reconciliation Act (COBRA) allows you to keep your health benefits (and your family's) for up to 18 months. The types of qualifying events are "voluntary or involuntary termination of employment for reasons other than 'gross misconduct'" or a reduction in your hours, according to the Department of Labor. You'll have 60 days after the qualifying event to accept the coverage. COBRA coverage is retroactive if elected and paid for within that 60-day period.

You'll probably have to pick up the tab for the coverage, including the portion your employer used to kick in, but health coverage under COBRA is still generally a lot less expensive than most individual policies and has the added benefit of not excluding preexisting conditions. The premium can't exceed 102 percent of the cost to your previous employer.

Under COBRA, your health coverage will remain identical to that provided by the plan under which you had been previously covered. Premiums are generally fixed for each 12-month cycle, but increase if the cost of the plan increases.

Breast cancer and the single woman

Some single women have additional challenges. While some have a network of family and friends to support them emotionally, others must go through the pain of breast cancer alone. Whether they have emotional support or not, they typically don't have any choice about getting back to work as soon as possible, even if they aren't feeling well.

"I was diagnosed two days before Christmas [in 1997] and I was all alone," says Sandra Cooley, a cancer survivor in her late thirties. "It's tough when you're all alone. You just want a shoulder to cry on and there's none there." Sometimes popular advice can't be carried out. For example, while it's advisable to take someone with you to doctor visits, Cooley

Bright Idea
Plan ahead—look beyond your treatment to what you want to do when you get well. Having goals will help you get through the hard days.

Bright Idea
If you have no one to provide encouragement, try to find others in your area in the same situation. They need your companionship as much as you need theirs. Ask your health-care team to help set up the match or join a few support groups and find others in your situation. You can also meet your "match" in chat groups and news-groups on the Internet, such as those listed in Appendix B at the end of this book.

notes, she had no one to bring along. So, she prepared herself to handle the visits on her own: Before each appointment, she wrote down questions for the doctor based on her own concerns and research she had done. Then, during each visit, she wrote down everything the doctor said so she could read her notes at home and make informed decisions. And she prepared herself to go through a mastectomy alone, too: There was no one with her when she awoke after 10 hours of surgery.

According to Cooley, "I just wanted to live and I wanted to get the best possible treatment that assured me the best possible outcome."

Although she didn't deal with the emotional aspects of her cancer at the time of diagnosis and treatment, Cooley learned to cope by creating a support network of family and friends. Even her clients supported her. Cooley, an insurance broker for small businesses, was scared to tell her clients for fear they'd think she was dying and wouldn't want her to handle their accounts. But they rallied around her. "I also got a lot of support from a church group," she says, who put her on their prayer list, and looked for other resources in the form of books and articles.

Many single women are not quite so alone. They have roommates, friends, and family living nearby on whom they can depend.

Yearning for bad hair days

When first dealing with a disease like breast cancer, most women put the issue of self-image on the back burner, focusing instead on decisions about surgery and treatment. Once "the dust settles," women have to confront the physical ramifications, such as hair loss or a change in the way their chest looks as a result of the treatment decisions they've made.

Some women lose their hair as a result of chemotherapy. This can be one of the most jarring side effects of cancer treatment. It is particularly difficult for those who must reenter the workforce. In younger women, breast cancer is typically aggressive, so they're treated in more aggressive ways, often with chemotherapies that result in complete hair loss.

"There's a lot of assault to the body image," says Carol Fred, licensed clinical social worker at the Rhonda Flemming Mann Resource Center for Women with Cancer, part of the Jonsson Comprehensive Cancer Center at UCLA. Fred also works at the Revlon UCLA Breast Center.

"For a lot of women, their [missing] hair is screaming to the public that they're ill," says Marsha Oakley, RN, BSN of the Breast Center at Mercy Medical Center in Baltimore. Many women don't have insurance coverage for wigs, which can cost $100 or more, Oakley says, adding that human hair wigs cost up to $1,000. Though there are less expensive wigs on the market, $50 wigs look like $50 wigs, she says.

But there are ways around this dilemma. The American Cancer Society (800/ACS-2345) sometimes has wigs on hand for to those who can't afford them. There are also stylish head wrappings available at shops at cancer centers and on the Internet that are less expensive than wigs.

Body image is also an issue after surgery. Women experience a profound sense of loss and lack of wholeness after breast surgery to remove cancerous tissue. A lumpectomy leaves behind an indentation and scar, which can be noticeable through snug clothing. A mastectomy takes the whole breast, leaving just a scar behind. The missing breast (or breasts) is obvious under most clothing without reconstructive surgery or a prosthesis.

Both of these surgical treatments are devastating to many women because breasts are a large part of what defines femininity and sexuality for them and for society as a whole. Many women undergoing mastectomies therefore opt for reconstructive surgery, which replaces the breast mound and can replace the areola and nipple, but not any sexual sensations. But other women do not want to have any more surgeries (or prolong the mastectomy surgery by scheduling reconstructive surgery to take place during the same operation), so many of them insert breast forms into their bras, and many women who have a lumpectomy insert breast enhancers into their bras. (Both of these options are discussed in greater detail in Chapter 15.)

The decision of whether to have reconstructive surgery or use breast forms may be difficult for many women who are faced with a mastectomy. (Some women choose to do neither.) "Those are big issues for these women," Oakley says. Indeed, there are many considerations to take into account when making this decision.

Diagnosed with ductal carcinoma in situ, Cooley had a simple mastectomy. She had two choices: reconstruction with a transverse rectus abdominis myocutaneous (TRAM) flap or saline implants, and had two months to choose between them.

She opted for a TRAM flap over saline implants. With the TRAM flap, the tram muscle is taken from the abdomen and placed in the breast to give it a blood supply. Fat is then taken from the abdomen and placed in the breast. Skin, typically from the abdomen, is used to cover the breast. To add authenticity, the areola can later be tattooed onto the breast. (TRAM flap reconstructive surgery is discussed further in Chapter 15.)

Following the reconstructive surgery, the whole breast is numb, according to Cooley. Since the skin is taken from the abdomen, the breast feels different, Cooley says. On the other hand, her stomach is flat, she jokes. Another benefit of this type of reconstructive surgery is that her new breast will age well, as do most reconstructed breasts. All in all, Cooley is very pleased with the outcome, she says, so much so that she went on a tropical vacation recently, got back into her bikini, and felt great. Add in the skiing and golfing she's been doing and she says, "I'm back where I wanted to be."

Cost, however, is a large factor in choosing whether to have reconstructive surgery or use a breast form. Prostheses are often covered by insurance, Oakley says, but you must pay the cost up front, file the insurance paperwork, and wait for reimbursement. The same goes for special prosthetic bras that have a pocket to hold the form in place. These special bras are more expensive than typical bras.

Behind the scenes on the dating scene

Some single women may find it hard to start dating again. When do you tell your date you have breast cancer, and when do you tell him you have only one breast or a reconstructed breast? How will you know when you should tell a prospective partner?

Although all women who go through mastectomy and breast cancer treatment experience at least some feelings of insecurity, single women who have been diagnosed with breast cancer typically have more concerns about attractiveness—Will men still want me? They have the potential for more anxiety than the woman who already has a partner with whom she feels secure, says Karen Donahey, Ph.D., director of the Sex and Marital Therapy program at Northwest University Medical School in Chicago, Illinois. She says sharing your questions and concerns with a support group made up of other single women may help.

You don't need to tell the men you date immediately, Donahey says. Think of it this way: Do you tell just anyone the most personal details about your life when you first meet? Get to know the person first and decide if he is one with whom you want to develop a relationship. Think of your new situation as a screening tool, weeding out the insensitive men and those who can't handle some of life's challenges. When you tell a new boyfriend about the breast cancer, if he shows concern and sticks around, he may be a good candidate for a long-term relationship. But if he backs off, consider yourself lucky. After all, do you really want a partner who will leave you if you get cancer again? Donahey reports that it does, in fact, tend to make women more discriminating about whom they date.

Telling your children you have cancer

Of course women want to protect their children from the diagnosis of cancer. But experts advise against this. The best advice is to frame the news in developmentally appropriate language, advises Mary Jane Massie, M.D., director of the Barbara White Fishman Center for Psychological Counseling at Memorial Sloan-Kettering Cancer Center's Breast Center in New York City.

Younger children know a whole lot more than you might think, Massie says. They learn about breast cancer from news reports, television programs, and school experiences. Massie suggests framing the news in a positive way, for example, "Mom has such a good doctor because he found this lump," shortly after you're diagnosed. Then, after surgery say, for example, "We have good news. The tissue the doctor removed had some ugly cells, but the doctor knows how to fix it. Mom will take medicine that will make her better." But don't lie to kids, Massie says. Don't say no one ever dies from breast cancer.

Dealing with children during treatment

Massie also suggests leaving kids out of the hospital setting, unless they're well prepared for what they'll see. Plus, for the most part, hospitals don't want kids there because some patients are immuno-suppressed. The hospital stay is usually short for surgery or adjuvant treatments, anyhow.

While hair loss is an issue for a woman, it's also an issue for her children. Kids are easily embarrassed by their parents' behavior and attire when they're out in public. In order to spare your child any embarrassment, Massie advises women to wear their wig at home, or some sort of head covering, when guests are over.

Another issue arises when you have children and you're going through treatments. Many women go to work, take chemo, and go to bed exhausted. Think through your priorities, Massie suggests. Family is important. Consider what you can ask others to do for you, such as grocery shop or make meals, so you have more time and energy to spend with your children.

Older children, even if they're off at college or living in another city, also need to be informed. What annoys older children the most is when they're protected" from what's going on, Massie says. They perceive it as being left out of the loop.

Single moms

Being a parent is no easy task. Being a single mom with breast cancer is even harder. Not only is the single mom coping with her illness, she also has to deal with the children as well. Many of these women have separated or gone through a divorce while going through treatment, Oakley says, adding that, frequently, this occurs because there were already problems in the marriage before diagnosis. Dealing with such an emotionally taxing situation as breast cancer, or any illness, can be the straw that breaks the camel's back.

So, in some cases, single moms have to help their children cope with the disease process as well as an impending divorce. If you are a single mom, your children may need some extra help getting through this. They may act cranky, develop discipline problems, and experience anxiety. Tell other, supportive adults in your child's life about your illness, especially teachers, neighbors, coaches, and extended family. That will give them the opportunity to step in and provide companionship, support, understanding, and help maintain your child's scheduled activities.

Some communities have support groups especially for children of cancer patients. The Internet can also be a source of support, especially for children in rural areas where support groups may not exist. Kids Konnected (www.kidskonnected.org) was founded by children whose parents had cancer. The Web site provides friendship and a support network for kids with parents who have been diagnosed with cancer.

Straight talk on sex

All components of the sexual response cycle (desire, arousal, and orgasm) have both psychological and physiological factors.

How a woman views herself after surgery may affect her sexual desire because the breast is a symbol of femininity and sexuality. A disfiguring alteration of the breast as a result of lumpectomy or the loss of an entire breast or breasts can also result in a profound sense of loss and a feeling of not being whole.

"Many women lose interest in sex during breast cancer treatment," states Donahey. "This is normal." "When confronted with a life-threatening disease, sex is usually further down on the list of priorities and needs."

Women undergoing chemotherapy or radiation therapy will often experience side effects such as nausea and fatigue that can interfere with sexual desire. Chemotherapy and radiation therapy can affect hormone levels in women. "Lowered hormone levels can lower sexual desire, as well as make intercourse more painful," Donahey explains. "The reduction in estrogen leads to less lubrication, which can make intercourse uncomfortable. If sex is uncomfortable, it can affect one's interest in being sexual," she points out. After treatment ends, most women find that their sexual desire returns to their pre-surgery levels, Donahey says. However, the other side effects of the treatment—hair loss, weight loss or gain—may interfere with a woman's self-image and consequently, her sexual desire. Additionally, depression or anxiety about having cancer, losing your breast or having it altered, may affect sexual desire.

Another issue regarding sex is communication. "Most women want to discuss their feelings regarding the cancer, their fears of having a life-threatening illness, of going through the various treatments, how it will affect the marriage, and the husband's desire for and attraction to her," Donahey says. "Many men will try to reassure their wives that everything will be alright," she says. Men tend to believe that it is better not to 'dwell' on these frightening feelings. However, according to Donahey, many women do not find this approach helpful and report feeling alone during this time. "Sometimes couples pull away from one another at this time, not wanting to 'burden' the other," she says.

"Research and clinical work with these couples shows that if couples can communicate, they can avoid many of the misunderstandings that can develop," according to Donahey. With regard to their sexual relationship, they can discuss when to attempt being sexual, their worries about doing so—he may worry he is pushing her into having sex too soon, and she may worry about her attractiveness. Many couples wait for the other to make the first move, and when nothing happens, make erroneous assumptions such as "He's not interested in me," or "She's not ready to be intimate," Donahey says.

"To resume sexual contact, it's helpful for the couple to communicate concerns [and] fears prior to being sexual that is, if he worries about hurting her, if she worries about being hurt, if she is concerned about being undressed in front to him, if lubrication is necessary, or will be available if needed," Dohahey says. "Couples may need to try a different position if the one they commonly use is now uncomfortable. They may want to try easing into sexual activity by first having some massage sessions, or kissing [and] caressing prior to any attempts at having intercourse," she says. For some women it may take months to become interested in sex, but others are interested shortly after treatment. If you are having trouble resuming your sexual relationship, consult your doctor or consider getting a referral to a therapist who specializes in sexual problems. Contact the American Association of Sex Educators, Counselors, and Therapists (AASECT) at www.aasect.org.

Moneysaver
There are two good, free booklets that deal with the subject of sex and recovery from cancer: *"For Single Women With Breast Cancer"*, published by Y-ME (800/221-2141) and *"Sexuality and Cancer for the woman who has cancer and her partner,"* published by the American Cancer Society (800/ACS-2345).

Breast cancer and pregnancy

For women in their childbearing years who haven't started or completed their family, the diagnosis of breast cancer can be all the more emotionally devastating since it raises such heart-wrenching questions as "Can I have a child?," "Should I have a child?," and "How will a pregnancy affect my health?"

Approximately 25 percent of women with breast cancer are diagnosed during childbearing years and approximately 7 percent of these women have one or more pregnancies after breast cancer treatment. Many of these breast cancers contain estrogen (56.7 percent) and progesterone (61.1 percent) hormone receptors, according to David N. Danforth Jr., M.D., senior investigator, surgery branch, NCI, in an article in *Oncology* (November 1991).

Pregnancy increases the levels of estrogen in a woman's body, and estrogen plays a role in breast tumor development (see Chapter 1 for more information on that causal relationship). Breast cancer also tends to be more aggressive in younger women.

Even though most women who have been diagnosed with breast cancer have been through rigorous treatments, there is still a possibility that micrometastases (cancer cells too small to detect) exist. Doctors worry that the high level of estrogens during pregnancy may promote their growth.

There have been only a few studies on recurrence rates in women diagnosed with breast cancer who subsequently got pregnant, and some scientists question the results of those studies.

"All the studies are actually not worth the paper that they're printed on, since none have ideal study design," says Jeanne Petrek, M.D., surgical director of the Evelyn H. Lauder Breast Center at Memorial

Bright Idea
Do things you enjoy, like reading and watching movies, even if you don't feel your best. Pleasure and laughter can be powerful tools for better health.

Sloan-Kettering Cancer Center in New York. Why? Some of the studies are retrospective, based on the memories of physicians. Retrospective studies have a bias weakness, among other validity problems. That is, the physicians may have a more vivid recollection of the patients seen recently—those with better outcomes to date—and therefore they inadvertently weigh the study with results from these patients, making the outcomes more positive than they are in actuality.

66

The younger you are the more likely you'll have fertility after chemotherapy, but there's always a risk [of becoming infertile].
—Carol Fred, licensed clinical social worker at the Rhonda Flemming Mann Resource Center for Women with Cancer, part of the Jonsson Comprehensive Cancer Center at UCLA, and the Revlon UCLA Breast Center.

99

There are also prospective studies—in which subjects are enrolled at diagnosis and observed as time goes on, with pertinent data collected along the way—on women, breast cancer, and pregnancy. The ones from Scandinavia have good data (an identification number is given to everyone at birth—the nation's health services follows its citizens through every medical event). But that study is flawed, too, according to Petrek, who, along with a co-author, presented her findings in the journal *Cancer* (April 1997). The researchers didn't have much information on the specific tumors or recurrence rates and the researchers used a two-tier staging system versus the four-stage system used in the U.S.

Clearly all of these studies have design flaws. Nonetheless, it would be unwise to ignore this research because that data is all we have right now. Furthermore, we're not going to ever have an ideal study since the "gold standard" is a randomized, double-blind, placebo-controlled study. That study design isn't going to be done for practical and ethical reasons.

"Pregnancy is a massive hormonal event," Petrek explains. If there are micrometastases, "would that high hormone level be like pouring gas on a fire?" she asks. The problem is, researchers don't have a definitive answer.

There are also clinical data showing treating metastatic disease with high doses of estrogen or progesterone can cause remission in hormone-sensitive tumors, so we really don't know the effect of hormones on micrometastatic disease.

Petrek developed a prospective study funded by the U.S. Army. Women are registered when they are first diagnosed. Because the researchers need to watch these study subjects over a long period of time to see the "big picture," it could take 10 years to see meaningful survival rates.

This study will, potentially, give a definitive answer for women who become or wish to become pregnant.

In the meantime, if a woman is in this situation, there are no data at present to support the contention that pregnancy adversely affects breast cancer and survival. On the contrary, available data dating back to the 1960s up to 1999 show either no effect on survival or a slightly better survival for age, stage, node, and treatment-matched pregnant and non-pregnant women.

"While there is often a delay in diagnosis of anywhere from 1.5 to 6 months (for whatever reasons), when matched for age and stage of disease, patients with breast cancer during pregnancy have the same prognosis as non-pregnant patients; the most important predictor of survival is the stage of disease at time of diagnosis," Danforth wrote in the *Oncology* article. The prognosis of the tumor is what's important when deciding whether to have children after breast cancer treatment, he noted.

According to the results of several group studies on stage I, II, III with and without node involvement, Danforth adds, virtually all of the authors concluded that pregnancy after being treated for breast cancer doesn't alter the prognosis when the woman is considered disease free. More than one pregnancy after being successfully treated does not appear to affect the prognosis of the primary tumor, either. However, he noted, recurrence rates for breast cancer are highest during the first two years after treatment. So it may be wise to defer pregnancy for two years after completion of therapy in order to predict how healthy you'll be while raising your children.

The decision of whether or not to have a baby after being diagnosed and treated for breast cancer is a personal one. You may want to consider three factors:

1. Prognosis based on tumor type.

2. The amount of time that has lapsed since treatment ended (which is an indirect measure of risk of recurrence).

3. Your ability to deal with the psychological aspects of a cancer diagnosis while caring for young children.

However, women with stage IV tumors (metastatic) should not consider getting pregnant because of the poor 5-year survival rates, Danforth wrote. Women with stage III disease should defer conception for at least five years after treatment ends, if they consider having a baby at all, he said. Women with stage I or stage II disease whose tumor has recurred should not consider getting pregnant because of the poor prognosis and need for ongoing treatment, he adds.

Getting pregnant after breast cancer treatment

According to an article in the journal *Oncology* (May 1998), three University of Rochester researchers at Strong Memorial Hospital in Rochester, New York

> **"** Although breast cancer in younger women may be a more aggressive disease, the additional factor of pregnancy does not adversely influence outcome when patients are compared by age and stage.
> —Frankie Anne Holmes, M.D., Anderson Cancer Center in "Breast Cancer During Pregnancy" *The Cancer Bulletin* Vol. 46 No. 5, 1994 **"**

reported on the problems of women who would like to become pregnant. They searched English medical literature published between 1966 to 1997 and came to several conclusions regarding pregnancy after breast cancer diagnosis. Six are listed here:

Unofficially...
Researchers believe that between 1 in 3,000 to 1 in 10,000 women are diagnosed with breast cancer during pregnancy.

1. Sexual function is not adversely affected by breast conservation surgery (lumpectomy) or mastectomy.

2. The incidence rate of infertility resulting from breast cancer treatment is directly proportional to the woman's age and the use and dose of alkylating agents, chemotherapeutic drugs that work in a specific way. There isn't any conclusive information, though, on the effects of duration, dose intensity, schedule, or route of administration of chemotherapy on fertility.

3. There doesn't appear to be an increase in birth defects in children whose parents had chemotherapy earlier in life.

4. Milk production is often limited in an irradiated breast.

5. Breastfeeding seems to decrease the risk of breast cancer.

6. While pregnant, the recommendations made by the American Society of Clinical Oncology (ASCO) regarding monitoring in non-pregnant women for recurrence should be followed.

This last finding is of particular interest because in a study published in the Italian journal *Minerva Ginecol* (July-August 1998) the two authors found a significant decrease in the rate of breast examinations among pregnant women over age 30, the age group where breast cancer incidence rises during pregnancy. They surveyed 500 pregnant women about "non-instrumental" (manual) breast checks during the pregnancy. Only 7.4 percent of the women were examined during their pregnancy (most—67.6 percent—without incidence). To compound that, self-examinations decreased from 28.4 percent to 6.2 percent. They concluded that the possibility of breast cancer gets less attention during pregnancy, causing a delay in the diagnosis, and consequently a worse prognosis.

Diagnosing breast cancer during pregnancy

Whether a woman has been previously diagnosed with breast cancer or not, it's very difficult to detect cancerous growths in the breasts of a pregnant woman, Petrek says. That's because it's possible to have a 100 percent increase in breast size during pregnancy. Along with the larger breasts comes nodular growth, additional weight and density of the breasts, and increased blood flow to the breasts; all factors that make detection difficult through either physical examinations or mammograms. So a mass that can be felt in a woman who isn't pregnant can't be felt at the same stage of growth in one who is. Complicating matters further, malignant tumors are more aggressive in pregnant women, possibly due to the increased levels of estrogen, Petrek says. However, other scientists note that it's the delay in diagnosis, not tumor aggression, that causes women with cancer diagnosed during pregnancy to generally have more advanced disease—larger tumors and more frequent spread to the lymph nodes (metastatic cancer).

Timing of pregnancy and breast cancer risk

First pregnancies after age 30 increase breast cancer risk. Women who have waited until then before getting pregnant have an additional complicating factor. During pregnancy, the breast cells differentiate—they form and specialize to perform certain functions, such as lactation. This differentiation, when it occurs at a younger age, has a protective effect against breast cancer. At later ages, the risk of breast cancer increases for those women who have not had their first pregnancy because the cells, while in an undifferentiated state, have now had a prolonged exposure to estrogen, a tumor promoter, and then, possibly "weakened" (made more susceptible to mutation) by this exposure, they experience a significantly increased exposure to estrogen during the pregnancy. So if you wait until your 35, for example, before getting pregnant, your breast cells, in an undifferentiated state, have been exposed to estrogen for 10 years longer than someone who had their first pregnancy at age 25. The key here is how long your cells—in an undifferentiated state—are exposed to estrogen.

Breast cancer treatment during pregnancy

Those women who get pregnant after being diagnosed with breast cancer and those who are initially diagnosed during pregnancy can have mastectomies safely, Petrek says. Chemotherapy is modified. It's safer for the fetus after the first trimester when the limbs and organs have already been formed, she says. The short-term problems reside in inadequate nutrition with chemotherapy, she says. Short-term studies to date show no adverse effect on these children. There are no solid long-term studies, she says. (Radiation, which causes growth retardation and other adverse effects, is almost always avoided due to scatter. That is, some radiation escapes the breast area, Petrek says.)

Healthy intrauterine growth and development— as well as a normal delivery—can be accomplished without excessive complications, according to an article published in the *Journal of Clinical Oncology* (March 1999). All of the women in an ongoing study have delivered healthy babies.

There's also the issue of the drug tamoxifen (Nolvadex), which is sometimes used prophylactically to keep cancer at bay or to keep a primary growth from forming. This drug is classified as one of those that causes birth defects. Ironically, it is theoretically possible that it may also increase a women's fertility, Petrek says, because that drug is related to clomiphene (Clomid), which increases ovulation.

Emotional consequences of breast cancer and pregnancy

"I think a lot of women are given misinformation about when it's okay to start a family," says Linda Larva, a social worker from the Cancer Caring Center in Pittsburgh, Pennsylvania. For those women who haven't started or completed their family, hearing about the risks of breast cancer and pregnancy is devastating. There's a lot of stress and strain because the life of the mother is pitted against that of the baby.

And for those who are diagnosed during pregnancy, the question of aborting comes into play. These women are worried about what they're putting the fetus through, Larva says. "We've had some women give birth to healthy babies," she says, "and we've had some women who have lost babies." For them, it's devastating and heartbreaking. For some, "there is so much pain involved that they have not been able to discuss it," Larva says, so much so that they dropped out of their support group.

Although it's not much consolation to women who had their hearts set on the experience of pregnancy, there are other ways of starting a family. In

her *Cancer* article, Petrek and her co-author empha-
size the need for physicians to talk to their patients
about such alternatives as adoption, surrogacy, and
in vitro fertilization (for those women who become
infertile as a result of treatment).

Just the facts

- You may have job protection under the Americans with Disabilities Act as well as other laws.

- One method of breast reconstruction preserves
  the breast skin, save for the nipple.

- Your children need to know that you have a diagnosis of breast cancer.

- Studies evaluating the rate of recurrence once a
  woman becomes pregnant may be unreliable
  because of flawed research design.

Common Emotional Consequences

Chapter 14

The diagnosis of breast cancers elicits fear, not just for the woman with breast cancer, but her friends and family as well. And, much like the grieving process, she and others experience a host of emotions, ranging from denial to anger to acceptance. During the initial stage, the woman learns a lot about treatment alternatives and must make difficult decisions.

In this chapter, experts give advice and tips on how to get through the initial stages of diagnosis and treatment and how to get the support you may need.

Common emotional consequences of diagnosis and treatments

It doesn't take much to imagine what it might feel like to be diagnosed with breast cancer. "Most of these women are just scared to death that they're going to die. Most of the time that's probably not going to be the case...But they're really terrified," says Carol Fred, licensed clinical social worker at the Rhonda Flemming Mann Resource Center for Women with

Cancer, part of the Jonsson Comprehensive Cancer Center at UCLA. Fred also works at the Revlon UCLA Breast Center.

After learning of their diagnosis, women experience a host of emotions, one of the strongest being fear. Many women feel afraid of pain or dying, the effects of treatment, and becoming disfigured or helpless. Some women are afraid that the cost of treatment or the loss of income will cause financial problems.

According to a study published in the journal *Health Psychology* (March 1999), during the first year after breast cancer surgery, the top three fears women have are death, pain, and overwhelming bills, not the loss of attractiveness or sexuality, as is often thought. Those issues, along with loss of being self-sufficient, ranked as mid-level concerns. Adverse reactions from friends, family, partners, and others ranked at the bottom of their list of worries. Interestingly, the researchers concluded that "what may be easiest to discuss with a patient may not be what the patient is most worried about." They suggest therapists help women diagnosed with breast cancer increase healthy behaviors, plan for their children's future, and develop a plan for dealing with medical bills.

Statistics and averages can add to the emotional burden by causing unnecessary worry. For those with advanced cancer, statistics can have an even greater emotional impact. Keep in mind that even if the numbers look grim, there are those who survive. Your chances of survival are affected by many factors—how well your cancer responds to treatment, your general physical health, your immune system, possibly your mental health, and perhaps factors yet unknown—and these study outcomes don't account for every environmental and physical factor present

Unofficially...
Cancer treatments do not always cause hair loss, weight loss, or major changes in lifestyle.

in each woman studied.

Besides fear, other emotions women tend to experience after being diagnosed with breast cancer include the following:

- **Denial**—Some women simply refuse to believe the diagnosis, blaming it on misinterpreting the slides under the microscope or a laboratory mix-up. Not always a bad thing, denial can soften the impact of the diagnoses and let you deal with the reality a little at a time.

- **Anger**—"Why me?" is a common reaction for anyone who is suffering. You may feel angry at the cancer itself, your doctor, friends, and family.

- **Stress and anxiety**—These two emotional reactions can cause physical symptoms such as diarrhea, dizziness, and loss of appetite. Some studies have shown that stress can affect your body's immune system and its role in fighting disease. You can manage stress by exercising, listening to music, watching videos, laughing, or otherwise distracting yourself. Relaxation exercises or meditation help reduce stress as well. Attending support group meetings and getting individual therapy may also be helpful.

- **Loss of control**—Many women struggle with the feeling of losing control: They now face an uncertain future, confront medical terms they don't understand, and rely heavily on health-care providers. You can boost your sense of control by learning as much as you can about your type of breast cancer and its treatments. Many women, especially those who have maintained a healthy lifestyle, feel betrayed by their bodies. If that's the case, you may want to take on challenges—athletic or intellectual—to renew your confidence

Bright Idea
Run (or walk) to get back control of your body, help women like yourself in your community, and benefit breast cancer research and initiatives at the same time by entering the Race for the Cure®. This 5K race is held each spring in cities nation-wide. Seventy-five percent of the funds raised supports educa-tion, screening, and treatment of under-served women in your community. The remaining funds are used to fight breast cancer through the Komen Foundation National Grant Programs.

in your body's capabilities.

- *Depression*—More than just the blues, some women become clinically depressed. Some symp-toms of depression include a sense of helpless-ness, a sense of hopelessness, grief, a feeling that life is meaningless, a loss of interest in activities that were previously enjoyable, sleeping prob-lems, a marked decrease in physical energy, and crying spells. Note that some of these symptoms, (loss of appetite, for example) can be side effects of cancer treatment. Make sure to tell your doc-tor how you're feeling.

- *Guilt*—Some women blame themselves or events for causing the cancer, for upsetting their friends and families, or for causing financial problems. Some resent others' good health and then feel bad for feeling that way. One good way to deal with this guilt is to put it into perspective. (For instance, think of children who have cancer: Did they cause their disease? Of course not.) Some women fear they may have passed the gene onto a daughter—but remember, only a small per-centage of breast cancers are familial. Even if the gene was passed along, it doesn't mean it will mutate. Family members may experience guilt because they feel that they cannot do enough to help you. They may find themselves resentful or impatient and feel guilty about that, too.

- *Loneliness*—Some women, despite being sur-rounded by family and friends, feel isolated and lonely. On the other hand, sometimes friends and family have a hard time dealing with the cancer and drift away. Some women are isolated because they are too tired for their usual social activities, and others may feel that friends could not possibly understand their experiences, so why hang out with them? A good way to deal with this problem is to join a support group.

Despite these very real fears, many women find that a good way to control fear is to arm themselves with knowledge. Many people find that they are less afraid when they know what to expect. Therefore, consider learning as much as you can about your specific type of breast cancer and the treatments. Talk to your doctor about your concerns, ask questions, and do research. A good place to start is the National Cancer Institute's Cancer Information Center hotline at 800/4-CANCER, where you can speak to a cancer specialist from 9 a.m. to 4:30 p.m. weekdays. Cancer information specialists are available around the clock at 800/ACS-2345, which is one of the American Cancer Society's services.

In addition, Y-ME also provides a 24-hour hotline to both men and women diagnosed with breast cancer. Y-ME also runs a phone support group, complete with guest speakers and breakout groups, for women under age 40. The hotline phone number is 800/221-2141 (English) and 800/986-9505 (Spanish). You can also get useful information on breast cancer (male and female) from their Web site (www.y-me.org). Cancer Care (800/813-HOPE) provides resources to cancer patients and their families on psychosocial issues.

Eventually, the initial shock wears off and many women report that they are able to develop a sense of hope that helps them get through the physical and emotional struggles. And there are plenty of real reasons to have hope—8.2 million reasons, to be exact. There are currently (in 1999) 8.2 million Americans alive today who have been diagnosed with

Bright Idea
If you can't talk to somebody about your feelings, try expressing your feelings in a daily journal. It might be a good outlet for your emotions and help you to better cope with them.

cancer. That's 200,000 more survivors in 1999 than in 1998—just one year!

Coping: When to get therapy

Coping and dealing with all of the emotions and practical aspects of being diagnosed with breast cancer is not easy. You may want to consider seeking professional assistance to help get you though the rough spots, such as making difficult medical decisions, handling both the physical changes and emotional challenges, taking back control, venting your pent up emotions, and dealing with loss of the medical support team once the treatments are over.

Making decisions

One of the earliest issues after diagnosis is making decisions about medical treatments, says Sandra Haber, a psychologist who works with breast cancer patients in New York City. Women are often left to decide between different types of treatment, for example a lumpectomy or mastectomy. "How exactly do you decide when the medical alternatives are equal?" Haber asks. (Some treatments have similar medical outcomes for many patients.)

There are many psychological issues to take into account when making these big decisions about medical treatment, Haber says. For example, while some women would be devastated by the loss of a breast, others want to get rid of the breast to reduce the risk of recurrence, or at least the thought of the recurrence. A big part of the decision is based on what you need psychologically, not necessarily medically, when there are "medical equivalents," Haber explains.

Sometimes women are faced with a similar question of whether to take chemotherapy. For instance, the data show that for certain types of breast cancer, those with a favorable histology such as mucinous carcinoma, pure tubular carcinoma, and papillary carcinoma, only a small percentage of women actually benefit from it in terms of preventing a recurrence in later years. But since it is impossible to know which patients are cured with just surgery and which aren't, a cautious approach, adjuvant chemotherapy, is usually taken.

Therefore, for favorable histologies an individual discussion of potential risk is more important because data about risk reduction in these types of breast cancer are less firm.

Cure is a difficult issue. For ductal carcinoma in situ the risk of death from breast cancer is quoted as 2 percent. As tumor size increases, the risk increases. T I tumors (those less than or equal to 2 centimeters in greatest diameter) have a 20 to 30 percent the risk of death from breast cancer, and T II tumors (those greater than 2 centimeters but less than or equal to 5 centimeters in greatest dimension) pose up to a 40 to 60 percent risk. Overall risk depends on the tumor size and node status.

Another issue for some patients, those who will or have undergone mastectomy, is whether or not to have reconstruction surgery. Those who choose to have reconstruction may be faced with two more decisions: how and when. There are two common types of reconstructive surgery: saline implants and transverse rectus adominus myocutaneous (TRAM) flaps (a much more complex series of surgeries), though it's not always the patient's choice. (See Chapter 15 for more on reconstructive surgery.)

Haber notes that some women may benefit from getting psychological assistance to make these tough decisions.

Handling the changes

There are additional reasons to seek the aid of a professional psychologist. During the time between hearing the diagnosis and undergoing the initial treatments a woman experiences an enormous amount of anxiety. Then there's more anxiety when transitioning from active treatment to being a survivor. During treatment, there are plenty of other issues to deal with.

For example, perimenopausal women often (if treated with chemotherapy) abruptly enter menopause. And those on hormone replacement therapy abruptly taken off to undergo chemotherapy experience a huge hormonal disruption, and these women may end up with a lot of other issues, such as hot flashes and loss of bone density. Plus, postmenopausal bone loss and its treatment becomes an issue.

For many there are the physiological changes, including moodiness, depression, and night awakenings due to hot flashes to contend with. "For some women it can be a very disruptive part of the aftermath of treatment," Fred says.

Single women may have to be more dependent again on parents, which is often associated with a loss of privacy, loss of independence, and a sense of failure. Some women may become dependent on siblings, and some may suddenly feel old if they enter an early menopause.

An issue for those who have always lived a healthy lifestyle and have taken good care of themselves is a feeling that their bodies have betrayed them. Many of these women feel they can't trust their bodies again, Fred says. Recurrence is a big fear among breast cancer survivors. "Recurrence fears loom large in lots of women who have been treated for breast cancer,"

Fred says. They're "being thrust into this uncertain future," she says.

Taking back control

There are, of course, other reasons that women may need outside support from a therapist. Prior to surgery, many women are very anxious. A good therapist can teach them coping techniques, such as relaxation and self-hypnosis to make the surgery easier. Furthermore, with chemotherapy, there are good data on hypnosis reducing the likelihood of nausea and vomiting, according to Haber. There's also some scientific evidence that positive imagery can help people heal faster. Therapists can help teach methods and construct the personalized images that will help them heal. All of these things give the woman who has lost control over part of her life some power. It's "something you can do to help yourself," as well as take control, Haber says.

Venting

Sometimes partners, other family members, and friends aren't receptive to or comfortable with the amount of venting women recently diagnosed with breast cancer might need to do. Therapists and support groups provide good shoulders to cry on and empathic people with whom to vent your anger. And there's so much to be angry about. For one, the breast cancer itself. Then there's hair loss (for some). "To the women it's usually devastating," Haber explains. To make matters worse, women frequently sense they shouldn't express their anger about this issue. Hair loss is often minimized by their medical team because it's considered a small side effect for saving a life, she says. Even though the hair will grow back, for a woman hair loss is a public display of her condition, a breach of privacy. It's also a constant reminder of the cancer. "You can't get away from it," Haber points out. It also symbolizes the loss of femininity and sexuality. A good therapist would be there to give support, mourn the loss, even if it is temporary, and provide a place to vent that anger. Support groups can be a big help here, too.

And just when you think it's over...

After the woman has surgery and chemotherapy or radiation, you'd think that the post-treatment period would be celebratory, Haber says. But she points out that many women actually feel *more* anxiety as they end treatment. That reaction may be due to several things:

Unofficially...
There are 1.3 million breast cancer survivors in the United States today, according to Johns Hopkins University.

- The loss of a medical support team

- Delayed depression surfacing after having coped for so long during diagnosis and treatment

- Post-treatment issues—sexuality, fertility, social issues (fears of recurrence/awareness of mortality

Women don't go back to their lives and just feel normal, she says. There are still adaptations and adjustments that must be made. "Every headache becomes a brain tumor. Every ache becomes bone cancer," Haber explains. A good therapist can help them work through these issues and fears.

The ties that bind fray for some

"The general data are that cancer doesn't kill marriages," Haber notes. But, she adds, the situation causes additional stress on marriage. Some couples rally, and others find it too stressful when they already have a shaky foundation. Interestingly, very often it's the women who leave the men, Haber notes. They feel their time is more limited (whether or not it really is), and they want to use it more wisely. They feel "if you get though cancer, you can get through anything," Haber says. "It can give you a new found sense of strength," she adds.

Take one teaspoon of laughter...

Science is just beginning to understand how the brain and emotions can play an important role in preventing and fighting disease. Laughter may be one of your best defenses. One of the biggest emotional issues of cancer patients is the loss of control. Seeing the humor in events by changing your perception of them can give you a sense of controlling the situation. By taking such "medicine" you can actually lower your stress hormones and strengthen your immune system.

Increased levels of stress hormones are produced by the body in response to stress. These hormones are corticotropin, cortisol, catecholamines, beta-endorphin, growth hormone, and prolactin. The increased levels of these hormones is associated with distress, a release of stress hormones into the bloodstream.

"We know that stress hormones can suppress your immune system. If you want to enhance your immune system, you can potentially do that with laughter," says Lee Berk, DRPH, MPH, a neuroimmunologist and associate director of the Center for Neuroimmunology at Loma Linda University's School of Medicine.

Laughter is also a stress, but it is a good stress, a eustress, Berk explains. Neuroendocrine and stress hormone responses are different from those observed in distress situations (whether physical or psychological).

In his studies, Berk found that mirthful (happy) laughter produced measurable biochemical changes

Bright Idea
If you're having marital problems, consider seeking professional help for both you and your husband as well as your children. Stronger families can be a source of strength.

that had a positive effect on central nervous system activity. Indeed, there is biology in the brain that affects the immune system, he says, noting that just as stress appears to play a role in some heart attacks and cancers, so can happiness benefit the immune response. Mirthful laughter appears to have an impact on the body by modifying or attenuating some hormone levels associated with distress.

In the *American Journal of Medical Sciences* (December 1989), Berk and his colleagues reported on a study in which they showed a humorous videotape to a group of healthy men. Five control subjects did not get to view it. Blood samples were taken and analyzed for measurable biological responses. The medical researchers found that mirthful laughter appears to decrease serum levels of cortisol and growth hormone as well as dopac, the major serum neuronal cetabolite of dopamine and epinephrine (adrenaline), also stress hormones. The control group did not have a significant change in hormone levels.

"These biological changes have implications for the reversal of the neuroendocrine and classical stress hormone responses," they wrote. So, it appears, mirthful laughter can play a role in the preventive and healing processes.

Berk's other research findings show the body's response to mirthful laughter include:

- An increase in the number and activity of natural killer cells. NK cells are among the body's immune response tools. They seek out aberrant cells and kill them before they become cancers. (See Chapter 1 for the stages a cell must go through to become cancerous.) They attack cells infected with viruses and have been noted to attack malignant tumor cells. NK cells play a role in tumor immune surveillance.

■ An increase in activated T cells (T lymphocytes). T cells facilitate many immune functions and enhance the activities of B cells in the production of antibodies and destruction of antigens. The same T-cell activation response can be elicited by moderate exercise (by someone who's conditioned). Moderate exercise is another eustress state, Berk notes. Excessive exercise is a distress state and causes the same reaction other negatives emotional stresses cause.

■ An increase in immunoglobulin A (IgA), an antibody that is produced in response to the presence of foreign antigens.

■ An increase in gamma interferon, a cytokine that activates certain components of the immune system, such as NK cells.

■ An increase in immunoglobulin G (IgG), the main antibody produced in response to viral and bacterial attacks. It is idiospecific, that is it is tailor made to fit the specific antigen. Berk's data suggest that it has a protective effect from the immune system, even into the next day with the study subjects. An increase of IgM (another immunoglobulin) that starts the first stages of an immune response. Both of these immunoglobulins are produced by B lymphocytes (B cells). IgG does the follow-up work and gives us an immunity to that microbe which was attacked. B cells have a memory.

■ An increase in complement C, which serves as an aid to antibodies to infiltrate infected and unhealthy cells. This increase, too, lasted into the next day on the subjects studied. (The complement system is one component of the immune system. It is made from a number of proteins that react in a cascade fashion to effect an immune response. Enhancing the components may enhance responsiveness.)

Improving the system with a good laugh

There is evidence that mirthful laughter reduces stress at a molecular level as well, so the immune system can work better, Berk says. He cites one study in *Brain Behavior and Immunity*, (Vol.12 1998) animals were given a human lung tumor and subsequently given the drug cyclophosphamide (Cytoxan), which is known to cure these tumors in animals. The results were positive. Next, the researchers placed a simple stress on the animals by restraining a leg. Then the researchers gave them the tumor again and gave them the same drug. The drug was no longer as effective. The stress and resultant stress hormones and suppressed immune response reaction actually interfered with the drug's efficacy.

Does stress affect breast cancer treatment response?

Three studies are currently investigating whether stress reduction can alter immune function in a way that influences cancer progression.

If stress adversely affects your response to treatment for breast cancer or helps your body resist the progression of the disease, then perhaps you can reduce it with mirthful laughter (and other methods such as progressive relaxation, positive imagery, and moderate exercise) and help your body fight the cancer, or at least be more receptive to the treatment. Recent study results show promise of a connection between stress and recovery from breast cancer.

Ohio State University researchers demonstrated

that the psychological stress women experience after being diagnosed with breast cancer and undergoing surgery can weaken their immune responses based on at least three different biochemical indicators. The findings were reported in the *Journal of the National Cancer Institute* (January 1998).

Barbara Anderson, professor of psychology and researcher at Ohio State's Comprehensive Cancer Center and Institute of Behavioral Medicine, and colleagues studied a group of 116 women who underwent surgery for stage II or stage III invasive breast cancer. Before the women completed follow-up therapy, they completed a questionnaire that assessed their levels of stress. Based on their responses, they were placed in either a high- or low-stress group. Blood samples were taken and measured for the breakdown extent of NK cells (the researchers also checked how effectively the NK cells responded to gamma interferon, which normally enhances NK cell activity and inhibits virus replication) and T-lymphocyte responses.

The authors concluded that data from their study showed that the physiologic effects of stress inhibit cellular immune responses that are important to the prognosis. These immune response include NK cell toxicity and T-cell responses, specifically:

- In the high-stress group, 15.4 percent more of the NK cells were destroyed compared with those of the low-stress group.

- The response to gamma interferon in the high-stress group was 20.1 percent less than it was in the low-stress group.

- The T-cell responses to two plant chemicals and monoclonal antibodies (tests for intact immune system responses) were 19.8 percent less in the

Bright Idea
Reduce your stress. Make exciting plans for the future. Think about what would make you happy—a fun-filled vacation to a sun-drenched beach? New furniture for your home? New paint for the walls? A closet full of new clothes? A night out on the town?

high-stress group than in the low-stress group.

(Note: The bullets above are tests of intact immune system responses.)

Ten years ago, David Spiegel, M.D., a psychiatrist at Stanford University, and his colleagues studied two groups of women with breast cancer. One group received support from group members; the other did not. The investigators found that long-term survival rates for the 50 women in the support were almost twice that of the 36 women in the control group after 10 years. (The average survival for the women in the intervention group was 36.6 months from the time of randomization. The average survival rate for women in the control group was 18.9 months.) In 1990, Spiegel and his colleagues began another larger trial with a total of 125 study participants to replicate their findings. In this study the investigators are monitoring endocrine and cellular markers of immune function and recurrence and survival rates.

Additional studies are important and necessary to determine if there was selection bias in Spiegel's studies.

In Canada, investigators are trying to replicate Spiegel's trial. A total of 235 women are being studied in seven centers. The investigation is being led by Pamela Goodwin, M.D. at Mount Sinai Hospital, Toronto.

All three studies currently under investigation "support the hypothesis that cancer-related stress is associated with cellular immune responses that may play a role in tumor growth," according to a news report by Caroline McNeil in the *Journal of the National Cancer Institute* (January, 1998). All three studies are randomized, controlled trials of support group interventions with breast cancer patients. Complete results should be in by 2000.

As in other research, the current study findings are causing controversy. Other researchers say there may be other factors affecting the immune system, such as the chemotherapy or unknown factors. There's also a question of whether support leads to better compliance.

Incorporating more laughter into your life

Bursting into fits of laughter at such a difficult time in life may seem easier said than done. However, working on the funny bone may just be a matter of timing. Ask any comedian, and he or she will tell you that timing plays an important role in the delivery of humor (if you want to get a laugh and not a pie in the face). Timing plays an especially important role for those who have been diagnosed with cancer. During the initial stage of diagnosis, when terror reigns, comedy may be the last thing on your mind. Eventually, as the initial impact lessens, though, it will become easier to bring comedy—and laughter— back into your daily life again. In fact, it may be imperative.

> **"**
> The most wasted of all days is one without laughter.
> —e. e. cummings
> **"**

Besides lifting your spirits, "cancer comedy," finding the humor in cancer, can be put to practical use. It can be used to reduce anxiety over getting a mammogram, so your fears don't interfere with getting preventive care, says Jane Hill, a cancer comedian and breast cancer survivor of eight years. Humor also can be used for other healing, from a job loss or the loss of relationship, she says. Humor distances the situation and allows you to gain perspective.

There are many cancer survivors who have turned their experience into humorous routines, jokes, and books. For a glimpse at the works these people have

Bright Idea
Need a laugh? Head over to http://www. humorinst.com/ video/videos.htm. Comedian Dave Fitzgerald will have you in stitches about his bout with cancer. He also gives some wise advice to cancer patients.

done, point your browser to www.canceronline.com. There Sydney Love introduces you to cancer humor, including jokes, books, cancer humor speakers, and research.

According to Berk, perception plays a role in how people respond to events. Try the following exercise. Read aloud the statement below:

OPPORTUNITY

ISNOWHERE

What you see depends on your perception. Some people will see "Opportunity is now here" while others will see "Opportunity is nowhere."

As demonstrated above, eustress for one person is distress for another person. "The biology is different because the response is different," Berk says. He and neurologist colleague Barry Bittman, M.D., created a computer software program called SMILE that devises a personalized humor profile and gives a humor "prescription" by telling patients what tools will work for them. These can be purchased by calling 909/796-4112.

Bottom line? If laughter is indeed contagious, you might consider exposing yourself to it on a regular basis. After all, ancient Biblical wisdom has tells us that "A merry heart does good like a medicine," Berk points out.

So how do you tickle your funny bone? Rent a funny movie, read a humorous book, go see comedians perform at a comedy club, read joke books, read jokes on the Internet, read a humorous book, and play with young children (they know how to laugh a lot). You can also try your hand at writing a humorous story or comedy routine about your experience with cancer. That will help you see your situation differently.

Accentuating the positive

Laughter is not the only medicine, Berk says. There are several other ways to elicit an eustress response and lower stress hormones, enhance the immune system, and help with treatment outcomes, Berk explains.

Overall, maintaining a positive outlook is extremely helpful in lowering stress. A positive attitude is something you can develop through cognitive restructuring techniques (rewording what you say to yourself and others), positive imagery, assertiveness training, and taking actions that make you proud (volunteer work, helping friends, family, and strangers). You can also change your attitude with the discipline necessary to master the martial arts. Or you can improve your appearance—wear make-up, change your wardrobe, and smile when you see people—which may in turn make your outlook more positive.

Music has also been found to help reduce distressful responses in the body.

Moderate exercise is another excellent way to reduce your stress and maintain a healthy immune system. It has been found to elicit a response similar to mirthful laughter in the body. Moderate exercise has also been shown to help break negative conditioned responses. This is important, since Pavlovian conditioning also plays a role when it comes to success with chemotherapy, Berk says. For instance, if you're conditioned to vomit before chemotherapy from anxiety, this is a distressful biological response, one that increases the amounts of stress hormones circulating in your blood. You need to lower stress hormones that adversely affect the immune system and elicit those with a positive effect to enhance the

> **"**
> When Sandy saw her surgeon following her re-constructive surgery, she placed a balloon under her blouse and asked the doctor if he had put too much saline in her implant! The hardy laugh she and her surgeon shared broke their tension, lifted their spirits, and made the experience memorable. Laughter is the best medicine!
> —Excerpted from comedian Sandy Baker's web page at www. leavemlaughing. com.
>

Watch Out!
Although
moderate exercise
is highly recom-
mended for
lowering stress
levels, strenuous
exercise is equat-
ed with distress
and lowered
immune response.

effects of the chemotherapy. Moderate exercise may be a great way to do this.

Team spirit

Getting enough support is also important in reducing stress. Psychologist Sandra Haber recommends organizing buddy teams for breast cancer survivors. Usually the partner and a friend organize the group to help the woman with breast cancer get through it. The team works out a schedule and divvies up jobs such as picking up children, picking up the slack at jobs, grocery shopping, and, of course, helping get to and through treatments. The team also can be structured to help gather medical information to help with making medical decisions.

You're anxious and scared and probably at your least capable self during treatment, Haber says. Maybe your husband or boyfriend isn't helpful in life, not competent, or just plain too scared. The team can help. In her role as therapist, Haber organizes buddy teams and helps find each member's strength and comfort level. Even long-distance relatives can play a vital role by keeping track of the bills and insurance claims or by doing medical research, which can be relayed quickly over the Internet. The therapist stays in touch with a "coordinator" to ensure everything gets done.

It may not seem possible in the beginning, but with the proper support and outlook, eventually some women are able to use their cancer to make better life decisions.

Bright Idea
ENCOREplus is an
exercise program
and support group
for women with
breast cancer. Call
800/95-EPLUS.

"Part of the work is to take this truly lousy experience and turn it into something that's going to make your life meaningful," Haber advises. Many cancer patients have changed jobs or made their marriages better as a result of this life changing experience.

Some families find a deeper level of communicating can lead to the sense of closer family ties.

Getting support

While you might have been alone when you got the diagnosis, it is unnecessary to go through the treatment process alone. Family and friends are good sources of support. However, those who are close to you may also be dealing with their own fears and confusion regarding your illness, so you may have to look for additional support in the following areas.

Getting support from those that have been there

For some women, talking with family and friends isn't enough because they don't understand completely—they haven't been in your situation. A support group can help you cope with the emotional as well as the practical aspects of breast cancer, because some of its members have already traveled down that road. Support groups can be useful in other ways. They are a good source of information about doctors, hospitals, and insurance providers. Group members sometimes share medical research and tips on managing treatment side effects. They may also share tips for dealing with finances.

Family and friends also may benefit from support groups. In addition to getting emotional support, they may need help finding ways of supporting you, dealing with disruptions in family schedules, and handling financial worries. Some support groups are designed just for family members.

Support groups come in a variety of setups and sizes. Some are led by therapists, others by survivors. Some are tailored for the older woman with breast cancer, others are geared toward teens and young adults with cancer, and still others are for family and

Bright Idea
Some hospitals have patient advocates or patient service representatives that may be able to identify ways to deal with financial concerns.

friends. Some are large groups, some small. Some meet frequently, others less often. Many groups are free, but some require a fee that your insurance may cover.

If you want to locate a support group, ask a member of your healthcare team or the hospital. Sometimes meetings are also listed in the health section of newspapers.

Religious support

Clergy are another good source of support. While they may not have walked a mile in your shoes, they can offer you spiritual support, guidance, and hope. Some studies show that people with cancer have less anxiety, depression, and pain when they feel spiritually connected, according to the NCI. In addition, many churches and synagogues offer other kinds of practical support as well. Religious organizations lend a helping hand with everything from financial aid to arranging for volunteers to help you with transportation or errands. They may also add you to their prayer list, which can also be a considerable comfort.

Practical support

While you're going through treatments, you may need more than emotional support; you may need practical support. If your career and family demand most of your energy, you may want to consider hiring a maid or maid service. If you're single or your family has too many other demands, and you're not feeling well, you may want to explore the possibility of getting home health care for help with food preparation and household chores. Most private insurers and managed health care plans don't reimburse for a home health aid unless nursing care is involved. For information on selecting an aide call the

Timesaver
If you're too tired to travel to a support group, or simply don't have the time, hook up with others on the Internet, either through a breast cancer survivor chat room or newsgroups. Or just read and post messages on bulletin boards. If you're not hooked into cyberspace, or would rather hear a friendly voice, let your fingers do the walking—Y-ME runs a phone support group for women under age 40. The hotline phone number is 800/221-2141 (English) and 800/986-9505 (Spanish).

National Association of Home Care at 202/547-7424. Some state Medicaid programs will pay for an aide, if they are supervised by a nurse.

If you've undergone a mastectomy, you will probably need physical therapy to help you rebuild muscles in your arm and shoulder. A few physical therapists specialize in helping women who suffer from lymphedema, discussed in Chapter 9. Check to see if this type of therapy is covered under your insurance plan. Also note, some cancer and social service organizations may provide you with free rehabilitation services if you're not insured for them.

Many women lose weight during and after chemotherapy. If this happens to you, you may need dietary/nutritional services. A dietitian can suggest ways for you to get enough calories and nutrition and can give you tips on how to deal with nausea, vomiting, heartburn, or fatigue so you can eat. Some women also have indigestion after radiation treatments and after taking some cancer drugs. (See Chapter 8 for more on getting enough nutrition during cancer treatments.)

Your pharmacist is a good source for practical support. He or she can give you information about your cancer treatment and your medications. A pharmacist can also explain how each medication works, describe possible side effects and how to deal with them, and tell you if you need to avoid certain foods or exposure to the sun.

There are many national organizations that offer help to people with cancer and their families. For a listing, see Appendix B.

Giving support

Your children will need help getting through this, too. They may act cranky, develop discipline prob-

Bright Idea
If you or someone you know has been diagnosed with breast cancer and live in an area where you don't have family and friends close by, ask a minister or rabbi to gather a team from his congregation to help. Or, ask a therapist to do that for you.

lems, or experience anxiety. Tell other, supportive adults in your child's life about your illness, especially teachers, neighbors, coaches, and extended family. That will give them the opportunity to step in and provide companionship, support, understanding, and help maintain your child's scheduled activities.

Some communities have support groups especially for children of cancer patients. The Internet can be a source of support, especially for children in rural areas where support groups may not exist. Kids Konnected (www.kidskonnected.org) was founded by children whose parents had cancer. The Web site provides friendship and a support network for kids with parents who have been diagnosed with cancer.

Just the facts

- Mirthful laughter appears to help in the healing process by boosting the immune system.

- There are many places to find support for yourself, your family, and your friends.

- Churches and synagogues can help you if you don't have family and friends to rely upon—or even if you do.

- Support groups have an added benefit—you can talk to women who really understand what you're going through.

Breast Reconstruction Methods

As much as cancer treatments, specifically, mastectomy and chemotherapy, are difficult to contend with emotionally as well as physically, there is another area that you'll have to deal with as well: how you look. As with any part of your body, losing a breast can be traumatic. How do you contend with this? In addition, chemotherapy treatments sometimes cause hair loss—also not an easy thing to accept. There are, however, things you can do to feel more like yourself again. Sometimes a boost in how you look is a boost in self esteem, which in turn makes you just feel better in general.

In this chapter we'll tell you about programs that can help you enhance your appearance while you're undergoing treatment. We also give you information on breast prostheses—used to enhance the affected breast area and to add balance to your posture—and we'll tell you about breast reconstruction surgery methods.

Chapter 15

Look better, feel attractive

Going through chemotherapy can not only make you nauseous and tired, but it may also result in the loss of your hair. Although the physical discomforts will eventually go away and your hair *will* grow back after the treatments end, there are things you can do to help yourself feel better during treatment. One of those things is looking better. You've heard the old phrase "if you look good, you feel good." It applies here. Although it's challenging for women who are in treatment to look good, it's far from impossible.

Some women who lose their hair lose their feeling of femininity, notes Marilyn Robinson, a headwear consultant and designer and creator of Headwear, Etc. (www.headwear-etc.com, 800/416-8224) in Houston, Texas. "They become devastated at the idea of losing their hair," says Robinson, who is also a six-year breast cancer survivor. "[They] don't want to be looked at as a sick person."

Many women use stylish headgear, like scarves, to cover up. Scarves are much softer on the scalp than wigs, and therefore more comfortable to wear. But there are certain times you may want to have a wig on hand, such as when you are having company or if you have children and they bring friends home. "It helps [women] to feel more like themselves again when they see their hair in the mirror," says Julie Durmis, manager of the Friends Boutique at the Dana-Farber Cancer Institute in Boston. If there are small children around, it also helps the children feel more comfortable. Typically, the wigs women undergoing chemotherapy wear are made mostly from synthetics and blends because they're easier to care for, she says. Human hair is good for long-term use, but these women are short-term users, she points out.

(Human hair wigs are also very expensive.) There's a variety of hairpieces with bangs available, as well.

In addition to boutiques at cancer centers, there are quite a few sites on the Internet selling wigs, hairpieces, hats, and scarves for women undergoing cancer treatment. And some savvy women have turned to the Jewish community to find head coverings. Married orthodox women must keep their heads covered in public by Jewish law. As a result, many wear wigs and some wear head coverings. Some shops that cater to this religious group have expanded their business to serve the chemotherapy community, reports Marsha Oakley, a registered nurse at the Breast Center at Mercy Medical Center in Baltimore. Contact an orthodox synagogue to find one of these shops.

It's interesting to note, however, that some women don't want to cover up their heads. According to Sandra Haber, a psychologist who works with breast cancer patients in New York City, "Some women don't want to appear like nothing is wrong when, in fact, everything is wrong."

Femininity is defined by clothes as well. Finding lacy lingerie and bathing suits to help enhance the area of loss is difficult but not impossible. There are more and more companies recognizing the needs of women who have undergone lumpectomies and mastectomies. For instance, one manufacturer Ladies First, Inc. (http://www.wvi.com/~ladies1/ nuproducts. html), sells a post-mastectomy camisole that is cut lower under the arms, has a small pocket on the underside of the garment to hold a drainage bulb in place, two removable, adjustable breast forms secured in place along a hidden Velcro strip.

Women who have recently had a mastectomy often have a problem finding comfortable clothes.

Unofficially...
Many organizations are ready and waiting to lend a helping hand, though some, reportedly, need a bit of prodding.

The breast area is swollen and sore and it may be difficult to lift the arm. Women who've had a TRAM flap (discussed later in this chapter), also experience pain in the abdomen or back. Special clothes are helpful. For example, Robinson sells a T-shirt held together with Velcro to wear to doctor's visits, for instance. This item is more easily removed than a shirt that is pulled over the head.

The American Cancer Society has a catalog, called "tlc," which has lingerie, including some pocketed for prostheses, as well as hats, turbans, kerchiefs, hair-pieces, and mastectomy bras and breast prostheses. There's also a soft mesh sleep cap to catch hair lost at night and a "hat sizer" used to make hats fit more snugly. (Note: Products in the "tlc" catalog are not endorsed by the American Cancer Society.) To order a copy of the "tlc" catalog call toll-free 800/850-9445.

Help is on the way!

Many cancer centers have programs to help cancer patients perk up their looks and camouflage their hair loss. In addition, the American Cancer Society has a free nationwide program called "Look Good...Feel Better." It teaches women with cancer beauty techniques specific to the treatment periods. The "Look Good...Feel Better" program is done in a small group setting (eight to ten women), which is led by trained beauty professionals. The group is taught a 12-step make-up program, and participants are given tips on make-up, hair, turbans, scarves, and wigs. Each woman also receives free make-up. (Note: Volunteers do not promote cosmetic product lines or specific manufacturers.)

The program takes place in cancer centers, hospitals, American Cancer Society offices, community centers, and in some beauty salons after hours. A free consultation in a participating salon may be more your style. This consultation does not come with free sample make-up.

If the "Look Good…Feel Better" program is not available in your area, you can order free pamphlets and a videotape. For more information, call 800/395-LOOK or the American Cancer Society at 800/227-2345.

The "Look Good…Feel Better" program is also offered in conjunction with the "I Can Cope" or "Reach to Recovery" programs sponsored by the American Cancer Society. Reach to Recovery is a one-on-one visitation program. A volunteer, matched to the patient based on surgery and treatment, age, and marital status, provides information, support, and practical tips. The volunteers are available to talk with you before or after breast surgery, reconstruction, or a recurrence of breast cancer. "I Can Cope" is a family education program about living with cancer. Doctors, nurses, social workers, and others provide information on cancer to everyone dealing with the day-to-day issues of living with cancer. For more information call the American Cancer Society at 800/ACS-2345 or visit their Web site at www.cancer.org.

Bright Idea
If you have private insurance, check your policy to see if the cost of breast prostheses is covered. If you have Medicare, call 800/MEDICARE. Medicare coverage varies from state to state.

Filling in the gaps—breast forms

Another issue of femininity is body shape. Women who have undergone a mastectomy (or two) or a lumpectomy are left misshapen. Clothes no longer fit right, and bras ride up. Plus, for those who want their medical history to remain discreet, it's hard to cover up a missing breast without some aid.

Aid can come in the form of a breast prosthesis (or two) or reconstructive surgery. Women who don't want reconstructive surgery often wear a breast prosthesis to simulate the weight, movement, and shape of the missing breast. A properly weighted breast form provides balance for correct posture and anchors your bra, preventing it from riding up. If you've had only one breast removed, it is important to wear a weighted breast form. Otherwise, you could end up with neck and back strain and pain because the weight of the natural breast will pull your spine in that direction.

Breast forms are typically worn inside a specially designed bra. Many pocketed bras, used to hold the breast form in place, are just as stylish as regular fashion bras. Many have lace accents and seamless design. Some attach to a camisole.

But everyone will not need a special mastectomy bra. Some high-tech breast forms attach directly to the body and others attach to the body with a special adhesive (described below), making pocketed "mastectomy" bras unnecessary. But if you use a fashion bra, you'll need support to keep your breast form in place. Consider wearing an underwire bra.

Getting into shape

There are two types of breast prostheses: lightweight and weighted. Weighted breast prostheses are for everyday wear. Lightweight breast forms are for swimming, leisure, and aerobic activity. Breast prostheses are made out of several materials, including the following:

Moneysaver
If your insurance won't adequately cover a mastectomy bra, or you just need a few extras, you can buy pre-made pockets and sew them into fashion bras.

- **Silicone gel**—Considered the top of the line material, silicone gel is typically the material of choice for weighted breast prostheses. Available in a variety of skin-tone shades, silicone gel simulates the weight, movement, and feel of a natural breast and warms to body temperature. (The silicone in breast forms is similar to but not the same as that found in breast implants. The silicone in external breast forms has been "cured" and is not in a liquid state.) Silicone breast forms are expensive. They can cost several hundred dollars. They typically have a two-year warranty.

Unofficially...
Breast prostheses are classified as medical devices and are regulated by the Food and Drug Administration.

■ **Rubber/latex**—Second in quality to silicone, rubber/latex also simulates the weight, movement, and feel of a natural breast, but doesn't match it as well as the silicone. But it does warm to body temperature and is less expensive than silicone.

■ **Foam**—These prostheses are primarily used for shape. Although some are weighted, most do not match the weight or movement of a natural breast. But they are inexpensive, and you can make them yourself if your budget is tight.

■ **Cotton batting**—Although it can be used to simulate shape, these prostheses usually serve more as a tool to estimate cup size. They are inexpensive and can be made at home. But this form will leave the weight of your chest unbalanced if you had a single mastectomy.

Breast form lingo
There are two main types of breast prostheses:
1. **Symmetrical**—These forms are interchangeable, that is, they can be worn on either the right or left side of the chest.

2. **Asymmetrical**—These forms are designed to fit either the right or left side of the chest.

Mix and match
Symmetrical breast forms come in three basic shapes:
1. **Triangle**—This shape has three corners and is

Moneysaver
If your insurance will only pay for one breast form in a lifetime, you may be able to successfully argue that breast size and shape change over time.

considered the most natural for a good bra fit.

2. **Teardrop**—Shaped like a teardrop, the tapered end fits under the arm. It can also be placed on the upper part of the chest.

3. **Heart shape**—Shaped like its name, the top part of the heart fits under the arm and the upper chest wall.

Stick to one side or the other

There are two types of asymmetrical breast forms:

1. **Curved teardrop**—This form is an extension of the symmetrical teardrop shape but has a slight extension for the upper chest wall.

2. **Extended triangle**—Again, a spin-off of the symmetrical form, one of the lower corners of this shape has an extension that fits under the arm.

But if you're looking for a perfect fit, right down to your scar, there is another option. Bio Portraits (www.bio-portraits.com; 800/655-4963) makes custom breast prosthetics. By taking a mold of the chest wall and the natural remaining breast they create a true prosthesis. There's even an inverse scar on the back to match your scar for a perfect fit. It's like making a limb, Durmis says. The manufacturer matches the skin tone, weight, slope, and shape of the breast as well as the areola, nipple size, and color. (A photo is available at their web site.) They're made of medical-grade silicone, which allows your skin to breathe. They are pricey, though—several thousand dollars, according to Durmis, but they can last a lifetime. (However, your natural breast size and shape may change, leaving you somewhat lopsided.) The prosthesis doesn't break down from exposure to natural body salts or water and can be worn in a pool, hot tub, or at the beach. Some insurance plans do cover

Watch Out!
If you decide to wear a low-cut dress or blouse, be careful about leaning forward—gravity will separate your form from your chest.

it, she says.

For some women, cost is an issue when choosing a breast form. Prostheses tend to be covered by insurance, Oakley says, but you have to file the paperwork. However, some policies won't cover special prosthetic bras that hold the form. These bras are more expensive than regular bras, she says.

Adding on

Not all women undergo mastectomies, but even breast-sparing surgeries can leave them disfigured. To make bras fit better, there are breast enhancers and attachable forms:

1. **Breast enhancers**—These fit over the breast and can be used to enhance the size of smaller breasts as well. These forms are shells or smaller shapes.

2. **Attachable forms**—Usually made of silicone, these triangular forms attach by Velcro; the soft side is attached to the chest using adhesive or surgical cement. With these forms you can wear a regular bra. The form can be used even during strenuous activity, including swimming.

Note: Most breast forms do not have nipples. However, you can purchase nipples that attach by suction.

Make your own breast form

Whether you've had a mastectomy or a lumpectomy, good breast forms are expensive, costing a few hundred to several thousand dollars. Because insurance and Medicare may not foot the entire bill, some women decide to make their own breast form. Here's one method of construction:

1. Find an old pair of panty hose and cut them off at the knees or get a pair of knee-high nylons that match your skin color. This will serve as the outer layer.

Moneysaver
If your insurance won't pay for a form after a lumpectomy, use a shoulder pad or the extra padding from breast-enhancer bras for symmetry.

Unofficially...
There is a new adhesive that can be applied to any breast form, including breast enhancers, to keep them in place. This adhesive, manufactured by Nearly Me, is placed on the back of the form and washed off at night. Whether used with breast forms or breast enhancers, this adhesive makes it easier to wear fashion bras.

2. Get a sturdy bra, one that has an appealing shape to you.

3. Purchase or make a form from foam or cotton. You can add weight inexpensively by tossing in fishing sinkers, dried peas, dried corn, dried barley, or similar-weighted product.

4. Fill the nylon and twist to close. Now place the filled ball back through the nylon to create a double layer. Knot it. Cut off the excess nylon. The knot can be shaped to serve as the nipple.

5. Place the form into an underwire bra.

Tips and tidbits

While a breast form is easy to slip in and out of, it requires care.

- **Keep it clean**—Wash your breast form with a mild soap every day after each use.

- **Keep it fresh**—Use antiperspirant (which, like the name implies, helps you to perspire less), not deodorant (which "deodorizes" the smell of perspiration). Perspiration can damage the form. Place a cotton pad—a soft cotton cloth—behind the form to absorb sweat.

- **Keep it safe**—Keep sharp jewelry away from a silicone form so as not to puncture it. Don't hold active animals against your chest. If a pet's claw pierces your breast form, the warranty is voided. That can be a costly accident.

To find out more about buying breast forms or hair gear, contact your local American Cancer Society for a list of stores. The American Cancer Society also may have wigs available free of charge. The Cancer Information Service at (800/4-CANCER) may be able to provide a list of local stores for these and other cosmetic aids.

Reconstructive surgery

Some women opt for reconstructive surgery rather than breast forms. Nearly all women who have had a mastectomy are candidates for reconstructive surgery. That surgery by a plastic surgeon can take place either at the time of the mastectomy or at a later date. Some women choose to get it at the same time to reduce the trauma of losing the breast and reduce exposure to more general anesthesia.

Although many women are satisfied with the results, the surgery is not perfect, Haber says. In addition to sometimes undergoing several procedures, women feel no sensation in the reconstructed breast, she notes. Some women anticipate they're getting their old breast back, she says, and frequently the new breast doesn't match the old breast. Often another surgery is needed to enlarge or reduce the other breast to make it match. Some women, for this reason, have found that a double mastectomy with reconstructive surgery is at least an equal match, Haber says, noting that surgeons may not like this resolution.

Some women Haber works with and who underwent breast reconstruction surgery didn't take the extra steps to get a nipple. It was a way for them to say enough is enough, Haber says. Some women, on the other hand, don't want reconstructive surgery—they don't want to appear like everything is okay. It appears that mastectomy, for them, symbolizes the loss, she says.

But there are many women who want to feel "whole" again, and for them reconstructive surgery (rather than a prosthesis) may be a good alternative. There are different ways for a plastic surgeon to perform a mastectomy in terms of incisions. Location of

Watch Out!
High-priced breast forms may not fit you right. Buy what feels good.

the biopsy scar influences the design of the incision used for the mastectomy, according to David Hidalgo, M.D., Chief of the Plastic and reconstructive Surgery Service at Memorial Sloan-Kettering Cancer Center in New York. Sometimes it's possible to preserve most of the skin, with the exception of the nipple, he says.

His team's newest approach is "skin-sparing" mastectomy, which leaves virtually no scars. Using this surgical technique, the surgeon removes the inner breast tissue, including the nipple, but leaves the shell of surrounding skin. A new breast is then constructed using tissue from the abdomen or buttocks.

In order to be a candidate for this type of surgery, you must have enough tissue to construct a new breast and your biopsy scar must not be too close to the nipple.

Your body type, age, and cancer treatment will also help to determine which type of reconstruction procedure will give you the best result. Hildalgo suggests consulting with a plastic surgeon before getting your biopsy.

There are two main types of breast reconstruction: One uses implants and the other uses tissue from another part of your body, as seen in the skin-sparing mastectomy.

Watch Out!
Women can opt for a double mastectomy under several circumstances, including having a BRCA1 or BRCA2 mutations, LCIS, or personal preference. This is a difficult discussion and decision for both the patient and doctor. Goals of treatment and expectations need to be CLEARLY defined.

Breast implants

Saline-filled (a salt-water solution) implants encased in silicone are used to make the breast mound for this type of reconstructive surgery. The saline sacs are placed under your skin behind the chest muscle.

The surgery may cause pain, swelling, bruising, and tenderness. These problems should disappear in several weeks or months and the scars will fade over time.

Saline implants have a lifetime of about 10 years. They deflate as the saline spills out. (It is absorbed into the body.) The implant can be replaced fairly easily, but it still requires general anesthesia, which carries risk.

For more information about breast implants, contact the following:

- NCI's Cancer Information Service (CIS): 800/4-CANCER

- The Food and Drug Administration (FDA): 800/532-4440

- The American Cancer Society (ACS): 800/ACS-2345

- Breast cancer survivors who have had reconstruction

TRAM flaps

Transverse rectus abdominis myocutaneous (TRAM flap) surgery is another option. This surgical technique creates a breast mound with tissue taken from another part of your body. This method creates a soft breast with a natural shape that ages similar to a natural breast. This type of surgery, however, leaves a new scar at the site where tissue is taken to form the mound.

There are two types of TRAM flaps: tunneled and free. When the tissue is taken from the abdomen, a section (flap) of skin, muscle, and fat, typically while still partially connected to its blood supply, is moved under the surface of the skin from the abdomen to the breast to create the breast shape. The abdominal muscle continues to supply blood to the skin and fat tissue forming the new breast. This is the tunneled method.

There are risks, though small, related to this

Unofficially...
Women who have radiation treatments aren't good candidates for implants because radiation adversely affects the skin's circulation and decreases elasticity.

method of breast reconstruction. If there is poor blood supply to the flap tissue, part or all of the tissue in the breast area may not survive the transplant. This type of surgery can result in abdominal weakness, causing back strain. Most women do not have this complaint, but those who undergo reconstructive surgery on both breasts are more at risk for having muscle weakness because portions of both abdominal muscles are removed in that case. The other type of TRAM flap—the free flap—reduces the likelihood of abdominal weakness. With this method only a small part of the abdominal muscle is needed. It is completely detached and reattached using microsurgery to reconnect the blood vessels, which results in better blood circulation to the newly reconstructed breast. However, there is a small risk with this type of surgery, too. The microsurgery fails to reestablish blood circulation to the transplanted tissue in one to three percent of patients, and the transferred tissue cannot be saved. Smoking, obesity, and diabetes increase the risk of microsurgery failure. If failure does occur, you'd have to choose another method of reconstructive surgery at a later date.

Most women who have had radiation therapy are good candidates for TRAM flaps, but generally are not candidates for implants because that reconstruction method involves expanding the tissue. (A skin-sparing mastectomy usually is not done with an implant. Therefore, there is no extra skin to cover the site, so stretching is required.) Radiation therapy reduces the skin's circulation in the treated area and, as a consequence, it's ability to expand.

Alternative reconstructive techniques

For those women who are not candidates for a TRAM flap because of an existing scar on their abdomen (a scar alters the anatomy and blood supply) or their abdomens are flat (you must have enough tissue in your abdomen to be a candidate for the reconstructive method because a flat abdomen does not have the fat and skin necessary for this procedure) or for implants, and for those who don't want implants, there's another type of reconstructive surgery that uses your own body tissue. With a gluteal free flap, tissue is taken from the upper or lower buttock, detached, and placed in the breast. (There is a slight flattening in the area where the tissue is taken from.) Because the tissue and fat is completely detached before it is moved, microsurgery to reconnect blood vessels is necessary. There is a one to three percent chance adequate circulation will not be restored and the tissue will be lost. (Additional surgery may be required at that point to restore viability of tissue, if possible, or to reconstruct a non viable graft. Usually tissue from another site is used.) Typically, this surgery is for women under age 45.

Women who have had radiation therapy may also be candidates for the latissimus dorsi flap reconstruction procedure, which uses muscle and skin from the upper back. While still partially attached, the tissue is slid underneath the skin to the breast. The transplanted skin is stretched using a tissue expander, which is later replaced with a permanent implant. In women who've had radiation, the skin that is stretched is skin that was not exposed to radiation, since stretching skin that's been exposed to radiation treatment usually is not possible because radiation can cause the skin to become fibrous.

Nipple and areola reconstruction typically take place two to three months after the reconstructive surgery so that the new breast has time to settle into place. The areola is generally made from skin grafted from the upper thigh and the nipple is usually reconstructed from skin and fat of the reconstructed breast, according to Hidalgo. (Skin from the breast can also be used to make a new nipple, as well.) This procedure is done as an outpatient surgery. Color is added by a tattoo procedure performed at the doctor's office several months after the nipple/areola reconstruction. According to Hidalgo, most breast reconstruction patients do not have complications.

Whether or not to have reconstructive surgery, when to have it, and which type to have are all issues you should discuss with your doctor. Table 15.1 lists other questions you should ask your physician.

Most women who have this and other breast

TABLE 15.1: QUESTIONS TO ASK YOUR PLASTIC SURGEON ABOUT BREAST RECONSTRUCTION

1. What is the latest information about the safety of breast implants?

2. How many breast reconstruction surgeries have you done?

3. Which type of surgery would give me the best results?

4. How long will the surgery take? What type of anesthesia is used?

5. When do you recommend I begin breast reconstruction?

6. How many surgeries will I need?

7. What are the risks at the time of surgery? Later?

8. Will there be scars? Where? How large?

9. Will flap surgery cause any permanent changes where tissue was removed?

10. What complications should I report to you?

11. How long will my recovery take? When can I return to my normal activities? What activities should I avoid?

12. Will I need follow-up care?

13. How much will it cost? (Read you health insurance policy and verify with your provider if it will pay for breast reconstruction.)

Source: National Cancer Institute

reconstruction surgery are pleased with the results.

Just the facts

- Some women with breast cancer need to look good to feel better and there are many programs available to help.

- There are a variety of breast form materials and shapes.

- You can make your own breast form.

- One method of breast reconstruction preserves the breast skin, save for the nipple.

Surviving
Breast Cancer

PART VII

How to Get Good Medical Care

Chapter 16

O nce you feel a lump or have a mammogram reading that indicates there might be a cancer growing, you need to find a good doctor. How do you find one who uses the most up-to-date techniques to make an accurate diagnosis using a method that has the least chance of limiting your choices for treatment? You also need to find a good hospital. And you have to pay the bills, which can get pretty messy, to say the least.

In this chapter you'll learn what qualities and factors to consider when picking your doctor and hospital. And you'll get expert tips on how to deal effectively with insurance companies. You also learn about alternatives to getting health coverage if your insurance runs out. Plus, you'll want questions to ask your doctor and you'll learn how to remember the answers accurately.

Choosing a doctor

Many city and state magazines have them—"Best Doctor Surveys." Those who make it onto the list proudly hang a copy of the article in their office for patients to see. Many people use this listing to choose their physicians. This may be a good strategy, or it may just be an easy one. It all depends on whom you pick. The validity of most of these surveys has not been evaluated by objective measures, the most important of which is patient outcomes. As most of the articles introducing these surveys explain, the choices are typically doctors' picks of doctors—doctors pick their colleagues, friends, and those who have published works or who lecture. So the listings may, in part, be popularity contests.

It's nice to have a doctor who's popular among his or her peers, but if you or someone you love has been diagnosed with breast cancer, you'll probably want to use a physician noted for good outcomes, not necessarily one who's well-liked by his or her colleagues.

"Reputation depends on a lot more than clinical skill," says Arthur Hartz, M.D., a University of Iowa professor of family medicine. Reputation is often a result of public presence—the physician's status, his or her professional position, and ability as a lecturer, researcher, or administrator, he explains. These qualities reflect reputation much more so than clinical skill, according to Hartz. A good researcher does not necessarily make a good clinician.

Hartz and his colleagues (Jose Pulido, M.D. and Evelyn Kuhn, Ph.D.), studied best doctor lists and compared them with those doctors who had measurable good patient outcomes. They concluded that there isn't any scientific evidence that best doctor surveys identify good clinicians. Results from this study, as well as those from a subsequent one, showed that the best measure of a good doctor is experience, which they defined by the number of patients a doctor treats. Their research was published in the *American Journal of Public Health* in October 1997.

In the first study, Hartz and his colleagues rated doctors in accordance with patient outcomes and compared that list with those voted best doctors in both *The Best Doctors in America* (a reference book) and community magazines.

The researchers chose a specialty—coronary artery bypass graft surgery—as it requires technical skill needed for surgery. In contrast, for other specialties like internal medicine, more intellectual skill may be a better indicator of a doctor with good outcomes. Hartz and his colleagues tabulated patient outcomes of physicians in New York, Pennsylvania, and Wisconsin. The failure rate for each physician was measured by his or her mortality ratio—that is, the actual number of deaths divided by the average number of deaths among patients with similar risk. The higher the ratio, the worse that physician's performance record.

Hartz and his colleagues found there wasn't much difference in the mortality ratio between the heart surgeons voted best doctors and others. Some physicians who were voted by their peers as best doctors had low mortality ratios, but others had high mortality ratios.

What factors have a positive impact on mortality ratio? The researchers found that the number of surgeries the physician performed was an important factor, and one that you might consider using as a screening criterion. In this study, physicians who performed more than 400 bypass surgeries in a three-year period had the lowest mortality ratio.

They also wanted to see if by choosing one of the "best doctors" the patient was any more likely to eliminate those doctors who had the worst performance records. But they found that those doctors were just as likely to be bad surgeons as those not identified as the best.

"[Ranking doctors is] a very difficult process to do correctly," Hartz says. There are no good resources for journalists or incentives for the magazines to do a careful analysis of the best area doctors. Because no good method has been established for conducting meaningful listings, these best doctor surveys are done in the least expensive way rather than a valid way, Hartz explains. Even with the research he conducted he did not believe the available data was adequate to identify individual doctors who were very good or very bad. To do so would take a very large number of patient outcomes. But, he says, it was good enough to identify groups of doctors that were very good or very bad.

Because they didn't find anything useful in choosing a doctor from the best doctor surveys, the research team decided to look at other characteristics to see if they might be important. The results of that study were published in the journal *Medical Care* (January 1999).

Hartz and his colleagues looked for physician characteristics that might be related to quality care, such as:

- The number of surgeries he or she performed in the previous year

- Where the surgeon had gone to medical school, and whether it was here or abroad (some medical schools outside of the United States have lower educational standards, though some have higher standards)

- The place where the doctor had trained (residency or fellowship)

> **"**
> The life so short, the craft so long to learn.—Hippocrates
> **"**

- The number of years of experience of the surgeon

- Whether he or she was affiliated with an academic institution and, if so, what his or her rank was (assistant professor, professor, department chair, etc.)

Their survey found, again, that of overwhelming importance in terms of patient outcome was the number of surgeries performed in the previous few years. They also found that there seems to be a decline in quality of the doctor's performance with age (after the mid-50s). Interestingly, they did not find that academic affiliation was related to outcome for bypass surgery, though many people use academic affiliation as a selection criterion because teaching hospitals are thought to be on the cutting edge of the latest treatments.

Be tentative in generalizing results—they're not definitive, Hartz concludes. "There are many limitations to this kind of study," he says.

Bottom line? Look for someone who has a lot of recent experience in the specific area of breast cancer for which you need treatment. Ask each doctor how many biopsies/surgeries/radiation or chemotherapy treatments they've done in the last three years. Ask for patient outcomes, that is, how well they faired. Make sure the doctor you choose is accessible to you and is someone with whom you feel comfortable. Cancer is not one of those things that you fix and it's done, like gallbladder surgery. Your relationship with your oncologist is ongoing. Finally, based on Hartz's findings, you may want to consider taking the physician's age into account.

Qualities of a good doctor
Your healthcare team will be made up of several

Timesaver
Keep up-to-date medical records, not just of your cancer care, but your entire medical history. Contact the medical records office to get a copy. If you go to several different doctors, or if you move out of town, you'll have everything handy.

doctors—your oncologist, perhaps a surgeon, a radiation oncologist, and pathologists (who work behind the scenes) as well as residents and interns (medical students) if you go to a teaching hospital. (Your primary care physician and gynecologist are kept in the loop, but many do not want to have primary responsibility for cancer-related decisions.)

You can't pick some members of your medical team, such as the pathologist (although you can choose one for a "second opinion" to confirm the biopsy results), but you can choose your oncologist and your surgeon. While many doctors perform breast cancer surgery, not many are true breast surgeons, according to Johns Hopkins University. There are surgeons, however, who do specialize in breast surgery. Breast surgeons will likely be more up-to-date on the latest surgical techniques, according to Johns Hopkins University. Furthermore, as noted earlier, those surgeons with more experience have better results and are more attuned to subtle differences in individual cases. Johns Hopkins University suggests seeking out a surgeon who does 50 or more breast cancer operations per year. How do you find out how many surgeries per year the surgeon has performed? Call his or her office and the hospital where the doctor performs surgeries and ask about case volume.

Consider choosing a breast surgeon who is board certified by the American Board of Surgery. The American Board of Medical Specialists can tell you names of surgeons who have this qualification in your area. To contact them, call 847/491-9091 or visit www.abms.org on the Web. Many of these surgeons are also members of the American College of Surgeons, according to Johns Hopkins University. In addition, an experienced, up-to-date surgeon typically belongs to the Society of Surgical Oncology, whose members have substantial training and/or experience in the management of cancer. They keep up with the latest developments in surgical management of breast cancer, in part, by attending annual educational meetings sponsored by the society, according to Johns Hopkins University.

Apply the same criteria for each of the other physicians on your team. Each should be board certified or board-eligible in his or her specialty. Then look for an oncologist who specializes in breast cancer.

Another way to find a physician: Talk to survivors who've been treated by any physicians you are considering. Listen hardest to women who've been treated in the last three years. Treatments advance rapidly, and their experience will be more relevant.

You may want to call the state medical board (locate your state board at the Federation of State Medical Board's Web site—http://www.fsmb.org/members.htm or see your local phone book) to find out if it has any information about the physician you are considering. It will have reports of any malpractice cases and quality of care complaints. Find out if there have been any complaints about your other physicians, too.

Note: The nonprofit consumer advocacy group Public Citizen (202/588-1000) publishes books by state listing doctors with blemishes on their records.

Experience counts

In the article "Impact of Hospital Volume on Operative Mortality for Major Cancer Surgery," published in the Journal of the American Medical Association (November 1998), Colin B. Begg, chairman of Memorial Sloan-Kettering's Department of Epidemiology and Biostatistics, and his colleagues found that

> 66
> Not all breast surgeons do breast cancer surgeries 100 percent of the time. But consider this— some full-time breast surgeons do surgery on only 25-30 new cancer cases each year but others who do only 75 percent breast surgery treat over 200 new cases per year.
> —Johns Hopkins University
> 99

Bright Idea
Doctors often give conflicting opinions, says Sandra Cooley, a breast cancer survivor. One says you're a good candidate for radiation treatments, another says you'll have a 30 percent chance of relapse with radiation. She came up with a practical resolution. Cooley asked her doctors what they would do if she was their wife/mother/ daughter in this situation. She found she received more direct answers posing the question in this manner.

mortality rates for cancer surgeries studied were 40 to 80 percent lower in hospitals where surgeons had the most experience performing particular surgical procedures. (They looked at 5,013 patients aged 65 years or older diagnosed between 1984 and 1993 who underwent pancreatectomy, esophagectomy, pneumonectomy, liver resection, or pelvic exenteration.)

William J. Hoskins, M.D., deputy physician-in-chief, disease management, a co-author of the study, adds, "It boils down to the idea that is central to the disease management system: superspecialization. If you work in a place focused on cancer—with enough volume, such as Memorial Sloan-Kettering—you can specialize. And while this study addressed surgical outcomes, the same principle applies to chemotherapy, radiation therapy, and the other modalities we use to treat cancer: When people do something day in and day out, they're going to do it better."

"The more experience the surgeon has in doing a specific procedure and managing patients with a specific cancer, the better that patient's chances that he or she will have a better outcome after the operation," says Murray F. Brennan, M.D., chairman of the Department of Surgery at Memorial Sloan-Kettering, another co-author of the article. The high-volume hospitals performed these surgeries about four times as often as the low-volume facilities.

Attitude counts

Consider choosing a doctor with the following personality qualities:

- Someone who will tell you the facts candidly

- Someone who will take the time to answer all your questions, one who will discuss treatment and results, and one who wants to educate you

■ Someone who will admit to his or her own short-comings—no doctor knows all— and who is willing to consider additional treatments that may not be standard

Talking to your doctor

Once you choose a doctor, your job as your own patient advocate isn't over. You must be ready to speak up for yourself. In other words, you must be prepared to ask for what you want rather than simply agreeing with the doctor and walking out the door. "If you don't ask for what you want you'll get what you don't want," says Mike D. Oppenheim, M.D., author of the article "7 Ways Doctors Torture Their Patients," which was published in *Hippocrates* magazine (October 1996). One way doctors cause their patients undue stress is by dragging things out, he says in his article. He tells of a friend who told him she had discovered a lump in her breast. The doctor had scheduled the biopsy for a week from then. Sensing her anxiety, Oppenheim suggested she call her doctor, tell him of her concern, and ask to have the biopsy sooner. "It hadn't occurred to her, as it doesn't to many patients, to question the doctor's schedule," he wrote. She made the call and her doctor rescheduled the biopsy for the following day.

Generally, physicians are not the best communicators, says Sandra Haber, Ph.D., a psychologist who works with breast cancer patients in New York City. It doesn't mean that they're not nice people, it just means they don't always know how to talk to their patients, she says. She suggests bringing someone with you to appointments, someone who can facilitate, if necessary, and serve as a second pair of ears. "Research shows that if you're traumatized, you're

Bright Idea
If you have a complaint against your doctor that you can't resolve, call the agency that licenses physicians in your state. If the complaint is against your hospital, contact your state's hospital association.

Unofficially...
You are entitled to be completely informed about your cancer, including information on the benefits and risks of procedures and treatments, any alternative treatments that may be available, and how the disease and the treatments may impact your life.

not going to retain the information," she says, adding that it's normal. Choose a buddy who will be calm and thoughtful.

Keep in mind that it's normal to be anxious, which means you might have trouble remembering what's said during an appointment. To help you keep track, Haber suggests the following tips:

■ Write down questions ahead of time and bring them along or fax them to the office ahead of time.

■ Start the appointment by telling your doctor how many questions you have. Avoid small talk so you have time to ask the questions.

■ Take notes. The writing helps you clarify what's being said as you jot down the doctor's comments. Keep all your notes together in one notebook for easy access. (See Worksheet 16.1 and 16.2. at the end of this chapter.)

■ Ask your doctor to give you a summary in writing. Take a tape recorder, too.

■ If your doctor makes a recommendation, ask questions. For example, if your doctor says tumors tend to respond well to a particular chemotherapy drug, ask if that translates to longer survival. Ask what the five- and ten-year rates of recurrence are for this treatment option. Sometimes quality of life, rather than survival, is the goal, making tumor shrinkage the measuring stick. If the tumor is pressing on a nerve, for example, ask if tumor shrinkage will occur and reduce any pain or discomfort. Ask if there are any studies with supporting data you can review. Haber cautions that it's preferable to look at data on women your age and with your type, stage, and histologic grade of tumor. You'll probably also want to know side effects—that is, how will the treatment affect the quality of everyday life (both in the short run, such as nausea or fatigue, as well as in the long run, such as increasing the likelihood of other cancers)? Radiation and chemo may also cause other cancers, fertility problems, etc.

- Ask whom you can call and when if you have any additional questions.

- If you're undergoing surgery, ask the doctor to give you a prescription for pain medication ahead of time so you don't have to wait for the prescription while you're in pain. Ask how to reach the physician on call if there's not one central number.

- Ask what side effects you might experience. Ask what you should do if the side effects are worse than anticipated and at what point should you contact the physician on call.

After you complete treatment, ask your doctor the following questions:

- What are the signs of the cancer's return?

- What changes might occur that are not danger signs?

Be sure to tell your doctor about any changes in your lifestyle. Even changes that seem minor to you, such as quitting smoking, could affect your treatment. (In that case, you may need a different dose of some medicines.) Use worksheets 16.1 and 16.2 to keep track of your appointment notes.

Choosing a hospital

U.S. News & World Report evaluated 6,400 hospitals to come up with "America's Best Hospitals," searchable by disease at www.usnews.com.

The rankings, which are reflective of patient care, are based on the following:

- **Mortality**—Death rates for each specialty were calculated and adjusted to reflect a patient's principal diagnosis as well as secondary problems.

- **Reputation**—150 randomly selected board-certified specialists each named the five hospitals in their specialty they consider to be the best, regardless of location or expense.

- **Other data**—The number of nurses at a hospital, the technology available to patients, and other medical information was considered.

Watch Out!
Don't set out to be a "good" patient, withholding any complaints. Your doctor needs to know how you're really doing in order to treat you properly.

(Note: If any data was missing or the survey was never filed, the hospital was dropped. So some good hospitals may have been left out of the rankings as a result. Furthermore, to be eligible for inclusion, a hospital had to be affiliated with a medical school, be a member of the Council of Teaching Hospitals, or have a minimum of nine of 17 specific technologies readily available.)

This is not to say you can't find a top-notch oncologist or radiologist at a hospital that may be on your insurance plan or in your city but didn't make the list. Remember, some hospital administrators didn't submit complete forms and some neglected to respond to the survey. Furthermore, good doctors can be found at hospitals that didn't qualify for the survey.

The Joint Commission on Accreditation of Healthcare Organizations (JCAHO) is an independent, nonprofit healthcare accrediting organization. Accreditation comes on many levels: accredited with commendation, accredited with recommendations for improvement, accredited without recommendations for improvement (accredited), provisional accreditation, conditional accreditation, preliminary non-accreditation, or adverse decision, in appeal. Accreditation with commendation is given to just a small percentage of all hospitals surveyed. Surveys include touring the hospital, visiting patient-care units, reviewing medical records, and meeting with patients and staff to determine the quality of care and to evaluate the overall management of the hospital. Check to see if the hospital you want to go to has the JCAHO seal of approval and, preferably, an accreditation with commendation.

Although many hospitals have an interdisciplinary team, some have only one such team (i.e., just one breast surgeon, one medical oncologist, etc.) But at some hospitals, typically teaching hospitals, there are several physicians for each specialty. In that setup, your specific case gets discussed and reviewed by your team as well as by the other physicians, which can lead to review and debate of each treatment step, possibly resulting in better treatment.

Be sure to check that the hospital has the most recent technology for diagnosing and treating breast cancer. Make sure it offers the latest treatment modalities, including clinical trials.

Cutting down the paper chase

There are two broad categories of health insurance coverage. The first is *fee-for-service*. The second is *managed care*. Under managed care there are *health maintenance organizations* (HMOs), *preferred provider organizations* (PPOs), and *point-of-service* (POS) plans.

Under a fee-for-service setup, your doctor will submit a bill to your insurance provider, or, if he or she does not have a relationship with your provider, you may have to pay the bill directly and get reimbursed from your provider. Under this type of plan, you can visit any doctor and go to any hospital. Under a fee-for-service structure, you'll be reimbursed for a percentage of the doctor or hospital bill. Usually, you're covered for 80 percent of the visit after satisfying the deductible.

There are three major types of managed care health plans: HMOs, PPOs, and POSs. Many of these plans charge a copayment.

If you're a member of an HMO, you are required to use the doctors and hospitals that participate in the plan or you'll have to pay for your medical care out of your own pocket. (However, certain exceptions may be made.) HMOs often have medical facilities where patient care is delivered. There is also a subcategory of HMOs called *individual practice associations* (IPAs). In this setup, individual practitioners are grouped together to provide patient care under an HMO.

If you're a member of an HMO, you must get an authorization to see a specialist or for any hospitalization. The request goes through a utilization review where plan administrators determine if the medical or surgical service you need is "appropriate" and/or "medically necessary."

Unofficially... While reputation may not be a reliable indicator, according to Arthur Hartz, M.D., a University of Iowa professor of family medicine, *U.S. News & World Report's* "Best Hospitals" is the best source of hospital rankings available.

PPOs and POSs (the latter usually has a primary care physician coordinating your care) are also considered managed care plans, but differ from HMOs in several ways. Like HMOs, these plans have a network of providers, but they also allow you to seek medical help from physicians outside the network. If you go outside of the plan, you'll typically be covered at 70 or 80 percent, like with the fee-for-service plans. You also may be responsible for annual deductibles if you choose a physician outside the network.

If you're a member of a fee-for-service plan or

you're a member of a PPO but using a physician or hospital outside of the network, you'll have to fill out some paperwork. Filing insurance claims can be tiring and frustrating, especially when you're in the midst of treatment. So it should come as no surprise that some cancer survivors don't take full advantage of their insurance. (Of course, that may be because you don't know exactly what coverage you have, so read your policy.)

Timesaver
For a list of the top hospitals in oncology, visit the U.S. News Web site at www.usnews.com

Sometimes insurance companies, for various reasons, deny claims, even though you may have coverage for them. If that happens to you, resubmit the claim or ask your doctor's office to do so. If it's rejected again, contact the company. The carriers have an appeal process and people on staff who can cut through the paper work, says a spokesperson for the Health Insurance Association of America. Work up the chain, he advises. Sometimes plans will appoint a case manager to help you.

If you don't get a positive response, take action. (See Table 16.1 to find out what government office oversees the type of insurance you have.)

Sometimes insurance companies deny claims for treatments on the grounds that they're experimental, says Audrey Selden, associate commissioner for Consumer Protection at the Texas Department of Insurance. But, she says, some previously experimental treatments may no longer hold this status at the time your claim is submitted. Recent research findings may help you update your insurance company. Ask your doctor if he knows of relevant journal articles or cancer centers where the treatment is being used, which shows acceptance by the medical community. (If you like, of course, you can take things into your own hands and search Medline at http://igm.nlm.nih.gov

Moneysaver
If you are required to get a referral before seeing a specialist, be sure to get one, and make sure you receive it on the proper form. A referral written on a prescription pad or other form may not qualify and may leave you holding the bill.

for journal articles. Sometimes it takes months for articles to get on Medline, so you might want to search journals at the hospital library.)

Other times, insurance companies deny claims based on specific language in the insurance policy. If that's the case, ask your insurance company for the specific language that supports their denial. See if the disagreement is a matter of interpretation of the policy.

If your claim is denied for any reason that does not seem right, ask your doctor's office or hospital claims staff for assistance. Some hospitals have knowledgeable people who can assist you if your coverage for claims is denied. Plus there's usually an

TABLE 16.1   FILING AN INSURANCE COMPLAINT IF YOU FEEL YOU HAVE BEEN TREATED UNFAIRLY

If your claims have been denied and you think the treatment is covered under your policy, here's where to complain.

If Your Insurer is...	It Is Regulated By...
A private company (e.g., Blue Cross, Prudential)	Your state department of insurance
A licensed healthcare service plan (e.g., Kaiser and other HMOs)	Your state department of insurance
Federal qualified Health Maintenance Organization	U.S. Health Care Finacing Administration, Office of Prepaid Health Care Operations and Oversight
Private Employer, union self-insurance, or self-financed plans	U.S. Department of Labor, Pension & Welfare Benefits Administration
Medicaid (sometimes called other names; e.g., in California it's known as MediCal)	Your state department of social services or medical assistance services
Medicare Supplemental Security Income	U.S. Social Security Administration
Veterans Benefits CHAMPUS	Department of Veterans Affairs, Veterans Assistance Service

Source: National Cancer Institute

appeal process if a benefit is denied, Selden says.

In addition, you can contact the complaint staff at your state insurance department. State insurance departments regulate insurance companies, Selden says. The state can fine insurance companies, make them pay restitution to consumers, or force them to close up shop in that state, though that's rare.

Your state insurance commissioner's office can often work with your insurance company, healthcare providers, and experts at major cancer centers to get procedures covered that insurance companies might normally refuse, claiming they're experimental, such as bone marrow transplants.

Many state insurance departments have complaint forms on their Web site that you can fill out and send by e-mail, or you can fax your complaint. In Texas you can walk in with all your paperwork, Selden says. (You can quickly locate your state insurance commissioner's office using the Web. The National Association of Insurance Commissioner's Web site at www.naci.org has links to most state regulators' sites.) The state will contact the insurance company and get account information. Why bother? State insurance departments have the history of complaints from other people covered by the same insurer. This helps them determine if an insurance company is paying or not. They also know which treatments other companies are paying for, which may help determine if a treatment is considered experimental.

Watch Out!
Before signing up for an HMO, consider whether you are willing to lose some control over the administration of your healthcare.

Setting the record straight

Keep a journal of your experience with doctors, hospitals, and insurance companies. It can serve as a quick reference should problems with insurance reimbursement arise. Your journal should include the following:

- A copy of your health insurance policy or certificate and benefit booklet. You need a copy of the actual policy to know what services and treatments are covered. (Be sure to read your policy. Don't rely on what your agent or benefits director says. If you have difficulty understanding the language, call your state insurance commissioner's office for help.)

- Copies of any materials you received when you enrolled in the plan and any updates you've received since then.

- Appointments. Note which doctor you saw, the date of the appointment, the treatment received, and the amount billed.

- A copy of all bills.

- Copies of all claims paid by the insurer as well as those that were denied.

- Phone calls. Include the name and title of the person with whom you spoke, the date and time of the call, and a detailed summary of the conversation. Record the length of the conversation and any long-distance costs incurred. Many insurance companies record their calls, too.

- Copies of all correspondence received and sent. Whenever possible, communicate in writing, by fax, or e-mail so that you have a written record. Don't rely on what was said over the phone.

Reaching your limit

Your policy has a cap. Once your reimbursements reach that limit, you'll have to foot the remaining medical bills. So it's important to keep tabs on your total medical bill. If you suspect your healthcare provider is overcharging in general, ask your insurer to audit the bills and verify that the right billing codes were used. If you just question one or two bills, call the provider first and ask them to verify the billing codes.

Before you reach the limit your insurance policy will pay, check with your state to see if you're eligible for health insurance coverage in a high-risk pool. Some states have these for people who have pre-existing conditions. Or ask if the state requires companies to issue policies to all applicants. Check with your county commissioner's office to see of they have an assistance program. Another good source is the following:

Health Insurance: Risk Pools
Pub. #HRD-88-66BR
U.S. General Accounting Office
P.O. Box 6015
Gaithersburg, MD 20884
Phone: 202/512-6000   Fax: 301/258-4066

Getting the maximum coverage for clinical trial costs

Besides hope and possibly a better treatment protocol, one of the benefits to being in a clinical trial (discussed in detail in Chapter 11) is that part, if not all, of the care is offered free of charge. However, some insurers won't cover certain costs when a new treatment is under study. If you are considering taking part in a clinical trial, take the following action:

- Ask your doctor about the coverage experience of other patients in the trial.

- Make sure your doctor is careful about the way he or she completes the paperwork submitted to your insurer. Often the way the doctor describes a treatment can help or hurt your chances of

Bright Idea
If you're covered by your employer's self-insured plan and your claim is denied, complain to the state insurance commissioner's office. Many of these plans respond to state regulators, even though they're not under their jurisdiction.

Moneysaver
Keep track of all non-reimbursable payments you make for medical care, prescription drugs, and medical equipment. These include gas mileage for trips to and from appointments, parking fees, and meals during long medical visits. If these costs exceed 7.5 percent of your adjusted gross income, you can deduct the portion that is greater than the 7.5 percent on your income tax.

insurance coverage.

- Read your policy to see if there's a specific exclusion for "experimental treatment." But remember, it may no longer be experimental at the time you submit your claim. However, in that case you'd be taking the risk on not being covered.

Getting financial help

Even if your insurance picks up 80 percent of the tab, 20 percent can still be a considerable out-of-pocket expense when it comes to medical bills for breast cancer. For financial help with treatment and other expenses, contact the following:

- **Local cancer support organizations.** They may be able to provide referrals to community sources for financial aid. Start with the American Cancer Society at www.cancer.org or 800/ACS-2345.

- **Your local office on aging**, if you're a senior citizen.

- **The county board** of assistance or welfare office.

- **The federal government's** Aid to Families with Dependent Children (AFDC) and Food Stamps Program.

- **Medicare,** a federal health insurance program administered by the Health Care Financing Administration, provides health insurance to people age 65 and over, those with permanent kidney failure, and certain people with disabilities. For more information visit www.medicare.gov or call 800/MEDICARE.

- **Medicaid,** which provides health insurance for the disabled and others. For more information visit www.hcfa.gov/medicaid/mcaicnsm.htm.

- **Social Security Administration.** It oversees Social

Security, Supplemental Security Income, and Medicare. Call 800/772-1213; TTY: 1/800-325-0778 (www.ssa.gov/SSA_Home.html).

■ **Department of Veterans Affairs**, if you or a member of your immediate family is a veteran. For more information, call 800/827-1000 or visit www.va.gov/benefits.htm.

■ **The Cancer Information Service of the National Cancer Institute**. Call 800/4-CANCER for information on all aspects of cancer.

■ **Your hospital**. Contact the patient advocate, the hospital's financial aid counselor, a hospital social worker, or a patient representative in the hospital business office to find out about setting up monthly payment plans for hospital bills.

■ **Hospitals that receive Hill-Burton funds** (construction funds from the federal government). They are required by law to provide some services to people who cannot afford to pay for their hospitalization. For more information call 800/638-0742 or visit www.hrsa.dhhs.gov/osp/dfcr/obtain/consfaq.htm.

■ **Drug companies.** Some pharmaceutical manufacturers have patient assistance programs to help pay for drugs for patients who can't afford them. To find out whether a specific drug may be available free or at a reduced cost, call the company that manufactures the drug, or ask your physician or a medical social worker.

■ **Transportation companies.** There are nonprofit organizations that arrange for free or reduced airfares for cancer patients who need to fly to cancer treatment centers. Financial need is not always a requirement. For more information, ask a social

"
In many cases the carriers often receive incomplete information from providers, and all too often, unfortunately, providers respond to this by simply billing the patients, which basically adds insult to injury.
—Spokesperson, Health Insurance Association of America
"

worker. Your local chapter of the American Cancer Society or state or local Department of Social Services may be able to arrange ground transportation or reimburse you for car mileage.

▪ **Community voluntary agencies and service organizations.** These groups may offer financial help to those in need.

▪ **Housing/Lodging.** Some organizations and private homeowners, through organizations, provide lodging for the family of a patient undergoing treatment. Check with the hospital social worker.

Keeping coverage

There may be a few ways for you to keep or increase your insurance coverage. You or your husband, if you are married, could try to get a new job at a large company with a group policy. Many of these companies don't screen for health coverage. You can join an HMO, again avoiding the screening. You may be better off, however, taking a new job with a lower salary, but that has better insurance coverage.

Some women, after going through something as serious as breast cancer, re-examine their lives and decide to leave their jobs to take a more fulfilling one. If this is the case, you may want to consider continuing your coverage with your company's group plan through COBRA after you leave. If a new job does not work out, you could be left with no coverage.

You can qualify for COBRA if you leave an employer either voluntarily or involuntarily, or lose your insurance coverage because the number of hours you work is reduced substantially. Federal law (Public Law 99-272), the Consolidated Omnibus Budget Reconciliation Act (COBRA), requires many employers to

Watch Out!
You can ask your insurer about coverage of specific therapies. But watch out— some patients say that their questions may have hurt their chances for coverage by raising a red flag, according to the National Cancer Institute.

allow employees to pay their own premiums for the company's group plan for up to 18 months, (up to 29 months if they lose their jobs due to disability and are eligible for Social Security disability benefits at the time they leave the job). It lasts 36 months for dependents. (COBRA applies to employers with 20 or more workers who already offer group health insurance.)

Just the facts

- There are many surveys that rank doctors and hospitals, but not all are reliable.

- Be sure to ask your doctor any questions you have about the diagnosis and treatment.

- Take notes during visits with your doctor—anxiety makes people forget exactly what was said.

- There are organizations and government services that may help you if you are in a tight financial situation.

Moneysaver
The American Association of Retired Persons (AARP) offers discounts on health care products and prescriptions to its members. Membership costs $8 annually. You must be 50 years old to qualify for membership. For more information call 800/424-3410 or write to AARP, 601 E St., NW, Washington, DC 20049.

WORKSHEET 16.1
VITAL INFORMATION ABOUT YOUR CARE

Use this form to record key facts about your care. Doctors may need this information to make future decisions about how to treat other illnesses or a recurrence of cancer. You can also use it as a reminder to get the follow-up care you need.

Cancer Treatment	Date	Hospital

Dose/Amount

Area(s) Treated

Complications

What to Watch For in the Future

Future Medical Tests Needed and When to Have Them

Cancer Treatment	Date	Hospital

Dose/Amount

Area(s) Treated

Complications

What to Watch For in the Future

Future Medical Tests Needed and When to Have Them

Source: National Cancer Institute

WORKSHEET 16.2
NOTES FROM VISITS TO YOUR DOCTORS

Keep a record of the questions you have about your care and the answers you receive. Date each entry for future reference.

Cancer Treatment	Date	Hospital

Cancer Treatment	Date	Hospital

Cancer Treatment	Date	Hospital

Cancer Treatment	Date	Hospital

Source: National Cancer Institute

GET THE SCOOP ON...
How and where to find good information on the
Internet ▪ The signs of a good Web site ▪
Finding support on the Internet

Using The Internet to Find Information And Support

Chapter 17

In cyberspace, there are scores of Web sites filled with useful information on breast cancer, cancer trials, and more. There are even thousands of women out there banded together in virtual support groups and newsgroups.

But if you're not careful, you can get sucked into a cancer quack's black hole. Many Web sites were developed by people with very little medical knowledge, but who speak like the pros. If you don't know much, it's easy to be swayed by their arguments. So the question is, how can you tell if the site that you're visiting contains valid information?

In this chapter, we'll tell you how to discriminate between sites that will inform you and sites that will misinform you. We'll also tell you about sites to see.

Sink or swim—how to surf the Net

Anyone in the world can open up shop on the Internet or World Wide Web. (Although the two terms are often used interchangeably, the Internet encompasses everything in cyberspace and the World Wide Web is the graphic component of the Internet.) All it takes is a few bucks (less than $100 a year) and perhaps a little programming skill. But even those who aren't computer savvy can fork over a few more dollars to pay someone to create an attractive Web site. Since there are no restrictions on who can open up shop, you have to be careful when you surf the Net. You have to learn how to "ride the waves," so to speak, and steer clear of the dangerous sites, especially when you're searching for information on a disease like breast cancer.

There are all sorts of medical sites on the Internet. Some are maintained by corporations, some by hospitals and medical schools, some by nonprofit organizations, and some by government agencies. Other sites are created by cancer survivors who simply want to share information, and some of those sites are top-notch. But there are also on-line entrepreneurs who engage in quackery, looking to sell their useless wares to those who don't know any better.

The problem is, most sites look professional. It's hard to discriminate the useful from the bogus.

Warning—the Internet can be harmful to your health

There's a lot of useful information on the Internet. But there's a lot of trash, too. Take time to consider the source of the material. Web sites posted and maintained by reputable U.S. medical schools, government agencies, professional medical associations, and major national disease-specific organizations can generally be trusted.

But watch out for sound-alike and authoritative sounding names. While the "American College of

Watch Out!
There is no magic answer on the Internet. A good doctor and a second opinion at a cancer center should answer 99 percent of your concerns, according to Lee Rosen, M.D., assistant professor of medicine and director of the Cancer Therapy Development Program at UCLA's Jonsson Cancer Center.

Surgeons" is a reputable organization, the "American College of _____ " may not be. Creating an authoritative-sounding name to attract visitors can be used as a strategy by those who aren't authorities on the subject or whose wares aren't proved by scientific testing.

Another trick is to get a Web address that closely resembles a reputable site's address. One spin is to change the last three letters of the address. For example, www.whitehouse.gov takes you to the White House's home page but www.whitehouse.com takes you to a sex site. A similar strategy—using an address similar to a reputable site but containing a common typographical error. For example, www.amazon.com goes to the well-known bookstore while www.amazone.com leads to a lesser known one.

Furthermore, even if you type in the right address, hackers can take over and catapult you into an entirely different one, though this rarely happens. Or, with the click of a button you might link to a Web site filled with unproven or false information. (Remember, they look authoritative.) Learn to tell when you've left your original Web site—look at the URL address. (The URL is the address beginning with *http://*). Learn to judge the validity of a site—consider the sponsors. If you are unfamiliar with the reputation of a specific organization, call a librarian or your doctor, and always discuss your search findings with your medical team.

In order to get more perspective on a too-good-to-be true claim, pick a key phrase or name and run it through a search engine to find other discussions of the topic, though you must take these discussions with a grain of salt since you don't know who's behind the posting. You can also post a query in a newsgroup, a

Moneysaver
If you don't have access to the Internet at home, you can access it free at public libraries as well as some restaurants and apartment complexes. Also many hospital libraries and office learning centers offer access.

virtual bulletin board, run a Medline search and, of course, ask your doctor.

Starting the search

If you don't know where to locate information on the Web, then you should start with a search engine. Today there are more than 50 search engines available. A few of the best-known search engines are:

- www.lycos.com

- www.excite.com

- www.yahoo.com

- www.infoseek.com

- www.hotbot.com

- www.altavista.com

- www.snap.com

- www.dogpile.com

- www.ask.com

- www.metacrawler.com

There are even search engines specific to certain industries. Some of the medicine-specific search engines are:

- www.achoo.com

- www.healthatoz.com

- www.medsitenavigator.com

There are two different kinds of search engines—indexes and directories. Directories are lists of Web sites that have been filtered by an editor or reviewer and placed into categories. Directories are more likely to point to relevant Web sites than an index, although this capability depends entirely on the quality of the reviewer. However, directories categorize only a fraction of documents available on the Web (a few hundred thousand at best). In addition,

Unofficially...
Cancer is the most frequently searched disease on the Internet, according to a Cyber Dialogue Survey in July 1998. Cancer was the number one search topic at Healthfinder.gov, the federal government's portal to health information links, according to the Department of Health and Human Services.

directories are often only aware of new sites when the site's author or administrator sends out a notice.

Indexes are large databases that contain keywords to the millions of Web pages on the Internet. These indexes contain software code, called "robots," that searches the Web for sites. The results of these searches are then placed into the search engine's database. When you enter keywords into this type of search engine, you are actually searching its database. But there is a drawback to this type of search. On average, they're only updated once a week or once a month, depending on the search engine.

You can use a directory the same way you use an index, searching by keywords, or you can click the mouse on a subject, such as "medicine" at Yahoo, then "oncology" (or "acupuncture" or "pain management") then "radiation oncology," and then you have a few sites from which to select. However, you'll often get more hits using a keyword search.

Each search engine has its own method of searching, which is why not all search engines come up with the same answers, and when search engines come up with the same "hits," they often aren't in the same order and are interspersed with additional sites. For example, using the keywords "breast cancer," one search engine returned 266 hits (sites containing the words "breast cancer") and another one had more than 167,000 hits. Making sure that the information is valid is harder than searching for the information.

Searching criteria

How do you navigate the seas in cyberspace? How do you know what to search for? The more specific you are when searching, the better your results will be. For example, if you are looking for information on

Timesaver
Ask your medical team what sites they use that have the information you're seeking. You can also ask librarians at public, hospital, and medical school libraries.

"breast cancer," you wouldn't want to search using just the word "cancer" because this will include many other forms of the disease.

Most, if not all, the search engines contain a help section to explain how they work. If you are having problems finding the information you want, read this section to see if you are inputting your query correctly. Remember, not all sites use the same criteria for inputting your requests. For example, if you enter the keywords "breast cancer," some search engines return hits that contain both words. However, other search engines return hits with one word or the other word or both. You can end up with some sites that may raise an eyebrow or two. Those search engines require you to place phrases in quotes ("breast cancer") if you want them to search for two or more words in a row. If you want to search for multiple words not necessarily in a row, you would connect them with "and." For example, "breast cancer and radiation." In addition, by being more specific in your search criteria, you will decrease the number of hits and increase your chances of finding the information that you need.

Because it gets difficult to remember each search engine's criteria many people find a couple of engines that they like and just stick with them.

Grading sites

Once you have found a site that has the information you need, how do you know if the information is current, reliable, and valid? An editorial by William M. Silberg, George D. Lundberg, M.D., and Robert A. Musacchio, Ph.D. published in The *Journal of the American Medical Association* (April 1997) suggested using the following guidelines:

- **Authorship**—Does the site list the authors and

contributors and their affiliations and relevant
credentials?

- **Attribution**—Are all references and sources for
  the content clearly listed and all relevant copy-
  right information noted?

- **Disclosure**—Is the Web site ownership promi-
  nently and fully disclosed, as well as any sponsorship, advertising, underwriting, commercial
  funding arrangements or support, and potential
  conflicts of interest?

- **Currency**—Are there dates to identify when the
  content was posted and updated?

There are other organizations trying, develop
standards for medical sites. The U.S. Food and Drug
Administration (FDA) currently regulates pharmaceutical advertising and promotion in the traditional
print and broadcast media. The FDA is, however, trying to figure out how to apply these regulations to the
Internet. The U.S. Department of Health and Human
Services (HHS) is also considering how to best promote quality in consumer health information networks, according to Mary Jo Deering, PhD, director,
Health Communication and Telehealth at HHS in
Washington, D.C.

The Health on the Net Foundation is a non-prof-
it organization in Geneva, Switzerland, whose mis-
sion is to build and support the international health
and medical community on the Internet and Web so
its potential benefits can be realized by health consumers and professionals. The Foundation suggests
medical Web sites adhere to the following eight prin-
ciples:

1. If medical/health advice is provided at the site,
   it should be given by health professionals unless
   clearly stated otherwise. In these cases, the indi-

vidual or organization giving medical or health advice must be highly qualified to do so.

2. The information provided at the site should be designed to support—not replace—the patient-physician relationship.

3. If the site requests information from visitors, that information should be kept strictly confidential. The site should have a disclosure saying what it will do with the information you provide. (Some sites may sell the information you provide to them.)

4. The site should provide references to information and data as well as html links to that data, where possible. The site should also post a date at the bottom of the page noting when a page containing clinical data was last updated.

5. If a claim is made about a specific treatment, commercial product, or service, it should be supported by balanced evidence including references and html links to that data, when possible.

6. The Web site designers should provide clear information and contact addresses for site visitors seeking further information or support. The Webmaster should display his/her e-mail address throughout the Web site.

7. Any financial support for the Web site should be clearly disclosed.

8. If the site is supported by any advertising, that information must be disclosed, along with a brief description of the site's advertising policy. Visitors must be able to tell the difference between the material created by the institution operating the site and advertising and other promotional material.

Deering suggests using consumer skepticism and asking yourself these questions:

- Is the Web site selling anything?

- Does the information conform with what you've seen elsewhere?

- Does the Web site link back to reputable sites?

- Did you find this Web site from a reputable site?

- What does the privacy statement say they will do with personal information you provide?

- Is there a disclaimer telling you to consult with your healthcare provider?

- Is there a disclosure from which to judge the credibility of the Web site?

Sites to see

There are some very useful general medical and oncology Web sites on the Internet. Here are a few good sites to visit:

- **The U.S. National Library of Medicine—www. nlm.nih.gov**—A part of the National Institutes of Health, this is the world's largest biomedical library. It offers free access to Medline, a database of abstracts and citations from peer-reviewed journal articles, publications, general information, news, and much more.

- **National Cancer Institute—www.nci.nih.gov**— This site contains information for patients, the public, health professionals, and the media, along with links to CancerNet, clinical trials lists, and current clinical trials.

- **The American Medical Association—www. amaassn.org**—This site contains a doctor finder—you can locate a specialist or check out a doctor's credentials. It also provides contact

Watch Out!
Because there are no set standards validating the accuracy of information on medical and health sites, you must be cautious. Be sure to talk to your doctor about *any* information you find on the Internet.

information. This site has links to the publications they produce, such as the *Journal of the American Medical Association.*

- **Medscape—www.medscape.com—**This is a commercial Web site for clinicians and health consumers. It contains a collection of searchable full-text, peer-reviewed articles. You can also search Medscape's database of full-text articles, DrugSearch, and more from this site. DrugSearch is a great tool to find out about medications, including any adverse reactions that have been reported and any drug-drug or drug-food adverse interactions that have been reported. Medscape also contains summaries of recent medical conferences.

- **Oncolink—www.oncolink.com—**This site is maintained by the University of Pennsylvania. It contains a wealth of information on many types of cancer, including causes, screening, prevention, personal experiences, and financial issues. By clicking on "Medical Specialty Oriented Menus" and then "Alternative Medicine," you will find a wealth of information on alternative therapies.

- **Massachusetts General Hospital's Cancer Resource Room—http://cancer.mgh.harvard. edu/resources—**This site has information on all aspects of cancer care. Most notably, it has treatment fact sheets on chemotherapy drugs and their early and late side effects as well as a fact sheet on diet modifications if you're taking steroids.

- **Massachusetts General Hospital's Treadwell Library Home Page—www.mgh.harvard.edu/ library/library.htm—**Click on "Consumer Health Information" to get to the Consumer Health

Watch Out!
Verify all drug information with your pharmacist. Editorial oversights occur and are part of the danger of using the Internet for finding medical information.

Reference Center and links to other health sites.

■ **American Association for Cancer Research—
www.aacr.org**—This site contains educational information, a public forum, links to journals, and
more.

■ **Cancer Cooperative Research Groups—http://
cancer.med. upenn.edu/resources/coop_groups**—
This Oncolink page has a listing of Cooperative
Research Groups.

■ **CancerGuide—http://cancerguide.org/tour.
html**—This site contains information and tips on
clinical trials, researching cancer, alternative medicine, and more from a patient's perspective.

■ **Cancer Research Institute—www.cancerresearch.
org/index.html**—This site provides information
about cancer and the immune system.

■ **Yahoo! Full coverage: Cancer Research—http://
headlines.yahoo.com/Full_Coverage/Tech/
Cancer_Research**—This page has links to recent
headlines in cancer research.

■ **Cancer Care, Inc.—www.cancercareinc.org**—This
is a comprehensive cancer site. It contains a page
on breast cancer and sexuality. It also contains
information on pain and fatigue as well as clinical
trials.

■ **Center for Alternative Medicine Research in
Cancer (University of Texas Houston Health
ScienceCenter)—http://chprd.sph.uth.tmc.
edu/utcam**—This site contains valuable information on alternative medicine, current investigations, and preliminary study findings.

■ **Healthfinder—www.healthfinder.gov**—This is
the federal government's consumer health portal. It contains selected links to Web pages creat-

ed by credible host institutions.

- **http://www.natlbcc.org**—The National Breast Cancer Coalition, a grassroots advocacy organization, offers Project LEAD, an educational and advocacy training program. This group is also active on Capitol Hill.

Cancer center Web sites are another good resource. Table 17.1 contains site addresses for those hospitals listed as the top 10 cancer Centers in 1998 by *U.S. News & World Report.*

TABLE 17.1: THE TOP 10 HOSPITALS IN THE NATION RANKED ACCORDING TO *U.S. NEWS & WORLD REPORT* (1998)

Cancer center sites are filled with useful information.

Cancer hospitals
1. Memorial Sloan-Kettering Cancer Center—www.mskcc.org
2. MD Anderson Cancer Center—www.mdanderson.org
3. Johns Hopkins Hospital—hopkins.med.jhu.edu
4. Mayo Clinic—www.mayo.edu
5. University of Washington Medical Center—www.washington.edu
6. Duke University Medical Center—www.mc.duke.edu
7. University of Chicago Hospitals—www-uch.uchicago.edu
8. Fox Chase Cancer Center—www.fccc.edu
9. University of Michigan Medical Center—www.med.umich.edu
10. Roswell Park Cancer Institute—rpci.med.buffalo.edu

While the general medical sites have information on breast cancer, there are also sites or pages on sites that are devoted solely to breast cancer, including the following:

- **Y-ME National Breast Cancer Organization**—**www.y-me.org**—This site provides health and support information to both men and women with breast cancer as well as toll-free crisis hotlines for both English and Spanish speakers.

- **National Alliance of Breast Cancer Organizations (NABCO)—www.nabco.org**—This site contains news updates, educational materials, information on clinical trials, and lists support group locations and phone numbers by state.

- **The Susan G. Komen Foundation—www.komen. org**—Sponsors of Race for the Cure®, the Foundation's Web site contains mostly advocacy information.

- **Doctor's Guide to Breast Cancer Information and Resources—www.pslgroup.com/Breastcancer. htm**—This site contains the latest medical news and information on breast cancer and breast cancer-related disorders and links to other breast cancer Web sites.

- **National Action Plan on Breast Cancer— www.napbc.org**—At this site, you can find information on breast cancer, clinical trials, and more.

- **American Cancer Society—www.cancer.org/ cancerinfo/res_home.asp?ct=5**—This page provides links to information about breast cancer.

- **INFO Breast Cancer—www.intranet.ca/~stancar/index.html**—This personal Web site contains a "Cyber Quilt." Each square tells another survivor's thoughts, feelings, suggestions, and comments.

Unofficially...
The Komen Race for the Cure®, a 5K run/walk, was held in almost 100 cities nationwide in 1999. Proceeds mostly fund local community programs related to breast health education, screening and treatment. Twenty-five percent of the proceeds fund national research efforts.

Other options to finding information

Besides Web pages, there are several other ways to find information on the Internet, including:

- E-mail
- Newsgroups
- Mailing lists
- Listservs

A quick word on netiquette

Before we get to interacting on the Web, first a quick primer on "Netiquette." For those of you making your maiden voyage into cyberspace, Netiquette is the informal code of conduct for sending messages. It's Web manners. Basic rules include the following:

- Be extra polite. Electronic messages have a way of seeming cold and impersonal and are easily interpreted in the wrong way.

- Do not overcapitalize. Using all capital letters is considered shouting. No one likes to be yelled at.

- Read old messages before posting new ones. Users who are new to a list or newsgroup should read messages for several days before taking part in a discussion. Read the archive of frequently asked questions for more tips.

E-mail

E-mail (electronic mail) is the simplest way to exchange information online and usually the first exposure most computer users, especially novices, have to the Internet.

E-mail is an easy-to-use, powerful communication tool that sends messages within seconds. In addition to text, you can send electronic files (including photos) and embed Web addresses (also known as hyperlinks) so that the recipient only has to click the colored link to go a Web site. You can also use e-mail to communicate with more than one person at a time by sending the same message to an entire group with one click of your mouse button.

A word of caution: When you send an e-mail message, you leave digital "bread crumbs" all over cyberspace. They can be picked up by "sniffers," people snooping to find out what you're doing. Chances are you're not being watched, but you should be cau-

Moneysaver
If you can't afford medication, hospital care, outpatient care, or nursing home care, visit The Institute at www.institute-dc.org. You can download free of charge the following publications: *Free and Low Cost Prescription Drugs*, *Free and Low Cost Hospital Care*, *Free and Low Cost Outpatient Care*, and *Free and Low Cost Nursing Home Care*.

tious when sharing sensitive or potentially embarrassing information, especially if you are sending those messages from work. Bosses and system administrators do snoop, and they have a legal right to do so. Some co-workers snoop, too. Furthermore, any e-mail message you send can be saved by the recipient.

Be wary of receiving attachments from people you do not know. They may contain viruses. Computer viruses are programs that infect your computer and can be executed and cause damage without your knowledge. Download and open an attachment only if you know what it is and who it is from. Have a virus scanner on your computer. Even friends and relatives can unintentionally send viruses through files.

Newsgroups

Newsgroups can be a good source of information. They are virtual bulletin boards open to anyone. In short, a newsgroup is an area where people ask and follow up on questions and talk about various topics, such as coping with an illness or medical news. Messages generally consist of plain text.

There are more than 15,000 newsgroups available on the Internet. Many of the online services like America Online and Compuserve also have their own message boards for members only.

How do you find a newsgroup? There are several Web sites devoted exclusively to newsgroups, including the following:

- **Deja News—www.dejanews.com**—A searchable database of newsgroup postings.

- **Reference.com—www.reference.com**—A searchable database of newsgroups and mailing lists.

- **Tile.Net/News www.tile.net/tile/news/med5. html**—A searchable database of newsgroups and mailing lists.

Watch Out!
Although it is a felony to open someone else's *snail mail* (the kind the postman delivers) without permission, it is legal for a system administrator to read a user's incoming and outgoing mail. If you must exchange sensitive information, consider encrypting it. Encryption codes the text, making it unreadable except to people who have the code to decrypt it. You can buy encryption software or download shareware programs from the Internet.

In addition, many online service providers and search engines provide ways for you to search for newsgroups. For example, on America Online, type in the keywords "Internet newsgroups" for information on how to find a newsgroup.

Many of the newsgroup sites also contain archives of recent postings to various newsgroups so you can go back and look at other messages. The more specific the focus of a newsgroup is, the more useful you'll likely find it. For example, the newsgroup "alt.cancer.breast." will more likely fit your needs than the group "alt.cancer."

All newsgroups are different. Some have thousands or millions of members, while others have only a few. The number of people who are members and how active they are will determine how many messages are posted a day or how many messages you will receive via e-mail (if you set up your access that way.) When you go to the newsgroup, you don't have to read each and every message. Just scroll through the subjects of the messages and read the ones that are of interest to you.

There are two different types of newsgroups:

■ Unmoderated

■ Moderated

Many newsgroups are unmoderated. That is, when you post a message, it will be sent to the newsgroup without someone reviewing it to determine if it is applicable or appropriate. As a result, some messages may contain irrelevant, rude, or commercial postings. If a group is moderated, then there is an administrator who screens the messages before they are posted onto the newsgroup.

There are seven major newsgroup categories:

1. **comp**—computer related

2. **misc**—miscellaneous

3. **rec**—recreation

4. **sci**—science

5. **soc**—social

6. **talk**—like talk radio

7. **alt**—set up using an alternative method

The categories are broken into subcategories. Some of the breast cancer newsgroups include:

- alt.cancer

- alt.cancer.breast

- news.sci.med.obgyn

- alt.support.cancer

- sci.med.diseases.cancer

- alt.support.cancer.breast

Mailing Lists/Listservs

Listservs are similar to newsgroups, but instead of being posted at a public location, the messages are delivered by e-mail to subscribers' computers. If you reply to a listing, then your response is sent to everyone who is a member of that list. (Sometimes people respond to each other personally.)

Mailing lists are designed to serve the needs of groups of people who want to exchange information on a common topic of interest. You can subscribe and unsubscribe to them at any time. These, like newsgroups, also come in moderated and unmoderated versions. The quality of the information probably will be better in a monitored list.

In order to be a part of a mailing list, you must apply by sending an e-mail message to the list owner. Note, however, some mailing lists have qualifications for membership, such as doctors practicing in a specific field.

Unofficially...
In good medical listservs, it is not uncommon for doctors, out of the goodness of their own hearts, to respond to patients' questions.

When you find a mailing list to which you'd like to subscribe, read the instructions for joining. They are usually pretty simple, such as typing "Subscribe" in the message section of an e-mail. Once you have signed up for a list, sometimes you'll receive an e-mail message asking you to confirm that you want to subscribe. This is just to ensure that the e-mail address that you typed in when registering is correct and that somebody didn't sign you up without your permission. That e-mail message should also contain information on how to unsubscribe if you want to stop receiving listserv postings.

Note: Some mailing lists give you the option of getting either a daily or weekly digest of the postings. If this option is available, the directions on how to sign up will be on the registration page.

You can find listservs at the following sites:

- **LISZT—www.liszt.com—**A directory of more than 90,000 mailing lists.

- **Reference.Com—www.reference.com—**A searchable database for newsgroups and mailing lists.

- **Tile.Net/News—www.tile.net/tile/news/med5. html—**A searchable database of newsgroups and mailing lists.

Breast cancer listservs include:

- **BMT-TALK—**This is a moderated discussion of bone marrow transplants.

- **BREAST-CANCER—**This is an unmoderated discussion list for issues relating to breast cancer.

- **CANCER-L—**Cancer-L is a support group.

- **CAREGIVERS—**This is an unmoderated discussion list for family and friends of cancer patients.

- **CaringKids—**For Kids Who Know Someone Who is Ill: This unmoderated list allows kids to share their thoughts, feelings, and experiences and establish friendships with other kids dealing with similar issues. While not moderated, the list is supervised by adult listowners.

- **CPCOS**—Cancer Patients Christian Online Support Group. A support group for Christians.

- **HOSPIC-L**—This list focuses on the general philosophy and approach to hospice care.

- **IBC**—Inflammatory Breast Cancer List. This list is a forum for friendly discussions about inflammatory breast cancer.

- **LT-SURVIVORS**—This discussion group focuses on the unique problems long-term survivors of cancer might have, such as challenges with insurance, employment, and emotions.

- **MaleBC**—This is an unmoderated discussion list for patients, family, friends, physicians, and researchers to discuss clinical and nonclinical issues regarding male breast cancer.

- **MOL-CANCER**—Consumer Discussion Group. This discussion group focuses on cancer treatment.

- **ONCONEWS**—This moderated list serves to broadcast oncology news.

To join any of these cancer groups, go to www. oncolink.com/forms/listserv.html for registration links.

Chatrooms

Chatrooms allow people around the world to "chat" with each other about a specific topic in "real time." That is, once you type and send the message, everyone in the chatroom can read it. These areas can be either a private room or a group room. Anyone can

Watch Out!
Newsgroups can be dangerous for children. You don't know what the messages may say and you don't know who's sending them. Be sure to supervise your children when they're on the Internet.

Watch Out!
Don't give out personal informa-tion in a chat-room. Anyone can hide behind a screen name.

enter group rooms and join in the conversation. Access to private rooms requires a password.

There are a wealth of chatrooms on the Web. To gain access to them, you will generally have to down-load software and install it on your computer. However, if your Internet service provider is provid-ing the chatroom, then you won't have to download any software to gain access to the conversation.

To locate a chatroom, enter the keywords "breast cancer chat room" into a search engine.

Medline

Medline is the electronic bibliography of the National Library of Medicine. It contains thousands of scientific journal article abstracts and citations from more than 3,800 journals. You can search Medline by keywords, authors, journal titles, and more. There are quite a few Web sites that offer free Medline access, including:

- **The National Library of Medicine—** http://igm.nlm.nih.gov

- **Medscape**—www.medscape.com

- **HealthGate**—www.healthgate.com

Note: Using the same search criteria at each of these sites will probably not return the same results because the sites update journal information at different times. Medline is usually updated every week by the National Library of Medicine. However, updates on some journals, those from foreign or smaller publications, take longer. And even though the site is updated frequently, it is still often months behind the actual publication dates. If you want current journal information, go directly to the publisher's Web site (some post full-text articles) or to the library.

Take note: Not all articles appearing in journals are cited on Medline. You can learn a lot from the correspondence and other sections. To read them, you must get a hard copy of the publication.

Just the facts

- The Internet is filled with valuable scientific information, but it is also speckled with quackery.

- You can distinguish a good site by authorship, attribution, disclosure, and its last update.

- Don't take advice from the Internet without first checking with your doctor.

- You can "talk" to others who are going through the same things you are through newsgroups, chatrooms, and listservs.

Bright Idea
Sometimes it's a good idea to learn about any medications you must take, including drug-drug and drug-food adverse interactions, possible side effects, and manufacturer information. One site containing drug information is Medscape (www.medscape. com). There you can search by drug name. This site includes study results. Be sure to verify what you find with a pharmacist.

Glossary

Antigen A protein, recognized as a foreign invader, which can induce an immune response.

Benign Not cancerous.

Biological therapy A treatment used to stimulate or restore the immune system's ability to fight infection and disease. Also called immunotherapy.

Biopsy The removal of a tissue sample, which is examined under a microscope to check for cancer cells.

Bone marrow transplantation Doctors replace marrow destroyed by high dose chemotherapy or radiation therapy. Reinfusion is done by a process similar to a blood transfusion. Also called BMT.

Cancer A term used for a collection of diseases in which abnormal cells divide uncontrolled.

Carcinogen A substance or agent that causes cancer.

Clinical trials Studies using human subjects.

Chemotherapy Anticancer drug treatment. Refers to a variety of drugs used to destroy cancerous tissue.

Colony-stimulating factors (CSF) Substances (granulocyte colony-stimulating factors (G-CSF) and granulocyte-macrophage colony-stimulating factors (GM-CSF) that stimulate the production of blood cells. This treatment may be used after chemotherapy or radiation therapy to help the blood-forming tissue recover from the effects of these cancer treatments.

CT or CAT scan Computerized x-ray photos. Also called computed tomography or computed axial tomography scan.

Estrogen A female sex hormone produced mainly by the ovaries and responsible for the development of the female secondary sex characteristics. During the menstruationit produces an environment to allow for fertilization and implantation of an egg and nutrition of an early embryo. Estrogen is used in oral contraceptives and hormone replacement therapy in postmenopausal women. Some breast tumors have receptors for estrogen and therefore are more susceptible to biological therapy.

Excisional biopsy The removal of the whole tumor for biopsy.

HER-2/neu and HER-2 Often used interchangeably to refer to the proto-oncogene HER-2/neu. This gene, present in normal breast cells, may cause cancer if overexpressed. HER-2 is the protein expressed by the HER-2 gene in normal breast cells that signals the cell to grow and divide. Overexpression of this protein is associated with the development of breast cancer. Also called C-erb B-2.

Hormone therapy A treatment that prevents hormone sensitive cancer cells from getting the hormones they need to grow.

Hormones Chemicals produced by glands in the body that control the actions of some cells and organs.

Immune system Cells and organs that defend the body against infection and disease.

Immunotherapy A type of cancer treatment that

helps a patient's immune system fight cancer. Also called biological therapy.

In vitro research Laboratory studies on a microscopic level.

Incisional biopsy The removal of only a sample of tissue for biopsy.

Lymph A fluid that carries cells that help fight infection and disease. Lymph travels through the lymphatic system.

Lymph nodes Small, bean-shaped organs located along the lymphatic system channels throughout the body. Cancer cells (and bacteria) that have entered the lymphatic system may be found in the lymph nodes. Also called lymph glands.

Lymphatic system The tissues and organs (bone marrow, spleen, thymus, and lymph nodes) that produce and store immune cells. Immune cells fight infection and disease. This system has channels that carry lymph.

Lymphocytes A class of white blood cells that are responsible, in part, for mounting an immune response. More specifically, B lymphocytes (B cells) produce tailor-made antibodies to bind antigens. T lymphocytes (T cells) help B cells manufacture antibodies and can directly kill cells that carry a specific antigen.

Malignant Cancerous.

Mammogram An x-ray of the breast.

Meta-analyses An analysis of a collection of research studies from peer-reviewed journal articles.

Metastasis The spread of cancer outside the primary site, in this case, the breast. The cells in the metastatic (secondary) tumor site are similar to those in the original (primary) tumor site, which is how the pathologist knows it is the spread of disease and not a new form of cancer.

Monoclonal antibodies Clones of human antibodies that target a single protein. The antibodies are isolated and cloned in the laboratory, grown and reinfused into the patient to stimulate an immune response. Monoclonal antibodies can be used alone or to deliver drugs, toxins, or radioactive material directly to the tumor cells.

Needle biopsy The removal of tissue or fluid with a needle for a biopsy. Also called needle aspiration.

Oncologist A doctor who is trained in the treatment of cancer.

Oncogene A gene that causes cancer.

Oncogenic Something that is capable of causing cancer.

Overexpression Overproduction of a protein molecule by a cell.

Pathologist A doctor who identifies diseases by studying cells and tissues under a microscope.

Peripheral stem cell support A method used to replace blood-forming stem cells destroyed by cancer treatment. Stem cells are formed in the bone marrow and circulate in the blood. In this process, stem cells are removed from the patient's blood before treatment and stored. The cells are reinfused into the patient after treatment in a process similar to a blood transfusion.

Progesterone A female sex hormone. It acts as an antagonist of estrogens. Some breast tumors have receptors for progesterone and therefore are more susceptible to biological therapy.

Radiation therapy A treatment using high-energy rays to kill or damage cancer cells. External radiation therapy uses a machine to aim high-energy rays at the cancer. With internal radiation, radioactive material is placed inside the body close to the tumor.

Remission   The disappearance of the signs (the tumor) and symptoms of cancer. Remission can be temporary or permanent.

Recurrence   The reappearance of the cancer.

Stage   The extent of the disease.

White blood cells   Immune cells that help the body fight infection and disease.

Resources

Helpful Web Sites

Breast Cancer Web sites

The Susan G. Komen Foundation

Web site: www.komen.org

Phone: 972/855-1600

Sponsors of Race for the Cure, the Foundation's Web site contains advocacy information.

Y-ME National Breast Cancer Organization, Inc.

Web site: www.y-me.org

Phone: 312/986-8338; 800/221-2141 (English); 800/986-9505 (Spanish)

E-mail: info@y-me.org

Provides information and support to anyone who has been touched by breast cancer. Holds a breast cancer phone support group for patients and survivors under age 40.

Doctor's Guide to Breast Cancer Information and Resources

Web site: www.pslgroup.com/Breastcancer.htm

This site contains the latest medical news and information on breast cancer and breast cancer-related disorders and contains links to other breast cancer Web sites.

INFO Breast Cancer
Web site: www.intranet.ca/~stancar/index.html
This Web site contains a "Cyber Quilt." Each square tells another survivor's thoughts, feelings, suggestions, and comments.

National Action Plan on Breast Cancer
Web site: www.napbc.org
At this site, you can find information on breast cancer, clinical trials, and more.

Living Beyond Breast Cancer
Web site: www.dvbiznet.com/lbbc
You can locate self-help groups at this site. You also can sign up to receive their newsletter and read past issues.

The National Breast Cancer Coalition
Web site: http://www.natlbcc.org
A grassroots organization involved in the fight against breast cancer. The site has legislative information and information on educational programs as well as breaking news.

UK Breast Cancer Awareness Campaign
Web site: www.easynet.co.uk/aware
This site has facts and figures on breast cancer and more.

Breast Cancer Updates
Web site: www.pgh.auhs.edu/bfisher
Comments and abstracts on breast cancer research by Bernard Fisher, M.D., scientific director, National Surgical Adjuvant Breast and Bowel Project (NSABP).

Breast Cancer Answers
Web site: www.medsch.wisc.edu/bca/bca.html

This site is sponsored by the University of Wisconsin Comprehensive Cancer Center (UWCCC) and provides current information from reliable sources on breast cancer research as well as prevention, detection, diagnosis, stage, and treatment.

Pathologia Paldion

Web site: http://www.erinet.com/fnadoc/index.htm
This site presents information on mammograms, biopsies, and the role of the pathologist as well as other important breast cancer-related information.

Family History of Breast & Ovarian cancer and Genetic Testing

Web site: www.familycancer.org
This site provides information on risk of hereditary breast cancer and genetic testing.

General medical and general oncology Web Sites

The U.S. National Library of Medicine

Web site: www.nlm.nih.gov
A part of the National Institutes of Health, this is the world's largest biomedical library. It offers free access to MEDLINE, a database or abstracts and citings from peer-reviewed journal articles, publications, general information, news, and much more.

National Cancer Institute

Web site: www.nci.nih.gov
This site contains information for patients, the public, health professionals, and the media, along with links to CancerNet and cancer Trials, which contains information on current clinical trials and news on clinical trials in progress.

The American Medical Association

Web site: www.ama-assn.org

This site contains a doctor finder—you can locate a specialist or check out a doctor's credentials. It also provides contact information. This site has links to the publications they produce, such as the *Journal of the American Medical Association.*

Medscape

Web site: www.medscape.com

This is a commercial Web site for clinicians and health consumers. It contains a collection of searchable full-text, peer-reviewed articles. You can also search Medscape's database of full-text articles, DrugSearch, and more from this site. DrugSearch is a great tool to find out about medications, including any adverse reactions that have been reported and any drug-drug adverse interactions or any drug-food adverse interactions.

Oncolink

Web site: www.oncolink.com

This site is maintained by the University of Pennsylvania. It contains a wealth of information about many types of cancer, including causes, screening, prevention, personal experiences, and financial issues.

Massachusetts General Hospital's Cancer Resource Room

Web site: http://cancer.mgh.harvard.edu/resources

This site has information on all aspects of cancer care. Most notably, it has treatment fact sheets that lists chemotherapy drugs and their early and late side effects as well as a fact sheet on diet modifications if you're taking steroids.

Massachusetts General Hospital's Treadwell Library

Web site: http://www.mgh.harvard.edu/library/library.htm

Click on "Consumer Health Information" to get to the Consumer Health Reference Center and links to other health sites.

Centers for Disease Control

Web site: www.cdc.gov

This site includes information on breast cancer-related projects.

American Association for Cancer Research

Web site: www.aacr.org

This site contains educational information, a public forum, links to journals, and more.

Cancer Cooperative Research Groups

Web site: http://cancer.med.upenn.edu/resources/coop_groups

This Oncolink page has a links to Cooperative Research Groups.

CancerGuide

Web site: http://cancerguide.org/tour.html

This site contains information and tips on clinical trials, researching cancer, alternative medicine, and more from a patient perspective.

Cancer Research Institute

Web site: www.cancerresearch.org/index.html

This site provides information about cancer and the immune system.

Yahoo! Full coverage: Cancer Research

Web site: http://headlines.yahoo.com/Full_Coverage/Tech/Cancer_Research

This page has links to recent headlines in cancer research.

Cancer Care, Inc.

Web site: www.cancercareinc.org

This is a comprehensive cancer site that includes a page on breast cancer and sexuality, information on pain and fatigue, and details of clinical trials.

Center for Alternative Medicine Research in Cancer (University of Texas-Houston Health Science Center)

Web site: www.sph.uth.tmc.edu/utcam

This site contains valuable information on what's currently being studied in alternative medicine.

Healthfinder

Web site: www.healthfinder.gov

This is the federal government's consumer health portal. It contains selected links to Web pages created by reputable, creditable host institutions. The sites are not reviewed for content validity by the federal government.

U.S. News & World Report "America's Best Hospitals"

Web site: www.usnews.com

Searchable by disease

THE TOP 10 CANCER CENTERS SELECTED BY *U.S. NEWS & WORLD REPORT* IN 1999

1. Memorial Sloan-Kettering Cancer Center—www.mskcc.org
2. MD Anderson Cancer Center—www.mdanderson.org
3. Johns Hopkins Hospital—hopkins.med.jhu.edu
4. Mayo Clinic—www.mayo.edu
5. University of Washington Medical Center—www.washington.edu
6. Duke University Medical Center—www.mc.duke.edu
7. University of Chicago Hospitals—www-uch.uchicago.edu
8. Fox Chase Cancer Center—www.fccc.edu
9. University of Michigan Medical Center—www.med.umich.edu
10. Roswell Park Cancer Institute—rpci.med.buffalo.edu

Organizations

American Cancer Society
1599 Clifton Road, NE.
Atlanta, GA 30329-4251
Phone: 404/320-3333; 800/ACS-2345
Web site: www.cancer.org
The site offers a variety of services to patients and
their families.

American Institute for Cancer Research
1759 R Street, NW.
Washington, DC 20009
Phone: 202/328-7744; 800/843-8114
E-mail: aicrweb@aicr.org
Web site: www.aicr.org
Provides information on cancer prevention through
diet and nutrition, including a toll-free nutrition hot-
line. It also has a pen-pal support network.

National Alliance of Breast Cancer Organizations
9 East 37th Street, 10th Floor
New York, NY 10016
Phone: 212/889-0606; 888/80-NABCO
E-mail: nabcoinfo@aol.com
Web site: www.nabco.org
Provides information about breast cancer, serves as an
advocate for the legislative concerns of breast cancer
patients and survivors, and maintains a list of phone
numbers for support groups organized by state.

National Coalition for Cancer Survivorship
1010 Wayne Avenue, Suite 505
Silver Spring, MD 20910
Phone: 301/650-8868; 888/650-9127
E-mail: info@cansearch.org
Web site: www.cansearch.org
A network of groups and individuals that offers

support and information and resources on cancer support, advocacy, and quality of life issues.

Sister Network
8787 Woodway Drive, Suite 4207
Houston, TX 77063
Phone: 713/781-0255
E-mail address: NATSIS4@aol.com
Web site: www.sistersnetworkinc.org
This site is a national, African-American, breast cancer survivors support group.

The Susan G. Komen Breast Cancer Foundation
5005 LBJ Freeway, Suite 370
Dallas, TX 75244
Phone: 972/855-1600
Sponsors of Race for the Cure, the Foundation's Web site contains advocacy information.

National Hospice Organization
1901 North Moore Street, Suite 901
Arlington, VA 22209
Phone: 703/243-5900; 800/658-8898
E-mail: drsnho@cais.com
Web site: www.nho.org
Provides hospice care and information about hospice care.

National Lymphedema Network
2211 Post Street, Suite 404
San Francisco, CA 94115-3427
Phone: 415/921-1306; 800/541-3259
E-mail: nln@lymphnet.org
Web site: www.lymphnet.org
Provides education, guidance, and a referral service to lymphedema treatment centers and health care professionals. The organization has a newsletter with medical updates, a list of support groups, and educa-

tional information. It also offers a pen-pal match up service.

The Wellness Community
10921 Reed Hartman Highway, Suite 215
Cincinnati, OH 45242
Phone: 513-794-1116; 888/793-WELL
E-mail: wellnessnational@fuse.net
Web site: www.brugold.com/wellness.html
Provides free psychological support to cancer patients and their families as well as support groups, stress reduction and cancer education workshops, nutrition guidance, exercise sessions, and social events.

Vital Options and "The Group Room" Cancer Radio Talk Show
P. O. Box 19233
Encino, CA 91416-9233
Phone: 818/508-5657; 800/GRP-ROOM
(Sundays, 4 p.m. to 6 p.m., EST)
E-mail: GrpRoom@aol.com
Web site: www.vitaloptions.org
Airs a weekly syndicated call-in cancer talk show on the Web.

Y-ME National Breast Cancer Organization, Inc.
212 West Van Buren Street
Chicago, IL 60607-3908
Phone: 312/986-8338;
800/221-2141 (English); 800/986-9505 (Spanish)
E-mail: info@y-me.org
Web site: www.y-me.org
Provides information and support to anyone who has been touched by breast cancer.

National Institutes of Health (NIH) information resources

The National Library of Medicine
8600 Rockville Pike
Bethesda, MD 20894
888/FIND-NLM; 301/594-5983
Web site: www.ncbi.nlm.nih.gov/PubMed
Interlibrary loans can be arranged through DOCLINE, an automated loan request and referral system. Information on and assistance with DOCLINE is available through the NLM at 888/FIND-NLM (888/346-3656) or 301/594-5983.

National Network of Libraries of Medicine
Phone: 800/338-7657
The National Network of Libraries of Medicine routes callers to regional medical libraries.

Combined Health Information Database
Web Site: http://chid.nih.gov
Produced by federal agencies, this Web site contains two cancer-related databases and more.

National Cancer Institute (NCI)
Phone: 800/4-CANCER
Web site: http://www.nci.nih.gov;
NCI's primary Web site, it contains information about the institute and its programs. Also includes news, upcoming events, educational materials, and publications for patients, the public, and the mass media on http://rex.nci.nih.gov. This site also contains information on cancer trials and epidemiological data.

CancerFax
Phone: 301/402-5874
NCI information about cancer treatment, screening, prevention, and supportive care.

Free Medline (an electronic database of journal abstracts and citations) access

The National Library of Medicine
Web site: http://igm.nlm.nih.gov

Medscape
Web site: www.medscape.com

HealthGate
Web site: www.healthgate.com

Medication information

Medscape
Web site: www.medscape.com
Search by drug name. This site includes study results, indications, food and drug interactions, and side effects.

Yahoo! Health
Web site: http://health.yahoo.com/health/drugs _ tree/medication_or_drug/
Search drugs by name. This site contains side effects, warnings, and what to do if you miss a dose.

Appearance tips

The American Cancer Society's "Look Good, Feel Better" program
Phone: 800/395-LOOK

Information on breast implants

NCI's Cancer Information Service (CIS)
Phone: 800/4-CANCER

The Food and Drug Administration (FDA)
Phone: 800/532-4440
The American Cancer Society (ACS)
Phone: 800/ACS-2345

Clinical trials

Clinical Trials and Insurance Coverage:
A Resource Guide
Web site: http://207.121.187.155/NCI_CANCER_
TRIALS/zones/TrialInfo/Deciding/insurance.html

Cancer Trials
Web site: http://cancertrials.nci.nih.gov
NCI's comprehensive information center on clinical
trials. It includes information on finding specific trials and research news.

CancerNet
Web site: http://cancernet.nci.nih.gov
Contains information from PDQ® about clinical tri-
als and CANCERLIT, where you can search literature.

Oncolink
Web site: www.oncolink.upenn.edu/clinical_trials
The University of Pennsylvania's OncoLink lists
cooperative cancer research group trials as well as
those open at the University of Pennsylvania. In addition, it has clinical trial news updates. This site also
has a feature to sign up for an moderated newsgroup
that alerts you to new trials.

UCSF Breast Care Center Clinical Trials
Web site: http://bcc-ct.his.ucsf.edu
The University of California at San Francisco Breast
Care Center Clinical Trials list.

Coalition of National Cancer Cooperative Group
Web site: http://bcc-ct.his.ucsf.edu

The Breast Cancer Answers California Clinical Trials Matching System

Web site: www.canceranswers.org/treat.htm

Site searches for breast cancer clinical trials in California to see if any are recruiting women with your medical history. You can also review the list of trials at the site.

CenterWatch

Web site: www.centerwatch.com

Clinical trials listing service. It also lists new FDA approvals and has a service that will notify you by e-mail when additional breast cancer (or metastatic bone cancer or brain cancer) trials are added to the site. In addition, it contains profiles of the centers conducting the research.

Clinical trials UK database

Web site: www.cto.mrc.ac.uk/ukcccr

A database of randomized clinical trials taking place in Great Britain.

CancerGuide

Web site: http://cancerguide.org/clinical_ trials.html

Information on clinical trials written from the perspective of a person with cancer.

Newly approved drugs

Web site: www.fda.gov/cder/ob

Part of the Food and Drug Administration's Web site, it allows you to access the FDA Electronic Orange Book, which lists newly approved drugs.

Trial buddy study

Contact: Allison C. Morrill, Ph.D.

New England Research Institutes

9 Galen Street

Watertown, MA 02172

Phone: 800/775-6374 x547; Fax: 617/926-8246

E-Mail: AllisonM@neri.org.

Web site: www.gis.net/~allisonm/gfx/buddies.html

Matches women considering participating in a trial with a buddy who has been through one.

DES Data

DES Cancer Network
514 10th Street N.W., Suite 400
Washington, DC 20004-1403
Phone: 800/DES-NET4, 202/628-6330
E-mail: DESNETWRK@aol.com
Web site: www.descancer.org.

DES Action USA
1615 Broadway, Suite 510
Oakland, CA 94612
Phone: 800/DES-9288, 510/465-4011
E-mail: desact@well.com
Web site: www.desaction.org.

The Registry for Research on Hormonal Transplacental Carcinogenesis (Clear Cell Cancer Registry)
University of Chicago
MC 2050
5841 South Maryland Avenue
Chicago, IL 60637
Phone: 773/702-6671
E-mail: registry@babies.bsd.uchicago.edu
Web site: http://bio-3.bsd.uchicago.edu/~obgyn/registry.html

Financial assistance

The Institute
Institute at Capitol Hill Office
611 Pennsylvania Ave., S.E., Suite 1010
Washington, D.C. 20003-4303
Web site: www.institute-dc.org
You can download free of charge or order a paper version (for a $5 fee) of *Free and Low Cost Prescription Drugs.* They also offer *Free and Low Cost Hospital Care, Free and Low Cost Nursing Home Care*, and *Free and Low Cost Outpatient Care.*

Cancer Care, Inc.
1180 Avenue of the Americas, Second Floor
New York, NY 10036
Phone: 212/302-2400; 800/813-HOPE
E-mail: info@cancercare.org
Web site: www.cancercare.org
Provides financial assistance for non-medical expenses, home visits by trained volunteers, referrals to community services, education, one-on-one counseling, and support groups. Services are free.

Patient Advocate Foundation
780 Pilot House Drive, Suite 100-C
Newport News, VA 23606
Phone: 800/532-5274, 757/873-6668
E-mail: patient@pinn.net
Web site: www.patientadvocate.org
Provides legal counseling to cancer patients and survivors on managed care, insurance, financial, and job discrimination issues as well as on debt crisis.

Medicare
Web site: www.medicare.gov

Medicaid
Web site: www.hcfa.gov/medicaid/mcaicnsm.htm

Social Security Administration and Medicare
Phone: 800/772-1213; TTY: 800/325-0778
Web site: www.ssa.gov/SSA_Home.html

Department of Veterans Affairs
Phone: 800/827-1000
Web site: www.va.gov/benefits.htm

Health Resources and Services Administration (HHS)
Phone: 800/638-0742
Web site: www.hrsa.dhhs.gov/osp/dfcr/obtain/consfaq.htm

Hospitals that receive Hill-Burton funds (construction funds from the federal government) are required by law to provide some services to people who cannot afford to pay for their hospitalization.

Checking legal rights

The Job Accommodation Network
West Virginia University
P.O. Box 6080
Morgantown, WV 26506-6080
Phone: 800/526-7234
Web site: http://janweb.icdi.wvu.edu

JAN provides information about job accommodations and employing people with disabilities. You can also find out information about the Americans With Disabilities Act at this site.

National Coalition of Cancer Survivorship
1010 Wayne Avenue, Suite 505
Silver Spring, MD 20910
Phone: 301/650-8868; 888/650-9127
E-mail: info@cansearch.org

Web site: www.cansearch.org
The National Coalition of Cancer Survivorship offers limited referrals to attorneys with experience solving on-the-job discrimination problems.

The Cancer Legal Resource Center
919 South Albany St.
Los Angeles CA 90015
Phone: 213/736-1455
E-mail: barbara.schwerin@lls.edu
Web site: www.lls.edu
This is a joint program of the Western Law Center for Disability Rights and Loyola Law School, can provide some legal direction.

"Cancer: Your Job, Insurance, and the Law"
This booklet is available free from the American Cancer Society at 800/ACS-2345.

Patient Advocate Foundation
780 Pilot House Drive, Suite 100-C
Newport News, VA 23606
Phone: 800/532-5274, 757/873-6668
E-mail: patient@pinn.net
Web site: www.patientadvocate.org
Provides legal counseling to cancer patients and survivors on managed care, insurance, financial, and job discrimination issues as well as debt crisis.

Additional contacts:
If you've been discriminated against, contact the organizations that enforce anti-discrimination laws: your state commission on discrimination; state affirmative action offices; U.S. Department of Health and Human Services, Office for Civil Rights; and U.S. Department of Labor, Office of Federal Contract Compliance, if your company contracts with the federal government.

Relationship concerns

Contact these groups for referrals to counselors:

American Association for Marriage and Family Therapy
1100 17th Street, NW
Washington, DC 20036
Phone: 202/452-0109

National Association of Social Workers
750 First Street, NE, Suite 700
Washington, DC 20020
Phone: 202/408-8600

American Association of Sex Educators, Counselors, and Therapists (ASECT)
435 North Michigan Avenue, Suite 1717
Chicago, IL 60611
Phone: 312/644-0828

Other sources

American Academy of Pain Medicine
4700 W. Lake Ave.
Glenview, IL 60025
Phone: 847/375-4731
Web site: www.painmed.org
Provides referrals to pain specialists.

National Cancer Institute, Cancer Information Hotline
Phone: 800/4-CANCER.
Cancer specialists answer questions about cancer. They'll also send you publications about cancer and copies of some scientific studies free of charge.

SMILE
Phone: 909/796-4112
SMILE computer software program devises a person-

alized humor profile and gives a humor "prescription" by telling patients what tools will work for them

ENCORE
YWCA
Office of Women's Health Initiative
624 Ninth Street, NW, Third Floor
Washington, DC 20001
Phone: 202/628-3636; 800/95E-PLUS
E-mail: Mcandreia@YWCA.org
Web site: www.ywca.org
A discussion and exercise program for women who have had breast cancer surgery.

National Association of Home Care
Phone: 202/547-7424

Kids Connected
Web site: www.kidskonnected.org
This Web site provides friendship and a support network for kids with parents who have been diagnosed with cancer.

National Association of Insurance Commissioners
Web site: www.naci.org
The Web site has links to the Web sites of most state regulators.

Recommended Reading List

Books

Breast Cancer Survival

Dr. Susan Love's Breast Book
Susan Love, MD
Price: $17.00
Paperback—627 pages (1995)
Perseus Press
ISBN: 020140835X

The Breast Cancer Survival Manual: A Step-by-Step Guide for the Woman with Newly Diagnosed Breast Cancer
John Link
Price: $15.95
Paperback—208 pages (1998)
Henry Holt & Company, Incorporated
ISBN: 0805055150

My Mother's Breast: Daughters Face Their Mothers' Cancer
Laurie Tarkan
Price: $14.95

Paperback—240 pages (1999)
Taylor Publishing Company
ISBN: 0878332278

***Spinning Straw into Gold: Your Emotional
Recovery from Breast Cancer***
Ronnie Kaye Designed by Chris Welch
Price: $11.00
Paperback—181 pages (1991)
Simon & Schuster, Inc.
ISBN: 0671701649

***Recovering from Breast Surgery: Exercises to
Strengthen Your Body and Relieve Pain***
Diana Stumm
Price: $11.95
Paperback—112 pages (1995)
Hunter House, Inc.
ISBN: 0897931807

General health

***A Different Kind of Health: Finding Well-Being
Despite Illness***
Blair Justice
Price: $22.00
Hardcover—310 pages (1998)
Peak Press
ISBN: 0960537643

***The Health Robbers: A Close Look at Quackery
in America***
Edited by Stephen Barrett MD and William T.
Jarvis, PhD, Foreword by Ann Landers
Price: $28.95
Hardcover—526 pages (1993)
Prometheus Books
ISBN: 0879758554

Complementary/integrative medicine

Spontaneous Healing: How to Discover and Enhance Your Body's Natural Ability to Maintain and Heal Itself
Andrew Weil
Price: $12.95
Paperback—309 pages (1996)
Ballantine Books (Trd Pap)
ISBN: 0449910644

8 Weeks to Optimum Health
Andrew Weil
Price: $13.95
Paperback—276 pages (1998)
Fawcett Books
ISBN: 0449000265

The Alternative Medicine Handbook: The Complete Reference Guide to Alternative and Complementary Therapies
Barrie R. Cassileth
Price: $19.95
Paperback—340 pages (1999)
W.W. Norton & Company
ISBN: 0393318168

Meditations for Enhancing Your Immune System: Strengthen Your Body's Ability to Heal
Bernie S. Siegel, MD
Audio
May 1992
Hay House, Inc.
ISBN: 1561700444

The Vitamin Pushers: How the "Health Food" Industry is Selling America A Bill of Goods
Stephen Barrett, MD, and Victor Herbert, MD
Price: $29.95
Hardcover—536 pages (1994)
Prometheus Books
ISBN: 0879759097

Laughter and medicine

Heart, Humor and Healing Quotes of Compassionate Comedy
Patty Wooten (Editor)
Price: $9.95
Paperback—294 pages (1994)
Commune-A-Key
ISBN: 1881394433

The Healing Power of Humor: Techniques for Getting Through Loss, Setbacks, Upsets, Disappointments, Difficulties, Trials, Tribulations, and All That
Allen Klein
Price: $11.95
Paperback—213 pages (1989)
J P Tarcher
ISBN: 0874775191

Don't Get Mad-Get Funny! Using Humor to Manage Stress: A Light-Hearted Approach to Stress Management
Leigh Anne Jasheway, Geoffrey M. Welles (Illustrator)
Price: $12.95
Paperback—128 pages (1996)
Whole Person Associates
ISBN: 1570251193

Gesundheit!: Bringing Good Health to You, the Medical System, and Society Through Physician Service, Complementary Therapies, Humor, and Joy
Patch Adams, Maureen Mylander (Contributor)
Price: $14.95
Paperback—227 pages (1998)
Healing Arts Press
ISBN: 089281781X

House Calls: How We Can All Heal the
World One Visit at a Time
Patch Adams (Introduction), Robin Williams,
Jerry Van Amerongen (Illustrator)
Price: $11.95
Paperback—159 pages (1998)
Robert D Reed
ISBN: 1885003188

Not Now...I'm Having a No Hair Day:
Humor & Healing for People With Cancer
Christine Clifford, Jack Lindstrom (Illustrator)
Price: $9.95
Paperback—110 pages (1996)
Pfeifer-Hamilton Publishing
ISBN: 1570251207

Journal articles—studies on use of alternative therapies

BR Cassileth, The social implications of questionable cancer therapies. *Cancer* 1989;63:1247-50.

BR Cassileth, EJ Lusk, TB Strouse, BJ Bodenheimer
Contemporary unorthodox treatments in cancer
medicine. *Annals of Internal Medicine* 1984;101:
105-12.

PD Cleary, Chiropractic use: A test of several hypotheses. *American Journal of Public Health* 1982; 72:
727-30.

DM Eisenberg, Advising patients who seek alternative medical therapies. *Annals of Internal Medicine* 1997;127:61-69.

DM Eisenberg, RB Davis, SL Ettner, S Appel,
S Wilkey, M Van Rompay, RC Kessler, Trends in
alternative medicine use in the United States,

1990-1997. *JAMA: The Journal of the American Medical Association* 1998;280:1569-1575.

JJ Kronenfeld, C Wasner, The use of unorthodox therapies and marginal practitioners. *Social Science and Medicine* 1982;16:1119-25.

WS Pearl, P Leo, WO Tsang, Use of Chinese therapies among Chinese patients seeking emergency department care. *Annals of Emergency Medicine* 1995;26:735-8.

U.S. Congress, Office of Technology Assessment. Unconventional cancer treatments. Washington, D.C. Government Printing Office, 1990 (OTA-H-405).

Booklets

The Cancer Information Service has booklets such as *What You Need To Know About Breast Cancer,* in addition to booklets on chemotherapy, radiation therapy, bone morrow transplants, dealing with pain, and more. These booklets are free. Call 800/4-CANCER.

Pending Legislation

Some women and their families become politically active as a result of breast cancer. In this appendix you'll find pending House and Senate bills from the National Cancer Institute (http://www.nci.nih.gov/legis/index.html.) Information in this database (cancer legislation) is changing constantly, so you should often check the web site for updates.

Breast cancer

H.C.R. 238, Resolution Authorizing Use of the Capitol Grounds for the National Race for the Cure

This concurrent resolution would authorize the use of the Capitol Grounds for a breast cancer survivors event sponsored by the National Race for the Cure. This resolution was introduced by Rep. Gerald Solomon (R-NY) on March 9, 1998, and referred to the House Committee on Transportation and Infrastructure. As of May 7, 1998, there are 4 co-sponsor of this resolution (3-D and 1-R).

S.Res. 198, Resolution Designating "National Breast Cancer Survivors' Day"

A resolution designating April 1, 1998, as "National

Breast Cancer Survivors' Day." This resolution was introduced by Sen. Connie Mack (R-FL) on March 18, 1998 and referred to the Senate Committee on the Judiciary. As of May 7, 1998, this resolution has 77 co-sponsors (36-D and 41-R).

Research

H.R. 1352, Consumer Involvement in Breast Cancer Research Act

This bill would amend the Public Health Service Act to provide, with respect to research on breast cancer, for the increased involvement of advocates in decision making at the National Cancer Institute. This bill was introduced by Rep. Nita Lowey (D-NY) on April 16, 1997 and was referred to the House Committee on Commerce. As of May 7, 1998 there are 13 co-sponsors (11-D, 2-R).

S. 67, Breast Cancer Research Extension Act of 1997

This bill would amend the Public Health Service Act to extend the program of research on breast cancer. This bill was introduced by Sen. Olympia Snowe (R-ME) on January 21, 1997 and was referred to the Senate Committee on Labor and Human Resources. As of May 8, 1998 there are 3 co-sponsor (1-D, 2-R).

S. 86, Breast Cancer Research Amendment of 1997

This bill would amend the Public Health Service Act to provide, with respect to research on breast cancer, for the increased involvement of advocates in decision making at the National Cancer Institute. On January 21, this bill was introduced by Sen. Olympia Snowe (R-ME). This bill was referred to the Senate Committee on Labor on Human Resources. As of May 7, 1998 there are 2 co-sponsors (1-D, 1-R).

S. Res. 85, Resolution Concerning Breast Cancer

This resolution expresses the sense of the Senate that an environment be encouraged where 1) the "family members and loved ones" of individuals affected by breast cancer should not be alone in their fight against the disease; and 2) everything possible is done to support both the individuals and their family through public awareness and education. This resolution was introduced by Sen. Judd Gregg (R-NH) on May 7, 1997, and was referred to the Senate Committee on Labor and Human Resources. As of May 7, 1998 there are 12 co-sponsors (4-D, 8-R).

Mammography

S. 999, (Untitled)

This bill would amend the Veterans Health Care Act of 1992 to require that screening mammograms be provided to women veterans in accordance with current recommendations of the American Cancer Society relating to the age of the recipient and frequency of screening. The bill was introduced on July 9, 1997 by Sen. Arlen Specter (R-PA) and referred to the Committee on Veterans Affairs. As of May 7, 1998. It has 2 co-sponsors, (1-D, 1-R).

S. 537/ H.R. 1289, Mammography Quality Standards Reauthorization Act

This bill amends Title III of the Public Health Service Act to revise and extend the mammography quality standards program administered by the FDA. The bill was introduced on Wednesday, April 9, 1997 by Sen. Barbara A. Mikulski (D-MD). The bill was passed by the Senate (by unanimous consent) on November 9, 1997 and referred to House Committee on Commerce. A companion bill, H.R.

1289, was introduced in the House by Rep. Nancy Johnson (R-CT) on April 10, 1997 and referred to the Committee on Commerce. As of May 7, 1998, it has 68 co-sponsors (44-D, 24-R).

H.R. 418, Breast Cancer Early Detection Act of 1997

This bill would amend Title XVIII of the Social Security Act to provide for coverage of annual screening mammography under part B of the Medicare Program for women age 65 or older. This bill was introduced by Rep. Carolyn Maloney (D-NY) on January 9, 1997, and referred to the House Committees on Commerce and Ways and Means. As of May 7, 1998, the bill has 114 co-sponsors (80-D, 33-R, and 1-I).

H.R. 421, Medicaid Mammography Coverage Act of 1997

This bill would amend Title XIX of the Social Security Act to require State Medicaid plans to provide coverage of screening mammography. This bill was introduced by Rep. Constance Morella (R-MD) on January 9, 1997, and the bill was referred to the House Committee on Commerce. As of May 7, 1998. It has 1 Democratic co-sponsor.

H.R. 617, Mammogram Availability Act of 1997

This bill would amend the Public Health Service Act and Employee Retirement Income Security Act (ERISA) of 1974 to require that group and individual health insurance coverage and group health plans provide coverage for annual screening mammography for women 40 years of age or older if the coverage or plans include coverage for diagnostic mammography. The bill was introduced on February 5, 1997, by Rep. Jerrold Nadler (D-NY) and referred to the House Committees on Education and the

Workforce, Committee on Commerce, and Committee on Ways and Means. As of May 7, 1998, it has 49 co-sponsors (42-D, 6-R and 1-I).

H.R. 760, Women's Preventive Health Care Act of 1997

The bill would amend the Public Health Service Act and the Employee Retirement Income Security Act (ERISA) of 1974 to require that group and individual health insurance coverage and group health plans provide coverage for screening mammography and pap smears. This bill was introduced by Rep. Jon Fox (R-PA) on February 13, 1997 and referred to the House Committees on Education and the Workforce and Commerce. As of May 7, 1998, there are 5 Democratic co-sponsors.

S. 90, Breast Cancer Screening Act of 1997

This bill would require studies and guidelines for breast cancer screening for women ages 40-49, and for other purposes. This bill was introduced by Sen. Olympia Snowe (R-ME) on January 21, 1997 and was referred to the Senate Committee on Labor and Human Resources. As of May 7, 1998, there are no co-sponsors.

S. 540, The Medicare Mammography Screening Expansion Act of 1997

This measure would amend title XVIII of the Social Security Act to provide annual screening mammography and waive co-insurance for screening mammography for women age 65 or older under the Medicare program. Introduced by Sen. Joseph Biden (D-DE) on April 9, 1997 and referred to the Committee on Finance. As of May 7, 1998, the bill has 4 Democratic co-sponsors.

S. 727, Public Health Service Act, Amendment; Employee Retirement Income Security Act of 1974, Amendment

This bill would amend the Public Health Service Act and Employee Retirement Income Security Act of 1974 to require that group and individual health insurance coverage and group health plans provide coverage for annual screening mammography for women 40 years of age or older if the coverage or plans include coverage for diagnostic mammography. This bill was introduced by Sen. Dianne Feinstein (D-CA) on May 8, 1997 and was referred to the Senate Committee on Finance. As of May 7, 1998, there are 8 co-sponsors (7-D, 1-R).

S.Res. 136, National Mammography Day

The resolution designates October 17, 1997, as "National Mammography Day." and requests that the President issue a proclamation calling upon the people of the United States to observe such day with appropriate programs and activities. This resolution was introduced on October 9, 1997 by Sen. Joseph R. Biden, Jr. (D-DE) and has 53 co-sponsors (27-D, 26-R). It was agreed to in the Senate by unanimous consent on the same day that it was introduced.

H.Res. 40, Resolution Concerning Guidelines for Breast Cancer Screening

This resolution expresses the sense of the House concerning the need for accurate guidelines for breast cancer screening for women between the ages of 40 and 49. This resolution was introduced by Rep. Edolphus Towns (D-NY) on February 5, 1997 and was referred to the House Committee on Commerce. As of May 7, 1998, the resolution has 33 cosponsors (32-D, 0-R, 1-I).

H.Res. 48, Resolution Regarding the Need for Studies and Guidelines for Mammography Screening

This resolution expresses the sense of the House of Representatives concerning the need for further studies and accurate guidelines regarding the use of mammograms and other technology to screen women between the ages of 40 and 49 for breast cancer. On February 11, 1997, this resolution was introduced by Rep. Jennifer Dunn (R-WA). This resolution was referred to the House Committee on Commerce. As of May 7, 1998, it has 47 co-sponsors (20-D, 27-R).

S.Res. 47, Resolution Concerning Guidelines for Breast Cancer Screening

This resolution expresses the sense of the Senate concerning the need for accurate guidelines for breast cancer screening for women between the ages of 40-49. On February 3, 1997, this resolution was introduced by Sen. Olympia Snowe (R-ME). As of May 7, 1998, there are 52 co-sponsors (38-D, 14-R).

Prevention

S. 1722, Women's Health Research and Prevention Amendments of 1998

This bill would amend the Public Health Service Act to revise and extend certain programs with respect to womens' health research and prevention activities at the National Institutes of Health and the Centers for Disease Control and Prevention. This bill was introduced by Sen. Bill Frist (R-TN) on March 6, 1998, and referred to the Senate Committee on Labor and Human Resources. As of May 7, 1998, this bill has 35 co-sponsors (12-D and 23-R).

H.R. 964, Unrestricted Marketing of Breast Self-Examination Pads, Provision

This bill would authorize the marketing of breast

self-examination pads without restriction. This bill was introduced by Rep. Richard Burr (R-NC) on March 6, 1997 and was referred to the House Committee on Commerce. As of May 7, 1998, there are 30 co-sponsors (8-D, 22-R).

Treatment

H.R. 616, Women's Health and Cancer Rights Act of 1997

This bill would require that health plans provide coverage for a minimum hospital stay for mastectomies and lymph node dissection for the treatment of breast cancer, coverage for reconstructive surgery following mastectomies, and coverage for secondary consultations. This bill was introduced by Rep. Susan Molinari (R-NY) on February 5, 1997 and referred to the House Committees on Education and the Workforce, the Committee on Commerce, and Committee on Ways and Means. As of May 7, 1998, there are 142 co-sponsors of this bill (84-D, 57-R and 1-I).

H.R. 135/S. 143, Breast Cancer Patient Protection Act of 1997

This bill would amend the Public Health Service Act and Employee Retirement Income Security Act of 1974 to require that group and individual health insurance coverage and group health plans provide coverage for a minimum hospital stay for mastectomies and lymph node dissections performed for the treatment of breast cancer. This bill was introduced by Rep. Rosa DeLauro (D-CT) on January 7, 1997 and referred to the House Committees on Education and the Workforce, and Commerce. As of May 7, 1998, there are 220 co-sponsors of this bill (196-D, 23-R and 1-I). A companion bill, S. 143, was introduced on January 21, 1997 by Sen. Thomas

Daschle (D-SD) and referred to the Committee on Labor and Human Resources. As of May 7, 1998, there are 22 Democratic co-sponsors of this bill.

H.R. 1374, Josephine Butler United States Health Service Act

This bill would establish a U.S. Health service to provide high quality comprehensive health care for all Americans and to overcome the deficiencies in the present system of health care delivery. As the measure relates to breast cancer, an area health board shall ensure before a mastectomy or other breast treatment that a women be provided with complete information about her options and the side effects of treatment. This bill was introduced by Rep. Ronald Dellums (D-CA) on April 17, 1997, and referred to the House Committees on the Budget, Commerce, Judiciary, and Ways and Means. As of May 7, 1998, there were no co-sponsors.

S. 249, Women's Health and Cancer Rights Act of 1997

This bill would require that health plans provide coverage for a minimum hospital stay for mastectomies and lymph node dissection for the treatment of breast cancer, coverage for reconstructive surgery following mastectomies, and coverage for secondary consultations. The bill was introduced by Sen. Alfonse D'Amato (R-NY) on January 30, 1997 and was referred to the Committee on Finance. As of May 7, 1998, there are 20 co-sponsors (11-D, 9-R).

Trust fund

H.R. 209, Taxpayers' Cancer Research Funding Act of 1997

This bill would amend the Internal Revenue Code of 1986 to establish and provide a checkoff for a breast and prostate cancer research fund, and for other purposes. This bill was introduced by Rep. Peter King (R-NY) on January 7, 1997 and referred to the House Committees on Commerce, and Ways and Means. As of May 7, 1998, there are 21 co-sponsors of this bill (11-D, 9-R and 1-I).

S. 726/H.R. 407, Breast Cancer Research Stamp Act

This bill would allow postal patrons to contribute to funding for breast cancer research through the voluntary purchase of certain specially issued U.S. postage stamps. On January 9, 1997, H.R. 407 was introduced by Rep. Vic Fazio (D-CA) and referred to the House Committees on Government Reform and Oversight and Committee on Commerce. As of May 7, 1998, there are 126 co-sponsors of this bill (96-D, 29-R and 1-I). The companion bill, S. 726, was introduced by Sen. Dianne Feinstein on May 8, 1997 and referred to the Committee on Government Affairs. The bill has 52 co-sponsors (32-D and 20-R).

H.R. 1585, Stamp Out Breast Cancer Act

This bill would allow postal patrons to contribute to funding for breast cancer research through the voluntary purchase of certain specially issued U.S. postage stamps. This bill was introduced by Rep. Susan Molinari (R-NY) on May 13, 1997, passed and signed into law by the President as Public Law 105-41 on August 13, 1997.

Research and environment

H.R. 832, Menopause Outreach, Research and Education Act of 1997

This bill would amend the PHS Act to provide for a program of research and education regarding menopause and related conditions. This bill was introduced by Rep. Clifford Stearns (R-FL) on February 25, 1997 and referred to the Committee on Commerce. As of May 7, 1998, it has 5 co-sponsors (5-D).

H.R. 1413/S. 631, New Jersey Women's Environmental Health Act

This bill would provide for expanded research concerning the environmental and genetic susceptibilities for breast cancer. This bill was introduced by Rep. Rodney Frelinghuysen (R-NJ) on April 23, 1997 and referred to the Committees on National Security and the Committee on Commerce. As of May 7, 1998, there are 8 co-sponsors (4-D, 4-R). A companion bill, S. 631, was introduced by Sen. Robert Torricelli (D-NJ) on April 23, 1997 and referred to the Senate Committee on Labor and Human Resources. As of May 7, 1998, it has 1 Democratic co-sponsor.

Further information

To review past legislation, or to check on recent developments, including the newest legislation, go to thomas.loc.gov or www.nci.nih.gov/legis.

If you want to write your congressperson or senator, you can find their e-mail address at either www.house.gov or www.senate.gov or call the Capitol at 202/224-3121.

Current Studies

NIH trials

To search for NIH research studies, go to cancernet. nci.nih.gov/prot/patsrch.shtml, the National Cancer Institute's search page for trials. Choose *Breast Cancer* and any other option to get a list of ongoing trials. Recent postings are listed in this appendix. Information in this data base (Cancernet) is changing constantly, so you should often check the web site for updates.

Dietary Intervention in Treating Women at High Risk for Breast Cancer (Ids: WSU-H-018296, NCI-P97-0123)

Diet And Estrogen Metabolism in Postmenopausal Women (Ids: UCLA-HSPC-950942302, NCI-P97-0112)

Doxorubicin in Treating Women with Advanced Breast Cancer (Ids: CRC-PHASE-II-PH2/038, EU-97028)

Diagnostic Study to Identify Sentinel Lymph Nodes in Patients with Stage I or Stage II Breast Cancer (Ids: FRE-FNCLCC-96008, EU-98055)

Exercise During Adjuvant Therapy in Women with Stage I or Stage II Breast Cancer (Ids: CAN-OTT-9605, NCI-V96-1084)

Pyrazoloacridine in Treating Women With Metastatic Breast Cancer (Ids: WSU-C-1148-93, NCI-T94-0003H)

Bryostatin 1 in Treating Patients with Stage IV Breast Cancer (Ids: UCHSC-97751, NCI-T97-0063)

Gossypol in Treating Women With Refractory Breast Cancer (Ids: MSKCC-95037, NCI-V95-0761)

Perillyl Alcohol in Treating Patients with Metastatic Breast Cancer (Ids: WCCC-CO-9611, NCI-T97-0068)

Prolonged Tamoxifen in Treating Patients Who Have Breast Cancer (Ids: UKCCCR-ATLAS, EU-96064)

Radiolabeled Tracer in Treating Patients With Breast Cancer (Ids: UCLA-HSPC-960629301, NCI-G97-1249)

Edatrexate Plus Paclitaxel in Treating Patients With Metastatic Breast Cancer (Ids: MSKCC-98026, NCI-G98-1447)

Gemcitabine in Treating Women with Metastatic Breast Cancer Previously Treated with Doxorubicin and Paclitaxel (Ids: MSKCC-98030, NCI-G98-1474)

Tamoxifen for the Prevention of Breast Cancer in Healthy Women (Ids: CNR-9508, EU-95026)

Eflornithine in Treating Patients with Breast Dysplasia (Ids: KUMC-HSC-6916-96, NCI-P97-0080)

Tamoxifen in Treating Women with Breast Cancer (Ids: CRC-TU-ATTOM, EU-98042)

Photodynamic Therapy in Treating Patients with Metastatic Breast Cancer (Ids: RPCI-DS-94-15, NCI-V97-1197)

Low-Fat Diet, Fish Oil, and Soy Supplements in Treating Women with Breast Cancer (Ids: UCLA-HSPC-9508339, NCI-V96-0940)

Pet Scans in Detecting the Extent of Cancer in Patients with Stage II, Stage III, Stage IV, Or Recurrent Breast Cancer (ID: NCI-94-C-0151)

Radiation Therapy after Surgery in Treating Patients with Phyllodes Tumor of the Breast (Ids: DMS-9801, NCI-V98-1442)

Docetaxel Combined with Estramustine in Patients with Metastatic Breast Cancer (Ids: CPMC-IRB-7929, NCI-V97-1325)

Pet Scans in Patients with Locally Advanced Breast Cancer (Ids: MSKCC-97046, NCI-G97-1308)

Antineoplaston Therapy in Treating Women with Stage IV Breast Cancer (ID: BRI-BR-12)

Antineoplaston Therapy in Treating Women with Advanced Breast Cancer (ID: BRI-BR-14)

Perillyl Alcohol in Treating Women with or without a History Of Breast Cancer (Ids: CCF-IRB-1193D, NCI-P97-0089)

Gene Therapy Plus Chemotherapy in Treating Patients with Breast Cancer (Ids: FCCC-97009, NCI-T97-0042)

Paclitaxel Plus Carboplatin in Treating Patients with Metastatic Breast Cancer (Ids: SUNY-HSC-2493, NCI-V97-1254)

Phase I Study of Recombinant Vaccinia Virus that Expresses DF3/MUC1 in Patients with Metastatic Breast Cancer (Ids: DFCI-97050, NCI-T98-0057)

Surgery with or without Lymph Node Removal in Treating Elderly Women with Stage I Breast Cancer (Ids: CNR-9502, EU-95020)

Tamoxifen for the Prevention of Breast Cancer in High-Risk Women (Ids: UKCCCR-IBIS, EU-94041)

Tamoxifen, Radiation Therapy, or No Further Therapy Following Surgery in Treating Patients with Node-Negative Breast Cancer (Ids: GER-ARO/AGO-GBSG-V, EU-93007)

Immunotherapy After Surgery in Treating Patients with Recurrent Breast Cancer, Colon Cancer, or Melanoma (ID: ARG-CO/BR-1)

Methotrexate with or without Antineoplaston Therapy in Treating Postmenopausal Women with Advanced Refractory Breast Cancer (ID: BRI-BR-10)

Gene Therapy with Autologous Tumor Cell Vaccine in Treating Patients with Advanced Breast Cancer (Ids: DUMC-93122, NCI-H96-1111)

Paclitaxel with or without Psc 833 in Treating Patients with Metastatic Breast Cancer (Ids: CHNMC-96002, NCI-H97-1137)

Interleukin-12 in Treating Women with Metastatic Breast Cancer Who Have Received High-Dose Chemotherapy and Peripheral Stem Cell Transplantation (Ids: BIH-L97-0252, NCI-T98-0002)

Monoclonal Antibody Therapy Plus Paclitaxel in Treating Women with Metastatic Breast Cancer (Ids: MSKCC-95086, NCI-V96-0832)

Raloxifene in Preventing Breast Cancer in Premenopausal Women (Ids: NCI-98-C-0123, MB-402)

Photodynamic Therapy in Treating Women with Recurrent Breast Cancer That Has Not Responded to Previous Radiation Therapy (Ids: PCI-P125-9702, NCI-V97-1314)

Chemotherapy in Treating Women with Previously Treated Metastatic Breast Cancer (ID: E-3197)

PSC 833 Plus Doxorubicin in Treating Patients with Metastatic Breast Cancer (Ids: MAYO-943001, NCI-V96-1077)

Hormone Therapy in Treating Women with Breast Cancer (Ids: MSKCC-98038, NCI-G98-1451, LILLY-H4Z-MC-JWWD)

Vaccine Therapy in Treating Women with Metastatic Breast Cancer (Ids: BIOMIRA-Stn-BR-104, NCI-V98-1489)

Epirubicin Alone or with Vinorelbine in Treating Patients With Advanced Breast Cancer (Ids: DAN-DBCG-94-03, EU-95008)

Venlafaxine In Treating Hot Flashes In Women Who Have Had Breast Cancer (Ids: NCCTG-979254, NCI-P98-0135)

Paclitaxel Plus Monoclonal Antibody Therapy In Treating Women With Recurrent Or Metastatic Breast Cancer (Ids: MSKCC-98028, NCI-G98-1473)

Immunotherapy In Treating Patients With Metastatic Breast Cancer (Ids: DUMC-97148, NCI-G98-1455)

MRI To Detect Breast Tumors In Women (ID: UPCC-ACR-6883)

Exemestane Compared With Tamoxifen In Treating Postmenopausal Women With Primary Breast Cancer (ID: EORTC-10967)

Ovarian Suppression In Treating Premenopausal Women Receiving Adjuvant Chemotherapy For Poor-Prognosis Nonmetastatic Breast Cancer (Ids: FRE-FNCLCC-9456, NCI-F94-0023)

Aminocamptothecin In Treating Patients With Advanced Or Recurrent Breast Cancer (Ids: UCCRC-9024, NCI-T97-0012)

Chemoprevention Therapy Plus Surgery In Treating Patients With Breast Cancer (Ids: MDA-ID-94029, NCI-P97-0113)

Combination Chemotherapy Compared With Mitoxantrone In Treating Older Patients With Advanced Breast Cancer (Ids: DUT-KWF-CKVO-9008, EU-92006)

Flavopiridol In Treating Patients With Refractory Cancer (Ids: NCI-97-C-0171C, NCI-T97-0064, NCI-97-C-0171B)

Combination Chemotherapy In Treating Patients With Recurrent Breast Cancer (Ids: CAN-OTT-9402, NCI-V94-0565)

Drug Resistance Inhibition In Patients With Recurrent Or Metastatic Breast Cancer (ID: E-1195)

Vaccine Therapy Plus QS21 In Treating Women With Breast Cancer Who Have No Evidence Of Disease (Ids: MSKCC-97123, NCI-H98-0015)

Paclitaxel With Low-Dose Fluorouracil In Treating Women With Metastatic Breast Cancer (Ids: URCC-U3196, NCI-G98-1441)

ICI 182780 Compared With Anastrozole In Treating Postmenopausal Women With Advanced Breast Cancer (Ids: RPCI-DS-97-29, NCI-G98-1412, ZENECA-9238IL/0021, ZENECA-RPCI-DS-97-29)

Pyrazoloacridine In Treating Patients With Metastatic Breast Cancer (Ids: OSU-9712, NCI-T96-0120)

Combination Chemotherapy In Treating Women With Metastatic Breast Cancer That Overexpresses Her-2 (ID: NCCTG-983252)

Vaccine Therapy In Treating Patients With Metastatic Breast Or Gastrointestinal Cancer (Ids: LAC-USC-OI972, NCI-T97-0061, LAC-USC-OC972)

Antibody Therapy In Treating Patients With Advanced Cancer That Expresses The Her2/Neu Antigen (Ids: NCI-95-C-0023L, NCI-MB-360, MDX-NCI-95-C-0023L)

Mitoxantrone Compared With Combination Chemotherapy In Treating Women With Good-Risk Metastatic Breast Cancer (Ids: GER-AIO-02/92, EU-93010)

Vaccine Therapy Following Dose-Intensive Chemotherapy In Treating Patients With Breast Cancer (Ids: NCI-95-C-0146D, NCI-T95-0021N, NCI-MB-374)

Phase I Randomized Study Of Vinorelbine Combined With Chronomodulated Fluorouracil In Previously Treated Women With Metastatic Breast Cancer (ID: EORTC-05971)

Vaccine Therapy In Treating Women With Metastatic Breast Cancer (Ids: PPMC-IRB-94-78, NCI-V98-

1379, OCC-ONC-9408-L)

Vaccination Therapy In Treating Patients With Previously Treated Breast Cancer (Ids: MSKCC-94130, NCI-H95-0628)

Evaluation Of Drug Resistance In Patients With Metastatic Breast Cancer (Ids: ONCOTECH-OTBR01, NCI-V98-1391, UCIRVINE-97-02)

Mitoxantrone Compared With Combination Chemotherapy In Treating Women With Metastatic Breast Cancer (Ids: GER-AIO-01/92, EU-93011)

Combination Chemotherapy In Treating Women With Breast Cancer (Ids: SCTN-BR9809, EU-98053)

Peripheral Stem Cell Transplantation In Patients With Advanced Breast Cancer Treated With High-Dose Chemotherapy (Ids: MCV-CCHR-9505-2S, NCI-G97-1326, BAXTER-302103, BAXTER-MCV-CCHR-9505-2S)

Docetaxel And Epirubicin With And Without G-CSF In Treating Patients With Metastatic Breast Cancer (Ids: CAN-NCIC-MA15, NCI-V96-1063)

Doxorubicin And Paclitaxel In Treating Patients With Locally Advanced Breast Cancer (Ids: GUMC-97018, NCI-V97-1276)

High-Dose Megestrol In Treating Patients With Metastatic Breast Cancer, Endometrial Cancer, Or Mesothelioma (Ids: SVMC-V89-0296, NCI-V89-0296)

Radiation Therapy Plus Paclitaxel In Treating Patients With Stage IIb Or III Breast Cancer (Ids: LAC-USC-1B972, NCI-G97-1304)

Her-2/Neu Vaccine With Adjuvant GM-CSF In Treating Patients With Stage III Or Stage IV Breast Or Ovarian Cancer (Ids: UW-100.1, NCI-V97-1259)

Adjuvant High-Dose, Sequential Chemotherapy In Treating Patients With Resected Breast Cancer (Ids: YALE-HIC-7374, NCI-V95-0720)

Pain Control In Patients With Recurrent Or
Metastatic Breast Or Prostate Cancer
(Ids: E-3Z93, NCI-P95-0068)

Adjuvant Combination Chemotherapy In Treating
Women With High-Risk Breast Cancer
(Ids: FRE-GFEA-09, EU-96015)

Chemotherapy And Radiation Therapy In Treating
Women With Stage I Or II Breast Cancer
(ID: NCCTG-953251)

Epirubicin And Cyclophosphamide Compared With
Epirubicin And Paclitaxel In Treating Women
With Metastatic Breast Cancer (Ids: MRC-
UKCCCR-AB01, EU-97002)

Combination Chemotherapy With Or Without
Epirubicin In Treating Women With Stage I Or
Stage II Breast Cancer (Ids: CRC-TU-NEAT, EU-
98041)

Irinotecan In Treating Patients With Metastatic
Breast Cancer (ID: NCCTG-963255)

Dolastatin 10 In Treating Patients With Metastatic
Breast Cancer (ID: NCCTG-983251)

Etoposide And Paclitaxel In Patients With Refractory
Metastatic Breast Cancer (ID: NCCTG-963254)

Lmb-9 In Treating Patients With Advanced Cancers
(Ids: NCI-98-C-0078A, NCI-T98-0005, NCI-MB-
400)

Chemotherapy In Treating Premenopausal Or
Perimenopausal Women With Node-Negative
Breast Cancer (Ids: IBCSG-VIII, NCI-F90-0001)

Combination Chemotherapy And Bone Marrow
Transplantation In Treating Women With
Metastatic Breast Cancer (Ids: JHOC-97101004,
NCI-G98-1404, J-9737)

Combination Chemotherapy In Treating Patients
With Advanced Breast Cancer (Ids: CHNMC-
IRB-93040, NCI-H96-1053)

Peripheral Stem Cell Transplantation, Busulfan, And
Cyclophosphamide In Treating Patients With

Metastatic, Recurrent, Or Refractory Breast Cancer (Ids: FHCRC-1213.00, NCI-G97-1332)

Chemotherapy Following Surgery In Treating Women With Early Stage Breast Cancer (Ids: SCTN-BR9601, EU-97013)

Identification Of Genes Associated With Cancer In Patients And Siblings Who Have Cancer (ID: E-1Y97)

Idoxifene Compared With Tamoxifen In Treating Postmenopausal Women With Metastatic Breast Cancer (Ids: SB-223030/010, NCI-V98-1383)

Vx-710 Plus Paclitaxel In Treating Women With Metastatic Or Locally Advanced Breast Cancer That Has Not Responded To Paclitaxel (Ids: VX-96-710-004, NCI-V97-1200)

Addition Of Paclitaxel To High-Dose Combination Chemotherapy In Treating Patients With High-Risk Breast Cancer (Ids: SLUMC-8038, NCI-V95-0607)

Addition Of Paclitaxel To High-Dose Combination Chemotherapy In Treating Women With Metastatic Breast Cancer (Ids: SLUMC-7915, NCI-V95-0608)

Gemcitabine And Cisplatin In Treating Patients With Metastatic Breast Cancer (ID: NCCTG-963251)

Vaccine Therapy With Or Without GM-CSF In Treating Patients With Recurrent Or Refractory Cancer (Ids: FCCC-97010, NCI-T97-0044)

Carcinoembryonic Antigen Peptide-1 In Patients With Metastatic Cancer (Ids: DUMC-96024, NCI-H96-1110)

Bispecific Antibody MDX-H210 Plus Interferon Gamma In Treating Patients With Metastatic Cancers Expressing The Her2/Neu Antigen (Ids: MDX-DMS-9318, NCI-V94-0450)

Vaccination Therapy In Patients With Cancer Of The Gastrointestinal Tract, Breast, And Lung (Ids: NCI-96-C-0139, NCI-T96-0058N, NCI-NMOB-9305)

High-Dose Combination Chemotherapy And
   Peripheral Stem Cell Transplantation In
   Treating Patients With Breast Cancer (Ids: MDA-
   DM-95156, NCI-V96-1017)

Breast Surgery With Or Without Lymph Node
   Removal In Elderly Women (Ids: IBCSG-10-93,
   NCI-F93-0008, EU-93013)

Tamoxifen And Radiation Therapy In Treating
   Patients With Early Stage Breast Cancer
   (Ids: UKCCCR-DCIS, CRC-PHASE-III-90001)

High-Dose Combination Chemotherapy Followed By
   Peripheral Stem Cell Transplantation In
   Treating Patients With Poor-Prognosis Breast
   Cancer (Ids: TUHSC-1992, NCI-V92-0205)

Tamoxifen With Or Without Combination
   Chemotherapy In Treating Postmenopausal
   Women With Operable Invasive Breast Cancer
   (Ids: SCTN-BR9402, EU-94003, UKCCCR-
   ABC/BR9402)

Tamoxifen Following Combination Chemotherapy
   In Treating Women With Operable Invasive
   Breast Cancer (Ids: SCTN-BR9403, EU-94004)

Vaccine Therapy In Treating Patients With Solid
   Tumors (Ids: MUSC-6124, NCI-T95-0044)

Combination Chemotherapy In Treating Patients
   With Stage III Breast Cancer (Ids: GOCS-08-BR-
   95-III, NCI-F95-0036)

Chemotherapy In Treating Patients With Advanced
   Cancer (Ids: NCI-94-C-0119I, NCI-T93-0123N,
   NCI-MB-330)

Peripheral Stem Cell Transplantation In Treating
   Patients With Advanced Breast Cancer (Ids: UIC-
   95-1011, NCI-V94-0573, LUMC-6728)

Interleukin-2 In Treating Patients With Hematologic
   Cancer Or Solid Tumors Who Have Received
   Stem Cell Transplantation (Ids: RPCI-DS-94-42,
   NCI-G98-1369)

Combination Chemotherapy Followed By Peripheral
   Stem Cell Transplantation In Treating Patients

With High-Risk Breast Cancer (Ids: CHNMC-IRB-95051, NCI-V96-1054)

Bone Marrow Or Peripheral Stem Cell Transplantation In Treating Patients With Breast Cancer (Ids: CCCWFU-95496, NCI-G97-1145)

Evaluation Of Breast Cancer Recurrence Rates Following Surgery For Ductal Carcinoma In Situ (ID: E-5194)

Sequential High-Dose Chemotherapy And Stem Cell Transplantation In Treating Patients With Chemotherapy-Sensitive Metastatic Breast Cancer (Ids: YALE-HIC-7372, NCI-V95-0721)

Surgery Plus Radiation Therapy In Treating Patients With Paget's Disease Of The Nipple Associated With In Situ Ductal Breast Cancer (ID: EORTC-10873)

Adjuvant Hormone Therapy In Treating Women With Operable Breast Cancer (Ids: CRC-PHASE-III-88002, UKM-CRC-BR-UNDER 50)

High-Dose Chemotherapy And Autologous Blood Cell Transplantation In Treating Patients With Primary, Locally Advanced, Or Stage IV Breast Cancer (Ids: UARIZ-HSC-9728, NCI-V97-1329, ALZA-UARIZ-HSC-9728)

Biological Therapy In Treating Patients With Metastatic Breast Cancer (Ids: STLMC-BRM-9503, NCI-V96-0902)

Paclitaxel In Treating Women With Metastatic Breast Cancer (Ids: THERADEX-B97-1250, NCI-V97-1365, BMS-TAX/MEN.01)

Dalteparin In Treating Patients With Advanced Breast, Lung, Colorectal, Or Prostate Cancer (Ids: NCCTG-979251, NCI-P98-0139)

Pain Control In Metastatic Breast Cancer, Non-Small Cell Lung Cancer, And Multiple Myeloma (Ids: E-4Z93, NCI-P93-0051)

Tamoxifen Compared With No Further Treatment Following Chemotherapy In Treating Women With Stage I Or Stage II Breast Cancer (ID: EORTC-10901)

Exemestane Compared With Tamoxifen In Treating Women With Locally Recurrent Or Metastatic Breast Cancer (Ids: EORTC-10951, PHARMACIA-EORTC-10951)

Vaccine Therapy In Treating Patients With Advanced Cancers (Ids: SVMC-ONC-222, NCI-V91-0075)

Standard Chemotherapy Compared With High-Dose Chemotherapy Plus Peripheral Stem Cell Transplant In Treating Women With Advanced Or Inflammatory Breast Cancer (Ids: SCTN-BR9810, EU-98054)

Chemotherapy In Treating Women With Advanced Breast Cancer (Ids: PHARMACIA-088050, NCI-V96-0828)

Tamoxifen, Ovarian Ablation, And/Or Chemotherapy In Treating Women With Stage I, Stage II, Or Stage IIIa Breast Cancer (Ids: UKCCCR-ABC, EU-94029, CRC-TU-BR3010)

Combination Chemotherapy In Treating Women Who Have Nonmetastatic Breast Cancer With Lymph Node Involvement (Ids: FRE-FNCLCC-PACS-01, EU-98044)

Chemotherapy And Stem Cell Transplantation In Treating Patients With Stage IIIb Breast Cancer (Ids: CHNMC-96139, NCI-G97-1288)

Amifostine Followed By High-Dose Chemotherapy In Treating Patients With Hematologic Cancer And Solid Tumors (Ids: SCRF-98014, NCI-V98-1396, ALZA-97-49-Ii)

Gemcitabine And Fluorouracil In Treating Patients With Cancer (Ids: UCCRC-8261, NCI-G97-1157)

Vaccine Therapy And Biological Therapy In Treating Patients With Advanced Cancer (Ids: NCI-95-C-0105A, NCI-T94-0096N)

Adjuvant Chemotherapy In Women Treated In The SWOG-8897 Clinical Trial (ID: SWOG-9342)

Chemotherapy Plus G-CSF Versus G-CSF Alone For Peripheral Stem Cell Transplantation In Women

With Breast Cancer (Ids: MDA-DM-95047, NCI-G96-1014)

High-Dose Chemotherapy And Peripheral Stem Cell Transplantation In Treating Patients With Recurrent Or Refractory Metastatic Breast Cancer (Ids: UNC-LCCC-9727, NCI-G98-1446, UNC-LCCC-970135)

Tamoxifen, Ovarian Ablation, And/Or Combination Chemotherapy In Treating Premenopausal Women With Operable Invasive Breast Cancer (Ids: SCTN-BR9401, EU-94002, UKCCCR-ABC/BR9401)

Marimastat Or No Further Therapy In Treating Patients With Metastatic Breast Cancer That Is Responding Or Stable Following Chemotherapy (ID: E-2196)

Lu-103793 In Patients With Breast Cancer Or Malignant Melanoma (ID: EORTC-16962)

Radiation Therapy Plus Gadolinium Texaphyrin In Treating Patients With Brain Metastases (Ids: PCI-P120-9801, NCI-V98-1470)

Adjuvant Therapy With Tamoxifen Alone Or With Octreotide In Treating Postmenopausal Women With Stage I, Stage II, Or Stage III Breast Cancer (Ids: CAN-NCIC-MA14, NCI-V96-1060)

Combination Chemotherapy And Peripheral Stem Cell Transplantation Followed By Interleukin-2 And GM-CSF In Treating Patients With Inflammatory Stage IIIb Or Metastatic Stage IV Breast Cancer (Ids: FHCRC-1229.00, NCI-G98-1399, PSOC-1605)

Carboxyamidotriazole And Paclitaxel In Treating Patients With Advanced Solid Tumors (Ids: NCI-95-C-0015F, NCI-T94-0006N, NCI-CPB-334)

High-Dose Combination Chemotherapy And Peripheral Stem Cell Transplantation In Patients With Advanced Cancer (Ids: CHNMC-IRB-95105, NCI-V96-1033)

Chemotherapy Plus Peripheral Stem Cell
Transplantation In Treating Women With
Metastatic And High-Risk Breast Cancer
(Ids: NCI-96-C-0104F, NCI-T95-0078N)

Gene Therapy In Treating Patients With Metastatic
Breast Cancer (Ids: NCI-93-C-0208I, NCI-T92-
0192N, NCI-MB-310)

Tumor Cell Vaccine In Treating Patients With
Advanced Cancer (Ids: CBRG-9212, NCI-V92-
0155, NBSG-9212)

Radioimmunotherapy In Treating Patients With
Advanced Cancers (Ids: VMRC-6366, NCI-V95-
0647)

Chemotherapy And Peripheral Stem Cell
Transplantation Compared With Standard
Therapy In Treating Women With Metastatic Or
Recurrent Breast Cancer (ID: CAN-NCIC-MA16)

Preoperative Compared With Postoperative
Combination Chemotherapy In Treating
Women With Stage II Breast Cancer (Ids: NCI-
90-C-0044F, NCI-T89-0118N)

Epoetin Alfa In Treating Anemia In Patients Who
Are Receiving Chemotherapy (Ids: NCCTG-
979253, NCI-P98-0133)

Paclitaxel Or Docetaxel In Treating Women With
Advanced Breast Cancer (Ids: RP-56976-TAX-
311, NCI-V95-0680)

Paclitaxel In Treating Patients With Advanced Breast
Cancer (ID: CLB-9840)

Hormone Therapy And Chemotherapy In Treating
Postmenopausal Women With Node-Positive
Breast Cancer (Ids: IBCSG-12-93, NCI-F93-0010,
EU-93015)

Chemotherapy Plus Surgery For Breast Cancer (Ids:
INT-23/96, EU-97001)

Hormone Therapy With Or Without Combination
Chemotherapy In Treating Postmenopausal
Women With Node-Negative Breast Cancer (Ids:
IBCSG-IX, EU-94040)

High-Dose Chemotherapy And Peripheral Stem Cell
Transplantation In Treating Patients With High-
Risk Breast Cancer (Ids: NCI-96-C-0032H, NCI-
MB-381)

Docetaxel In Patients With Solid Tumors And
Abnormal Liver Function (Ids: CHNMC-PHI-08,
NCI-T96-0028H, LAC-USC-PHI-08)

Combination Chemotherapy Plus Amifostine In
Treating Patients With Advanced Cancer
(Ids: CCF-IRB-1907, NCI-V98-1424, IMMUNEX-
001.G9701, IMMUNEX-CCF-IRB-1907)

Nutritional Intervention In Treating Patients With
Breast Cancer (Ids: AHF-WINS, NCI-H94-0001,
MRMC-CTCA-9604, WINS-1)

Combination Chemotherapy And Hormone Therapy
In Treating Premenopausal Women With Node-
Positive Breast Cancer (Ids: IBCSG-13-93, NCI-
F93-0011, EU-93016)

Combination Chemotherapy And Hormone Therapy
In Treating Perimenopausal And Postmeno-
pausal Women With Node-Positive Breast Cancer
(Ids: IBCSG-14-93, NCI-F93-0012, EU-93017)

Combination Chemotherapy Before Or After
Surgery In Treating Women With Breast Cancer
(ID: EORTC-10902)

High-Dose Combination Chemotherapy Plus
Peripheral Stem Cell Transplantation Compared
With Standard Combination Chemotherapy In
Treating Women With High-Risk Breast Cancer
(Ids: IBCSG-15-95, EU-96021)

Aminocamptothecin In Treating Patients With
Advanced Cancer Of The Peritoneal Cavity
(Ids: NYU-9753, NCI-T97-0123)

Repeated Autologous Bone Marrow Transplantation
In Treating Patients With Advanced Breast
Cancer (Ids: LSU-97447, NCI-V97-1341)

Peripheral Stem Cell Transplantation Compared
With No Intensification Therapy In Treating
Patients With Locally Recurrent Or Metastatic

Breast Cancer (Ids: FRE-FNCLCC-PEGASE03, EU-96032)

High-Dose Chemotherapy, Peripheral Stem Cell Transplantation, And Gene Therapy In Treating Women With Stage IV Breast Cancer (Ids: NCI-96-C-0007K, NCI-T95-0096N, NCI-MB-361)

Doxorubicin With Or Without DPPE In Treating Patients With Recurrent Or Metastatic Breast Cancer (Ids: CAN-NCIC-MA19, BMS-CA151-007)

Tamoxifen In Treating Patients With High-Risk Breast Cancer (Ids: CAN-NCIC-MA12, NCI-V93-0323)

Combination Chemotherapy Followed By Peripheral Stem Cell Transplantation In Treating Patients With Refractory Cancer (Ids: MRMC-CTCA-9711, NCI-V98-1446)

Combination Chemotherapy Followed By Autologous Peripheral Stem Cell Transplantation In Patients With Refractory Cancer (Ids: MCC-11310, NCI-V97-1327)

Standard Chemotherapy Versus High-Dose Combination Chemotherapy In Treating Women With Breast Cancer (Ids: SCTN-BR9405, EU-95048)

Medroxyprogesterone In Patients With Breast Cancer (Ids: SWOG-S9630, SWOG-9630)

Gene Damage Following Chemotherapy In Patients With Stage II Or Stage III Breast Cancer (ID: SWOG-9719)

Combination Chemotherapy In Treating Patients With Advanced Cancer (Ids: UCCRC-7341, NCI-T94-0082C)

Interleukin-2 Plus Monoclonal Antibody Therapy In Treating Patients With Solid Tumors (ID: CLB-9661)

Docetaxel In Treating Patients With Solid Tumors (ID: CLB-9871)

Combination Chemotherapy In Treating Women

With Breast Cancer (Ids: E-2197, SWOG-E2197)

Bay 12-9566 Plus Fluorouracil Or Doxorubicin In Treating Patients With Metastatic Or Recurrent Cancer (Ids: CAN-NCIC-IND113, BAYER-STR-C01)

Hydroxyurea And Fluorouracil In Treating Patients With Advanced Solid Tumors (Ids: LAC-USC-0C942, NCI-T95-0081H)

Biological Therapy Following Chemotherapy And Peripheral Stem Cell Transplantation In Treating Patients With Cancer (Ids: MRMC-CTCA-9801, NCI-V98-1449)

Gene Therapy Plus Chemotherapy In Treating Patients With Advanced Solid Tumors Or Non-Hodgkin's Lymphoma (Ids: CWRU-2Y97, NCI-T97-0060)

Correlation Of Menstrual Cycle Phase At Time Of Primary Surgery With 5-Year Disease-Free Survival In Women With Stage I Or Stage II Breast Cancer (Ids: NCCTG-N9431, NSABP-N9431)

Lymph Node Radiation Therapy In Patients With Resected Stage I, Stage II, Or Stage III Breast Cancer (Ids: EORTC-10925, EORTC-22922)

High-Dose Combination Chemotherapy With Peripheral Stem Cell Transplantation In Treating Patients With Advanced Cancers (Ids: CHNMC-IRB-94098, NCI-V96-1042)

Adjuvant Hormone Therapy In Treating Postmenopausal Women With Receptor-Positive Breast Cancer And Involved Axillary Lymph Nodes (Ids: E-EB193, INT-0151, SWOG-9514)

Prevention Of Graft-Versus-Host Disease In Patients Undergoing Bone Marrow Transplantation For Hematologic Cancers (Ids: MSGCC-9720, NCI-V98-1428)

Octreotide, Tamoxifen, And Chemotherapy In Treating Women With Breast Cancer (ID: NSABP-B-29)

Physician-Initiated Stop-Smoking Program For Early-Stage Cancer Patients (Ids: E-1Y92, NCI-P93-0042)

Standard-Dose Chemotherapy Compared With High-Dose Chemotherapy And With Peripheral Stem Cell Transplantation In Treating Women With Breast Cancer (Ids: SWOG-S9623, SWOG-9623, E-S9623)

Chemotherapy Compared With Combination Chemotherapy In Treating Patients With Breast Cancer (Ids: CLB-9741, NCCTG-C9741)

Docetaxel Before Or After Surgery Or No Docetaxel In Treating Women With Operable Breast Cancer (ID: NSABP-B-27)

Doxorubicin And Docetaxel In Treating Women With Locally Advanced Or Metastatic Breast Cancer (ID: NSABP-BP-57)

Combination Chemotherapy In Treating Women With Stage IIIb Or Stage IV Breast Cancer (ID: NSABP-BP-58)

Adjuvant Isotope Therapy In Patients With Stage I/II Breast Cancer (ID: RTOG-9517)

Radiation Therapy In Treating Patients With Bone Metastases From Breast Or Prostate Cancer (Ids: RTOG-9714, NCI-P97-0124, NCCTG-R9714)

Tamoxifen With Or Without Radiation Therapy In Treating Node-Negative Breast Cancer In Elderly Women (Ids: CLB-9343, E-C9343)

Chemotherapy In Treating Women With Resected Breast Cancer Following Tamoxifen Therapy (Ids: CAN-NCIC-MA17, JRF-CAN-NCIC-MA17, JRF-Vor-Int-10, NCCTG-CAN-MA17, NCCTG-JMA.17)

Clinical trials

For a list of other trials being conducted, go to www.centerwatch.com and click on the list of trials. Next, click on *oncology* and then find breast cancer.

Recipes*

Down Home Healthy Cookin' published by the National Cancer Institute

20-Minute Chicken Creole
4 medium chicken breast halves (1 1/2 lbs total),
skinned, boned, and cut into 1-inch strips**
1 14-oz can tomatoes, cut up***
1 cup low-sodium chili sauce
1 1/2 cups chopped green pepper (1 large)
1/2 cup chopped celery
1/4 cup chopped onion
2 cloves garlic, minced
1 tbsp chopped fresh basil or 1 tsp dried basil,
crushed
1 tbsp chopped fresh parsley or 1 tsp dried parsley
1/4 tsp crushed red pepper
1/4 tsp salt
Nonstick spray coating

1. Spray deep skillet with nonstick spray coating.
   Preheat pan over high heat. Cook chicken in hot
   skillet, stirring for 3 to 5 minutes or until no
   longer pink.

*A special thanks to the National Cancer Institute for permission to
print recipes from their cookbooks.

509

2. Reduce heat. Add tomatoes and their juice, low-sodium chili sauce, green pepper, celery, onion, garlic, basil, parsley, crushed red pepper, and salt. Bring to boil; reduce heat and simmer covered for 10 minutes. Serve over hot, cooked rice or whole wheat pasta.

Makes 4 servings

**You can substitute 1 lb boneless, skinless, chicken breasts, cut into 1-inch strips, if desired.

***To cut back on sodium, try low-sodium canned tomatoes.

Nutrition content per serving:
Calories: 255
Total fat: 3 g
Saturated fat: 0.8 g
Carbohydrates: 16 g
Protein: 31 g
Cholesterol: 100 mg
Sodium: 465 mg
Dietary fiber: 1.5 g

Garlic Mashed Potatoes

1 lb potatoes (2 large)
1/2 cup skim milk
2 large cloves garlic, chopped
1/2 tsp white pepper

1. Peel potatoes; cut in quarters. Cook, covered, in a small amount of boiling water for 20 to 25 minutes or until tender. Remove from heat. Drain. Recover the pot.

2. Meanwhile, in a saucepan over low heat, cook garlic in milk until garlic is soft, about 30 minutes.

3. Add milk-garlic mixture and white pepper to

potatoes. Beat with an electric mixer on low speed or mash with a potato masher until smooth.

Microwave Directions:

1. Scrub potatoes, pat dry, and prick with a fork. On a plate, cook potatoes, uncovered, on 100% power (high) until tender, about 12 minutes, turning potatoes over once. Let stand 5 minutes. Peel and quarter.

2. Meanwhile, in a 4-cup glass measure, combine milk and garlic. Cook, uncovered, on 50% power (medium) until garlic is soft, about 4 minutes. Continue as directed above.

Makes 4 servings.

Nutrition content per serving:
Calories: 141
Total fat: 0.3 g
Saturated fat: 0.2 g
Carbohydrates: 29 g
Protein: 6 g
Cholesterol: 2.0 mg
Sodium: 70 mg
Dietary fiber: 2 g

Hot `n Spicy Seasoning

1/4 cup paprika
2 tbsp dried oregano, crushed
2 tsp chili powder
1 tsp garlic powder
1 tsp black pepper
1/2 tsp red (cayenne) pepper
1/2 tsp dry mustard
Mix together all ingredients. Store in airtight container.
Makes about 1/3 cup.

New Orleans Red Beans

1 lb dry red beans
2 quarts water
1 1/2 cups chopped onion
1 cup chopped celery
4 bay leaves
1 cup chopped sweet green peppers
3 tbsp chopped garlic
3 tbsp chopped parsley
2 tsp dried thyme, crushed
1 tsp salt
1 tsp black pepper

1. Pick through beans to remove bad beans; rinse thoroughly. In a 5-quart pot, combine beans, water, onion, celery, and bay leaves. Bring to boil; reduce heat. Cover and cook over low heat for about 1 1/2 hours or until beans are tender. Stir and mash beans against side of pan.

2. Add green pepper, garlic, parsley, thyme, salt, and black pepper. Cook, uncovered, over low heat until creamy, about 30 minutes. Remove bay leaves.

3. Serve over hot, cooked brown rice, if desired.

Makes 8 servings.

Nutrition content per serving:
Calories: 171
Total fat: 0.5 g
Saturated fat: 0.1 g
Carbohydrates: 32 g
Protein: 10 g
Cholesterol: 0 mg
Sodium: 285 mg
Dietary fiber: 7.2 g

Sweet Potato Custard

1 cup mashed, cooked sweet potato
1/2 cup mashed banana (about 2 small)
1 cup evaporated skim milk
2 tbsp packed brown sugar
2 beaten egg yolks (or 1/3-cup egg substitute)
1/2 tsp salt
1/4 cup raisins
1 tbsp sugar
1 tsp ground cinnamon
Nonstick spray coating

1. In a medium bowl, stir together sweet potato and banana. Add milk, blending well. Add brown sugar, egg yolks, and salt, mixing thoroughly.

2. Spray a 1-quart casserole with nonstick spray coating. Transfer sweet potato mixture to casserole.

3. Combine raisins, sugar, and cinnamon; sprinkle over top of sweet potato mixture. Bake in a preheated 300°F oven for 45 to 50 minutes or until a knife inserted near center comes out clean.

Note: If made with egg substitute, the amount of cholesterol will be lower.

Makes 6 servings.

Nutrition content per serving:
Calories: 144
Total fat: 2 g
Saturated fat: 0.7 g
Carbohydrates: 20 g
Protein: 6 g
Cholesterol: 92 mg
Sodium: 235 mg
Dietary fiber: 1.4 g

Chillin' Out Pasta Salad

8 oz (2 1/2 cups) medium shell pasta
1 8-oz carton (1 cup) plain nonfat yogurt
2 tbsp spicy brown mustard
2 tbsp salt-free herb seasoning
1 1/2 cups chopped celery
1 cup sliced green onion
1 lb cooked small shrimp
3 cups coarsely chopped tomatoes (about 3 large)

1. Cook pasta according to package directions. Drain; cool.

2. In a large bowl stir together yogurt, mustard, and herb seasoning. Add pasta, celery, and green onion; mix well. Chill at least 2 hours.

3. Just before serving, carefully stir in shrimp and tomatoes.

Makes 12 servings.

Nutrition content per serving:
Calories: 140
Total fat: 1 g
Saturated fat: 0.1 g
Carbohydrates: 19 g
Protein: 14 g
Cholesterol: 60 mg
Sodium: 135 mg
Dietary fiber: 1.3 g

Garden Potato Salad

3 lbs potatoes (6 large)
1 cup chopped celery
1/2 cup sliced green onion
2 tbsp chopped parsley
1 cup low-fat cottage cheese
3/4 cup skim milk
3 tbsp lemon juice

2 tbsp cider vinegar

1/2 tsp celery seed

1/2 tsp dillweed

1/2 tsp dry mustard

1/2 tsp white pepper

1. Scrub potatoes; boil in jackets until tender. Cool; peel. Cut into 1/2-inch cubes. Add celery, green onion, and parsley.

2. Meanwhile, in a blender, blend cottage cheese, milk, lemon juice, vinegar, celery seed, dillweed, dry mustard, and white pepper until smooth. Chill for 1 hour.

3. Pour chilled cottage cheese mixture over vegetables; mix well. Chill at least 30 minutes before serving.

Makes 10 servings.

Nutrition content per serving:

Calories: 151

Total fat: 0.5 g

Saturated fat: 0.2 g

Carbohydrates: 30 g

Protein: 6 g

Cholesterol: 2.3 mg

Sodium: 118 mg

Dietary fiber: 3.1 g

Celebre La Cocina Hispana published by the National Cancer Institute

Picadillo

1 lb extra lean ground beef

1 medium onion, chopped

1 clove garlic, minced

1/4 cup sherry (optional)

1/2 tsp cumin
1/2 tsp oregano
1/8 tsp salt
Pinch ground red pepper
1/4 cup raisins
1 cup diced fresh or canned pineapple
1 16-oz can crushed tomatoes
1 medium green bell pepper, chopped
1/4 cup chopped pimiento or red bell pepper

1. In a large skillet over medium-high heat, brown the ground beef, onion, and garlic until the onion is tender and the meat is no longer pink and the juices run clear. Drain off all fat. Add all remaining ingredients except the green pepper and pimiento. Bring to a simmer and cook 5 minutes. Add green pepper and pimiento and heat through.

Serve with rice and bread.
Makes 4 servings.

Nutrition content per serving:
Calories: 324
Total fat: 14 g
Saturated fat: 6 g
Carbohydrates: 27 g
Protein: 24 g
Cholesterol: 70 mg
Sodium: 282 mg
Dietary fiber: 3 g

Chicken Tamales with all the Extras

30 corn husks or 20 pieces of aluminum foil cut into 10-inch squares
Dough:
4 cups (1 lb) masa harina
2 cups skim milk

1 1/2 cups low-sodium chicken broth (remove fat)
1/2 cup mashed potatoes
1 tbsp vegetable oil
1 tbsp lemon juice
1/2 tsp salt
Filling:
1/4 cup lemon juice
1/2 tsp salt
2 cloves garlic, minced
1/2 lb boneless, skinless chicken breasts, cut into
20 strips, 1/2-inch by 2-inches
Garnishes:
2 medium potatoes, peeled, halved lengthwise and
thinly sliced (20 slices)
40 raisins
2 tomatoes, halved and thinly sliced (20 slices)
1 onion, halved lengthwise and thinly sliced
1/2 red bell pepper, thinly sliced (20 slices)
2 fresh green chilies, thinly sliced (20 slices)
20 fresh mint sprigs

To make the dough:
In a large saucepan, stir together the dough ingredients with a wooden spoon. Cook the dough over medium-low heat for 20 to 25 minutes, until firm but still moist. Cool to room temperature and wrap in plastic until needed. The dough may be made one day in advance and refrigerated.

To make the filling:
In a medium mixing bowl, stir together the lemon juice, salt, and garlic. Stir in the chicken. Cover and refrigerate for at least 2 hours and up to 24 hours.

To assemble and cook:
1. If you are using packaged corn husks, separate them, put in large bowl, cover with water, and set aside to soak for several hours or overnight.

2. Divide the dough into 20 pieces. Form each piece into a cylinder about 3 inches long and place it in the center of a husk or foil wrapper. Press into the dough a piece of chicken, 2 raisins and a slice of potato. On top of the dough place a slice of tomato, some onion slices, and a slice each of pepper and chili. Top with a sprig of mint.

3. Fold the ends of each foil or husk wrapper over the filling and garnishes and then fold the sides of the wrapper in tightly. To tie them into waterproof packages, use thin strips torn from several husks or use 5-inch pieces of string. If you are using foil instead of husks, tying is not necessary.

4. Fill the bottom half of a large steamer with water. Stand all the tamales upright in the top of the steamer and cover them with corn husks. Cover the pot tightly, bring the water to a boil, adjust heat to maintain a simmer, and let the tamales cook for about 1 1/2 hours. To check for doneness, open a tamale; the dough should come away solidly from the husk or foil. As the tamales cook, check the water level occasionally and replenish if necessary.

5. Unwrap and serve immediately.

Makes 20 tamales.

Nutrition content per serving:
Calories: 354
Total fat: 7 g
Saturated fat: 1 g
Carbohydrates: 59 g
Protein: 17 g
Cholesterol: 20 mg
Sodium: 308 mg
Dietary fiber: 7 g

Vegetarian Beans with Rice

Beans:

2 cups pinto beans

1/2 medium onion, chopped

2 bay leaves

8 cups cold water

Very small amount of salt (optional)

1 tsp vegetable oil

3 cloves garlic, chopped

Rice:

1 small onion, chopped

2 medium tomatoes, peeled and seeded

2 cloves garlic

2 cups long-grain white rice

1 tsp vegetable oil

4 cups low-sodium chicken broth (remove fat)

Very small amount of salt (optional)

1 cup fresh or frozen peas

1 tbsp chopped fresh cilantro

To make the beans:

1. Pick over the beans to remove any stones and wash. Soak beans overnight. Put the beans into a large pot with the onion, bay leaves, and water. Bring the water to a simmer and cook the beans until they are tender, 1 1/2 to 3 hours. Add water as needed as the beans cook. Season to taste with salt (optional) and cook until very soft. Remove from heat and discard the bay leaves. Strain off any remaining liquid and set aside.

2. In a medium, nonstick skillet, warm the oil over medium heat. Add the garlic and cook until fragrant, about 1 minute. Add 2 cup of cooked beans to the skillet and mash them with the back of a wooden spoon. Gradually stir in the liquid

from the bean pot and cook until the paste is quite thick. Stir the mashed bean mixture back into the pot of beans and simmer together for 4 to 5 minutes.

To make the rice:

1. In a food processor or blender, puree the onion, tomatoes, and garlic.

2. In a medium, nonstick saucepan, warm the oil over medium heat. Add the rice and stir until light golden. Stir in the vegetable puree and cook until all the moisture has been absorbed. Stir in the chicken broth and season lightly with salt (optional). If you are using fresh peas, stir them in, too. Bring the rice to a simmer, reduce the heat to very low, and cover the pan. Cook until the rice is tender and the chicken broth is absorbed, about 20 minutes. If you are using frozen peas, stir them in at the last minute. Sprinkle cilantro over the top of the rice and serve.

Serve with salad and tortillas.

Makes 8 servings.

Nutrition content per serving:
Calories: 404
Total fat: 3 g
Saturated fat: 0 g
Carbohydrates: 78 g
Protein: 17 g
Cholesterol: 0 mg
Sodium: 42 mg
Dietary fiber: 6 g

Fruit Salad with Frozen Yogurt
3 tbsp honey
3 tbsp lemon juice

1 medium apple, cored and chopped
1 medium plum, pitted and sliced
1 large orange, peeled with a knife and sliced into
1/4-inch thick rounds
1 large grapefruit, peeled with a knife, and sectioned
1 medium banana, peeled and sliced into rounds
1 quart frozen nonfat vanilla yogurt
In a large bowl, whisk together the honey and lemon
juice. Stir in the fruit. Serve the fruit topped with a
scoop of frozen yogurt.

Makes 8 servings.

Nutrition content per serving:
Calories: 161
Total fat: 1 g
Saturated fat: 0 g
Carbohydrates: 38 g
Protein: 4 g
Cholesterol: 3 mg
Sodium: 73 mg
Dietary fiber: 2 g

Eating Hints for Cancer Patients published by the National Cancer Institute

Creamy Potato Salad

1/3 cup plain low-fat yogurt
1/3 cup mayonnaise
1/4 tsp finely minced or scraped onion
1 sprig of parsley, finely chopped
1/4 cup chopped celery or green pepper
(optional)
2 potatoes, boiled and diced
2 hard-boiled eggs, diced
Salt to taste

Blend yogurt, mayonnaise, onion, parsley, celery, and pepper. Stir in remaining ingredients. Cover and refrigerate for several hours.
Makes 4 servings.

Quick Barbecue Sauce

1/2 cup catsup
2 tsp salad style mustard
1/2 tsp lemon juice
1 tbsp brown sugar
1/2 tsp onion salt

Mix together in small saucepan. Heat until boiling, stirring as it cooks.

Serving suggestions: Make Sloppy Joes. Use as a barbecue sauce for hot dogs, chicken, or meatballs. (The sauce will easily coat eight pieces of chicken.) Use as a marinade for chicken or meat. Pour over pieces in a deep dish and refrigerate in marinade at least 12 hours to tenderize.
Makes 1/2 cup.

Sweet and Sour Sauce

1/4 cup vinegar
1 cup catsup
1 tbsp soy sauce
1/2 red or green pepper, cubed
1/2 cup honey or brown sugar (packed)
1/2 tsp salt
1 can (8 oz) pineapple chunks (optional)
Water
2 tbsp cornstarch

Mix all ingredients except cornstarch in saucepan. Bring to boil. Turn heat down to simmer, stirring occasionally and cook for at least 20 minutes to allow flavors to blend. Dissolve cornstarch in small amount of water. Add, stirring until thickened. (You can omit cornstarch and allow the sauce to thicken by cooking it longer.) Use on meat or chicken. Makes 2 cups.

Fresh Peach Sauce

1 large peach, peeled and thinly sliced
1 1/2 tbsp sugar
1/4 cup water
1 tsp cornstarch
Dash nutmeg

Combine ingredients in a small pan, stir until cornstarch is dissolved. Cook over medium heat until sauce boils and is thickened.
Makes 1 serving.

Peanut Butter Snack Spread

1 tbsp instant dry milk
1 tsp water
1 tsp vanilla
1 tbsp honey*
3 heaping tbsp creamy peanut butter

Combine dry milk, water, and vanilla, stirring to moisten. Add honey and peanut butter, stirring slowly until liquid begins to blend with peanut butter. Spread between graham crackers or milk lunch crackers. The spread can also be formed into balls, chilled, and eaten as candy. Keeps well in refrigerator but is difficult to spread when cold.
Makes 1/3 cup.
*For molasses taffy flavor, substitute molasses for honey

Granola I and II

1 1/2 cups quick oatmeal
1/2 cup regular wheat germ
1/2 cup coconut

1/2 tsp. salt
1/2 cup chopped nuts
2/3 cup sweetened condensed milk
Measure oatmeal, wheat germ, coconut, salt, and nuts into mixing bowl, stirring to blend. Add oil and mix thoroughly. Pour in condensed milk and blend well. Sprinkle a handful of wheat germ on a cookie sheet and gently spread mixture on top. Bake in 325° oven about 25 minutes. Check mix as it bakes-after the first 10 minutes, mix will begin to brown. Stir it on cookie sheet every 10 minutes until it is as brown as you like. Cool on pan; store in covered container in refrigerator.

Granola II: Omit milk. Add 1/2 cup honey. Bake as above.

Chocolate chip: Put hot mixture in bowl. Stir in 1/2 cup of chocolate chips.

Raisin: Stir in 1 cup of raisins after the mixture cools.

Granola Bars

3/4 cup quick cooking oatmeal
1/2 cup Granola II (see recipe)
1/2 cup coconut
1/2 cup brown sugar (packed)
1/4 cup melted margarine
1 egg
1/4 tsp vanilla extract
1 tbsp honey
1/4 tsp salt
1/4 cup flour

Measure oatmeal, granola, coconut, and brown sugar together in deep bowl. Mix well. Pour melted margarine over all and blend thoroughly. Beat the egg, vanilla, honey, and salt together. Pour this over dry ingredients, stirring to blend. Add flour, stirring until smoothly mixed. Press mixture onto greased, floured 11x7-inch shallow baking pan or cookie sheet. Bake at 325° for 35 minutes. Cool slightly, cut into bars, and remove from the pan while warm. Makes 18 bars.

Macaroni and Cheese

1 cup milk
1 tbsp flour
1-2 tbsp margarine
1 tsp minced onion
Salt and pepper to taste
1 tsp dry mustard (optional)
2 cups elbow macaroni, cooked and drained
1 cup shredded cheddar cheese
Measure milk into the pan and blend in flour until no lumps remain. Add margarine, onion, and other seasonings and cook until sauce thickens. Stir in macaroni and cheese. Bake uncovered in greased, 1-quart casserole at 400° for 15 minutes or until slightly browned and bubbly. May be kept frozen before baking.
Makes 4 servings.

Tuna Broccoli Casserole

2 packages (10 oz) frozen broccoli, whole or chopped
2 cans (7 oz) water-packed tuna broken into small pieces
1 can (10 oz) cream of mushroom soup diluted with 1/2 cup of milk
1 cup grated cheddar or American cheese
1/2 cup plain bread crumbs
2 tbsp melted margarine
Cook broccoli according to package directions, drain,

and place in shallow 2-quart casserole. Add tuna and cover with diluted mushroom soup. Sprinkle with cheese. Add bread crumbs to melted butter and sprinkle over casserole. Bake at 350° for 20 minutes. Makes 5 servings.
Contributed by a patient.

Cheese-Spinach Pie

1/3 cup chopped onion
1 tbsp margarine
1/4 lb sliced Swiss or Muenster cheese
1 cup cooked, chopped spinach (drained)
3 large eggs
1/3-1/2 cup of milk
1/2 tsp salt
Dash pepper
9-inch pie shell

Cook onion in margarine until tender; cool. Lay slices of cheese in pie shell, follow with spinach, then onions. Beat eggs, adding enough milk to make 1 cup. Add seasonings and pour over ingredients in the pie shell. Bake in 400° oven about 35 minutes, or until a knife comes out clean. Serve piping hot. (Can be frozen after baking.)
Makes 4 servings.

Variation: Substitute cooked, chopped broccoli, green beans, zucchini, or peas for spinach.

Chicken Skillet Supper

2-3 lbs frying chicken, cut up
1/2 can (10 oz) vegetarian vegetable soup
1 can water
2 sprigs of parsley
1 basil leaf (optional)

Place chicken, skin side down, in cold skillet. Brown

over medium heat, turning to brown inside. Remove from heat (chicken skin can easily be removed at this point). Pour off all fat remaining in skillet. Replace chicken, pour soup and water over chicken, and add seasonings. Simmer 1 hour in covered skillet, turning pieces once to keep them moist. May be frozen after cooking.

Makes 4 servings.

Tomato special: Substitute 1/2 can of cream of tomato for vegetarian-vegetable soup. Add 1 package (10 oz) of mixed frozen vegetables with the soup and water.

Creamy chicken: Substitute 1/2 can of cream of chicken for vegetarian vegetable soup. Add 1 package (10 oz) frozen peas and carrots.

High-Protein Pancakes

1/2 cup milk
2 tbsp dry milk
1 egg (2 for thinner, crepe-type)
2 tsp of oil
1/2-3/4 cups pancake mix

Measure milk, dry milk, egg, and oil into blender or bowl. Beat until egg is well blended. Add pancake mix. Stir or blend at low speed until mix is wet but some lumps remain. Cook on hot, greased griddle or frying pan. Turn when firm to brown the other side. These can be kept warm in a warm oven or in a covered pan on low heat.

Makes 7 four-inch pancakes.

Note: If there is batter left over, it will keep 1 day in the refrigerator, or it can be made into pancakes, cooled, and wrapped in foil to be frozen for later use. To reheat, leave in foil and place in 450° oven for 15 minutes. If using a toaster oven, unwrap them, brush with margarine, and toast as for light toast.

Low-Lactose Pancakes

1 egg (2 for crepe-type)

1/2 cup soy formula

2 tsp milk-free margarine, melted

1/2 cup milk-free pancake mix

Put egg, soy formula, and melted margarine into bowl or blender. Beat to blend. Stir in mix until wet but some lumps remain. Cook on greased or oiled pan (use only milk-free margarine, bacon fat, or shortening) until firm enough to turn over. Brown other side. Keep warm in oven or covered pan on low heat. If you wish to freeze pancakes, follow directions in recipe for High-Protein Pancakes.

Makes 6 four-inch pancakes.

High-Protein Milkshakes

1 cup fortified milk

1 generous scoop ice cream

1/2 tsp vanilla

2 tbsp of butterscotch, chocolate, or your favorite fruit syrup or sauce

Measure all ingredients into blender. Blend at low speed for about 10 seconds.

Citrus Fake Shakes

1 frozen citrus fruit juice bar (2 1/2 oz) or

2 bars (1 3/4 oz) same flavor

1/2 cup chilled soy-based milk substitute/nutritional supplement

1/4 tsp vanilla

Remove citrus bar from freezer and allow to thaw slightly (about 5-10 minutes until soft). Break bar into pieces. Place in blender. Add other ingredients and blend at low speed for 10 seconds.

Makes 1 serving.

Double Citrus: Add 1 tbsp frozen orange juice concentrate and 1 tbsp sugar to the lemon or orange flavor Fake Shake before blending.

Butterscotch Fake Shake

1/2 cup chilled or partially frozen soy-based milk substitute/nutritional supplement

1/4 tsp vanilla

2 tbsp milk-free butterscotch sauce

Blend all ingredients at low speed about 10 seconds. Using the partially frozen liquid will produce a much colder, thicker shake.

Makes 1 serving.

Variations:

Chocolate: Use 2 tbsp chocolate syrup in place of butterscotch. (Commercial chocolate syrups are often made without milk or lactose; always read the ingredient labels).

Butterscotch-Banana: Add 1/2 well ripened, sliced banana to ingredients for butterscotch shake.

Peanut Butter-Honey: Omit butterscotch sauce. Mix together in a cup: 1/4 cup soy formula or nondairy creamer, 2 tbsp smooth peanut butter, 1 tbsp honey, and 1/4 tsp vanilla. Place partially frozen liquid in blender, then add peanut butter mixture. Blend for about 10 seconds or until smooth.

Fake Shake Sherbet

Follow recipe for Peanut Butter-Honey (you can double or triple recipe). Pour shake into small container. Freeze 2 hours or until it begins to harden around edges. Scrape into bowl and mix thoroughly, until lumps disappear. Return to container and refreeze 2 hours or until firm.

Other Frozen Fake Shakes: The Butterscotch, Chocolate,

or Butterscotch-Banana shakes (see recipe) can be frozen using the same method as for Fake Shake Sherbet.

Instant Breakfast Shake

1 package instant breakfast mix
1 cup whole milk
1/4 cup instant nonfat dry milk
1 cup ice cream (2 to 3 scoops)*
1 egg (poached or soft-boiled), if desired
Mix or blend ingredients until smooth. Add more milk for a thinner shake. If shake tastes too sweet, add a few drops of lemon juice.
Makes 1 serving.
*(Sherbet may be substituted for ice cream.)

Make-Your-Own Shake

You can add any of the following to the Instant Breakfast Shake recipe:
1/2 large banana
1 to 2 tbsp chocolate sauce
1 tsp instant coffee plus sugar to taste
1 tbsp malted milk powder
1/2 cup canned fruit
1/2 tsp vanilla flavoring plus 1/4 tsp cinnamon
1 tbsp molasses
Fresh or frozen fruit, as allowed
Try something not listed, mix together to make new combinations, or ask a registered dietitian for suggestions.

Homemade Peanut Butter Shake

1 cup vanilla-flavored, soy-based, nutritional supplement
1 pint low-fat vanilla ice cream

1 cup water
1/4 cup ginger ale
1 banana
5 tbsp peanut butter
Put all ingredients in a blender and mix thoroughly until smooth. Refrigerate unused portion. Makes 4 servings.

Fruit Smoothie
2 tbsp blackberry or cherry cordial
3/4 cup chilled or partially frozen half-and-half
Mix or blend until smooth. Serve in a fancy glass, frosted if you like.
Makes 1 serving.
Panamanian Smoothie: Omit cordial; add 2 tbsp chocolate syrup and 2 tbsp rum.
Creme de Menthe Smoothie: Omit cordial; add 2 tbsp creme de menthe and 2 tbsp vanilla ice cream (omit ice cream for low-lactose diet).

Apple Brown Betty
4 cups thinly sliced pared apples or 1 can (16 oz) pie apples, drained
2 cups bread cubes or torn bread pieces
1/2 cup brown sugar, packed
1/8 tsp ground cinnamon
2 tbsp margarine
1/4 cup hot water
Grease 1-quart baking dish. Arrange half of apples on bottom of dish. Follow with half of bread, then half of sugar. Repeat layers. Sprinkle cinnamon over top, cut margarine in pieces and lay them on top, finish by pouring hot water over all. Cover and bake at 350° for 30 minutes, uncover and bake 10 minutes longer. Serve warm or chilled.

Makes 4 servings.

Apple Cheese Betty: Spoon 1 cup ricotta cheese over first layer of apples, bread, and sugar. Complete as above.

Banana-Nut Bread

2 eggs
3 medium well-ripened bananas, cut into chunks
1/4 cup of milk
1/4 cup of oil
1 tsp vanilla extract
2 cups all-purpose flour
3/4 cup sugar
1 tbsp baking powder
1/2 tsp baking soda
1/2 tsp salt
1/4 tsp nutmeg
1/2–1 cup chopped walnuts or pecans, or wheat germ

Blend eggs, bananas, milk, oil, and vanilla at medium speed until smooth, about 15 seconds. Measure rest of ingredients (except nuts or wheat germ) into bowl and stir to mix. Make a well in the center of the dry ingredients and pour in banana mixture. Mix just enough to moisten. Add nuts. Spread batter into well greased 9x5x3-inch loaf pan or three small 5x3x2-inch pans. Bake the bread at 350°, about 1 hour for the large loaf and 35-45 minutes for the smaller ones.

Makes 1 large loaf or 3 small loaves. Serves 16.

Peanut Butter Bars

1/4 cup margarine
1/4 cup smooth peanut butter
1 1/3 cups brown sugar, packed

2 eggs
1 1/2 cups flour
1 1/2 tsp baking powder
1/2 cup chocolate chips
1/2 cup finely chopped nuts (optional)
Cream margarine and peanut butter. Add brown
sugar and mix well. Add both eggs and mix until well
blended. Stir in flour and baking powder until blended, then chocolate chips and nuts. Spread batter in
greased and floured 9-inch square pan. Bake at 350°
for 30-35 minutes. Cool in pan. Cut when cooled into
36 bars.

Milk-Free Double Chocolate Pudding

2 squares baking chocolate (1 oz each)
1 tbsp cornstarch
1/4 cup granulated sugar
1 cup nondairy creamer or soy formula
1 tsp vanilla
Melt chocolate in small pan or on foil. Measure cornstarch and sugar into saucepan. Add part of the
creamer and stir until cornstarch dissolves. Add the
remainder of the creamer. Cook over medium heat
until warm. Stir in chocolate until mixture is thick
and comes to a boil. Remove from heat. Blend in
vanilla and cool.
Makes 2 servings.

Milk-Free Vanilla Pudding

1/4 cup sugar
2 tbsp cornstarch
2 cups soy protein formula
1 egg, beaten
1 tsp vanilla
Measure sugar and cornstarch into saucepan. Add a

little of the soy formula. Stir to dissolve cornstarch, then pour in the rest of the liquid. Add beaten egg. Cook over medium heat until it comes to a boil and is thickened. Add vanilla and cool.

Makes 4 servings.

Variations:

Maple Pudding: Omit vanilla and add 1/2 tsp maple flavoring.

Maple-Nut Pudding: Add 1/4 to 1/2 cup chopped walnuts or pecans to cooled pudding (not permitted on soft diet).

Coconut Pudding: Add 1/4 cup coconut. Read the ingredient listing on coconut to be sure it has no lactose added (not permitted on soft diet).

Super Frozen Delight

1 package instant pudding (chocolate, vanilla, butterscotch, or lemon)
2 cups of chilled soy protein formula
2 cups nondairy whipped topping

Read the label of pudding mix to see that no milk or other milk product has been included. Prepare pudding as directed, substituting soy protein formula for milk. Gently fold in whipped topping. Pour into freezer container, cover, and freeze until firm, about 3 hours.

Makes 1 quart. Serves 8.

Nut Delight: Fold in 1 cup of your favorite chopped nuts with the whipped topping (not permitted on soft diet).

The *Unofficial Guide*™ Reader Questionnaire

If you would like to express your opinion about Breast Cancer or this guide, please complete this questionnaire and mail it to:

The *Unofficial Guide*™ Reader Questionnaire
Macmillan Lifestyle Group
1633 Broadway, Floor 7
New York, NY 10019-6785

Gender: ___ M ___ F

Age: ___ Under 30 ___ 31-40 ___ 41-50 ___ Over 50

Education: ___ High school ___ College ___ Graduate/ Professional

What is your occupation?

_____

How did you hear about this guide?

___ Friend or relative

___ Newspaper, magazine, or Internet

___ Radio or TV

___ Recommended at bookstore

___ Recommended by librarian

___ Picked it up on my own

___ Familiar with the *Unofficial Guide*™ travel series

Did you go to the bookstore specifically for a book on Breast Cancer? Yes___ No___

Have you used any other *Unofficial Guides*™?
Yes___ No___

If Yes, which ones?

_____

_____

What other book(s) on Breast Cancer have you purchased?

_____

_____

Was this book:
___ more helpful than other(s)
___ less helpful than other(s)

Do you think this book was worth its price?
Yes___ No___

Did this book cover all topics related to Breast Cancer adequately? Yes___ No___

Please explain your answer:

_____

_____

Were there any specific sections in this book that were of particular help to you? Yes___ No___
Please explain your answer:

_____

_____

On a scale of 1 to 10, with 10 being the best rating, how would you rate this guide? ___

What other titles would you like to see published in the _Unofficial Guide_^{TM} series?

_____

_____

Are _Unofficial Guides_^{TM} readily available in your area? Yes___ No___
Other comments:

_____

_____

_____

Get the inside scoop...
with the *Unofficial Guides*™!

The Unofficial Guide to Alternative Medicine
ISBN: 0-02-862526-9 Price: $15.95

The Unofficial Guide to Conquering Impotence
ISBN: 0-02-862870-5 Price: $15.95

The Unofficial Guide to Coping with Menopause
ISBN: 0-02-862694-x Price: $15.95

The Unofficial Guide to Cosmetic Surgery
ISBN: 0-02-862522-6 Price: $15.95

The Unofficial Guide to Dieting Safely
ISBN: 0-02-862521-8 Price: $15.95

The Unofficial Guide to Having a Baby
ISBN: 0-02-862695-8 Price: $15.95

The Unofficial Guide to Living with Diabetes
ISBN: 0-02-862919-1 Price: $15.95

The Unofficial Guide to Overcoming Arthritis
ISBN: 0-02-862714-8 Price: $15.95

The Unofficial Guide to Overcoming Infertility
ISBN: 0-02-862916-7 Price: $15.95

All books in the Unofficial Guide™ series are available at your local bookseller, or by calling 1-800-428-5331.